# Oxford Handbook of
# Gastrointestinal Nursing

Edited by

**Christine Norton**

**Julia Williams**

**Claire Taylor**

**Annmarie Nunwa**

**Kathy Whayman**

The Burdett Institute of Gastrointestinal Nursing,
in partnership with King's College London,
Florence Nightingale School of
Nursing and Midwifery, and
St. Mark's Hospital, Harrow

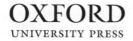

OXFORD
UNIVERSITY PRESS

# OXFORD
UNIVERSITY PRESS

Great Clarendon Street, Oxford OX2 6DP

Oxford University Press is a department of the University of Oxford.
It furthers the University's objective of excellence in research, scholarship,
and education by publishing worldwide in

Oxford New York

Auckland Cape Town Dar es Salaam Hong Kong Karachi
Kuala Lumpur Madrid Melbourne Mexico City Nairobi
New Delhi Shanghai Taipei Toronto

With offices in

Argentina Austria Brazil Chile Czech Republic France Greece
Guatemala Hungary Italy Japan Poland Portugal Singapore
South Korea Switzerland Thailand Turkey Ukraine Vietnam

Oxford is a registered trade mark of Oxford University Press
in the UK and in certain other countries

Published in the United States
by Oxford University Press Inc., New York

British Library Cataloguing in Publication Data

Data available

Library of Congress Cataloging in Publication Data

Data available

Typeset by Newgen Imaging Systems P Ltd., Chennai, India
Printed in China
on acid-free paper by
Asia Pacific Offset

ISBN 978-0-19-929865-5

10 9 8 7 6 5 4 3 2 1

# Preface

Each patient who a nurse cares for has a gut. Many diseases, illnesses, and their treatments can disrupt gut function. Nurses are at the forefront of recognizing, assessing, and treating gastrointestinal disturbances, whether or not this is the primary reason for the patient needing care.

This Handbook moves logically through the gastrointestinal tract, identifying the most common problems, and outlining investigations and treatments. We have brought together a leading team of nursing and medical authors who have written succinct, authoritative notes which should be accessible to the specialist and non-specialist nurse.

Christine Norton
London
August 2008

**The COMET Library**
Luton & Dunstable Hospital
NHS Trust, Lewsey Road
LUTON LU4 0DZ

**Tel: 01582 497201**
E-mail: library@ldh.nhs.uk

## Published and forthcoming Oxford Handbooks in Nursing

**Oxford Handbook of Mental Health Nursing**
Edited by Patrick Callaghan and Helen Waldock

**Oxford Handbook of Midwifery**
Edited by Janet Medforth, Susan Battersby, Maggie Evans, Beverley Marsh, and Angela Walker

**Oxford Handbook of Children's and Young People's Nursing**
Edited by Edward Alan Glasper, Gillian McEwing, and Jim Richardson

**Oxford Handbook of Nurse Prescribing**
Edited by Sue Beckwith and Penny Franklin

**Oxford Handbook of Cancer Nursing**
Edited by Mike Tadman and Dave Roberts

**Oxford Handbook of Primary Care and Community Nursing**
Edited by Vari Drennan and Claire Goodman

**Oxford Handbook of Cardiac Nursing**
Edited by Kate Johnson and Karen Rawlings-Anderson

**Oxford Handbook of Gastrointestinal Nursing**
Edited by Christine Norton, Julia Williams, Claire Taylor, Annmarie Nunwa, and Kathy Whayman

**Oxford Handbook of General and Adult Nursing**
Edited by George Castledine and Ann Close

# Foreword

Like many parts of our body we take our gut for granted until something goes wrong. From top to bottom it is a complex and remarkable structure fundamental to life and its quality. It plays a significant role in our activities of daily living, our socializing, and our health. Being able to eat, drink, and eliminate normally is basic but precious. Some problems with the gut are life threatening but many are not and remain hidden due to embarrassment or assumptions that 'these things are to be expected'. As a result quality of life suffers and, for some, is ruined without sensitive expert help and support largely from nurses.

Helping and caring for people with gut problems is becoming an increasingly specialized nursing role. As knowledge and technology grow so does the demand for evidence-based care that combines the art and science of nursing. The Burdett Institute of Gastrointestinal Nursing is making a significant contribution to the research base and, just as importantly, to the capacity building of nursing expertise. Professor Christine Norton and her team have marshalled impressive contributions for this comprehensive, easy to access handbook which exemplifies the high standard we have come to expect from the Institute.

Condensing a large amount of material into short informative notes is often more challenging than writing a book. This welcome addition to the Oxford Handbook series combines clarity with comprehensiveness and the provision of excellent links to further information. As well as symptomology, investigations, treatment, and care, the increasingly important, to patients, role of complementary therapies is addressed. The current and future health care environment points to more care for people in the community where they live rather than in hospital. This handbook will be a relevant and important contribution in both environments where the responsibilities and opportunities for nurses will undoubtedly grow for the benefit of patients.

Sue Norman
June 2008
London

# Contents

Contributors *xi*

Symbols and abbreviations *xiii*

| | | |
|---|---|---|
| 1 | Overview of the gut and its function | 1 |
| 2 | Nursing care of gastrointestinal (GI) patients | 9 |
| 3 | Nursing specialties in GI practice | 31 |
| 4 | Imaging the GI tract | 39 |
| 5 | Nutrition | 55 |
| 6 | Clinical nutrition | 97 |
| 7 | Endoscopy | 173 |
| 8 | Stoma care | 235 |
| 9 | Oesophagus and stomach | 327 |
| 10 | Small bowel | 371 |
| 11 | Liver | 395 |
| 12 | Pancreas | 427 |
| 13 | Gall bladder and biliary system | 439 |
| 14 | Colon | 447 |
| 15 | Rectum and anus | 505 |
| 16 | Inflammatory bowel disease | 595 |
| 17 | Neurological bowel care | 639 |
| 18 | Paediatric bowel care | 647 |
| 19 | Bowel care and vulnerable groups | 671 |
| 20 | Complementary therapies in bowel disorders | 679 |
| 21 | Pain management | 687 |
| 22 | Gastrointestinal emergencies | 701 |
| | Appendix | 713 |

Index *723*

# Contributors

**Mariann Baulf**
Endoscopy Unit,
St. Mark's Hospital, Harrow,
Middlesex

**Pat Black**
Coloproctology Department,
Hillingdon Hospital, Hillingdon,
Middlesex

**Francesca Bredin**
Department of Gastroenterology,
Addenbrooke's Hospital,
Cambridge

**Jennie Burch**
Physiology Unit,
St. Mark's Hospital, Harrow,
Middlesex

**Andrea Cartwright**
Basildon University Hospital
Nethermayne, Basildon, Essex

**Sonya Chelvanayagam**
The Burdett Institute
of Gastrointestinal Nursing,
St. Mark's Hospital, Harrow,
Middlesex

**Graham Clayden**
Sherman Centre,
Division of Medical Education,
School of Medicine,
King's College London, London

**Maureen Coggrave**
The Burdett Institute
of Gastrointestinal Nursing,
St. Mark's Hospital, Harrow,
Middlesex, and
The National Spinal Injuries
Centre, Stoke Mandeville Hospital

**Lynne Colagiovanni**
Nutrition Support,
University Hospital Birmingham
NHS Foundation Trust
Edgbaston, Birmingham

**Angie Davidson**
Lennard–Jones Intestinal Failure
Unit, St. Mark's Hospital,
Harrow, Middlesex

**Julie Duncan**
The Burdett Institute
of Gastrointestinal Nursing,
St. Mark's Hospital, Harrow,
Middlesex

**Anton Emmanuel**
University College Hospital London,
London.

**Simon Gabe**
Department of Gastroenterology
St. Mark's Hospital, Harrow,
Middlesex

**Helen Griffiths**
Department of Gastroenterology
Hereford Hospitals NHS Trust,
Hereford

**Fiona Hibberts**
Department of Colorectal Surgery
St Thomas' Hospital, London

**Warren Hyer**
Paediatric Department,
Northwick Park Hospital, Harrow,
Middlesex

**Diane Laverty**
Palliative Care
Royal Marsden Hospital, London

**Michele Marshall**
Intestinal Imaging,
St. Mark's Hospital, Harrow,
Middlesex

**Isobel Mason**
Centre for Gastroenterology,
Royal Free Hospital, London

**Kay Neale**
The Polyposis Registry
St. Mark's Hospital, Harrow,
Middlesex

**Jeremy Nightingale**
Gastroenterology Department
St. Mark's Hospital, Harrow,
Middlesex

**Marion O'Connor**
IBD Unit
St. Mark's Hospital, Harrow,
Middlesex

**Vashti Perry-Woodford**
St. Mark's Hospital, Harrow,
Middlesex

**Zarah Perry-Woodford**
Pouch care
St. Mark's Hospital, Harrow,
Middlesex

**Theresa Porrett**
Homerton Hospital, Hackney,
London

**Gillian Schofield**
The Prince Charles Hospital,
Chermside, Queensland,
Australia

**Graeme Smith**
School of Health, University
of Edinburgh, Edinburgh

**Lynn de Snoo**
Ashford and St. Peter's Hospitals
NHS Trust, Chertsey, Surrey

**Catherine Stansfield**
Salford Royal Hospitals NHS Trust

**Julian Stern**
Psychological Medicine Unit
St. Mark's Hospital, Harrow,
Middlesex

**Anna-Marie Stevens**
Palliative Care,
Royal Marsden Hospital, London

**Deep Tolia-Shah**
Broomfield Hospital, Chelmsford
Essex

**Sarah Patricia Varma**
Stoma Care Department,
St. Mark's Hospital, Harrow,
Middlesex

**Angela Vujnovich**
Stoma Care Department,
St. Mark's Hospital, Harrow,
Middlesex

**Fran Woodhouse**
Department of Colorectal Nursing,
John Radcliffe Hospital, Oxford

**Sue Woodward**
The Burdett Institute
of Gastrointestinal Nursing,
St. Mark's Hospital, Harrow,
Middlesex

**Lisa Younge**
The Burdett Institute
of Gastrointestinal Nursing
St. Mark's Hospital, Harrow,
Middlesex

# Symbols and abbreviations

| | |
|---|---|
| ↑ | increase |
| ↓ | decrease |
| ~ | approximately |
| ∴ | therefore |
| ♂ | male |
| ♀ | female |
| 5-ASA | 5-aminosalicylic acid |
| 5-FU | 5-fluorouracil |
| ACBS | Advisory Committee on Borderline Substances |
| ACE | antegrade continence enema |
| AFLP | acute fatty liver of pregnancy |
| AFP | α-fetoprotein |
| ALT | alanine aminotransferase |
| AMA | anti-mitochondrial antibody |
| ANA | antinuclear antibody |
| APER | abdominoperineal excision of the rectum |
| ASMA | anti-smooth-muscle antibody |
| AST | aspartate aminotransferase |
| BMD | bone mineral density |
| BMI | body mass index |
| BMR | basal metabolic rate |
| BSG | British Society of Gastroenterology |
| Bx | biopsy |
| CAM | complementary and alternative medicine |
| CBD | common bile duct |
| CD | Crohn's disease |
| CEA | carcinoembryonic antigen |
| CJD | Creutzfeldt–Jakob disease |
| CMV | cytomegalovirus |
| COSHH | Control of Substances Hazardous to Health |
| CPD | continuing professional development |
| CRP | C-reactive protein |
| CS | Caesarian section |
| CT | computed tomography |
| DAC | dispensing appliance contractor |
| DBE | double-balloon enteroscopy |
| DEXA | dual-energy X-ray absorptiometry |

| DN | district nurse |
| DOH | Department of Health |
| EAR | estimated average requirement (nutrients) |
| EAS | external anal sphincter |
| ECF | enterocutaneous fistula |
| EMG | electromyography |
| EN | enteral nutrition |
| ENT | ear, nose, and throat |
| ERAS | enhanced recovery after surgery |
| ERCP | endoscopic retrograde cholangiopancreatography |
| ESR | erythrocyte sedimentation rate |
| EUA | examination under anaesthetic |
| FAP | familial adenomatous polyposis |
| FBC | full blood count |
| FI | faecal incontinence |
| FOBT | faecal occult blood test |
| g | gram(s) |
| GI | gastrointestinal |
| GIST | gastrointestinal stromal tumour |
| GIT | gastrointestinal tract |
| GORD | gastro-oesophageal reflux disease |
| GP | general practitioner |
| GTN | glycerine trinitrate |
| h | hour(s) |
| H&E | haematoxylin and eosin |
| HAV | hepatitis A virus |
| HBV | hepatitis B virus |
| HCC | hepatocellular carcinoma |
| HCV | hepatitis C virus |
| HDV | hepatitis D virus |
| HETF | home enteral tube feeding |
| HEV | hepatitis E virus |
| HIDA | hepatobiliary iminodiacetic acid |
| HIV | human immunodeficiency virus |
| HNPCC | hereditary non-polyposis colorectal cancer |
| HPV | human papilloma virus |
| HRT | hormone replacement therapy |
| HSE | Health and Safety Executive |
| HV | health visitor |
| IAS | internal anal sphincter |
| IBD | inflammatory bowel disease |
| IBS | irritable bowel syndrome |

| IF | intestinal failure |
| IM | intramuscular |
| IRA | ileo-rectal anastamosis |
| ISO | International Organization for Standardization |
| IV | intravenous |
| IVF | *in vitro* fertilization |
| IVH | intravenous hyperalimentation |
| JP | juvenile polyposis |
| L | litre(s) |
| LD | learning disabilities |
| LOCM | low-osmolar contrast media |
| LRNI | lower reference nutrient intake |
| MAP | *MYH*-associated polyposis |
| MC&S | microscopy, culture, and sensitivity |
| MDT | multidisciplinary team |
| mcg | microgram(s) |
| mg | milligram(s) |
| min | minute(s) |
| ml | millilitre(s) |
| MMC | migrating myoelectric complex |
| MRI | magnetic resonance imaging |
| MRSA | methicillin-resistant *Staphylococcus aureus* |
| MS | multiple sclerosis |
| MSI | microsatellite instability |
| NAFLD | non-alcoholic fatty liver disease |
| NASH | non-alcoholic steatohepatitis |
| NBM | nil by mouth |
| NCD | nutrition-related non-communicable disease |
| NCJ | needle catheter jejunostomy |
| ND | nasoduodenal |
| NHL | non-Hodgkin lymphoma |
| NHS | National Health Service |
| NICE | National Institute for Health and Clinical Excellence (formerly National Institute for Clinical Excellence) |
| NJ | nasojejunal |
| NMC | Nursing and Midwifery Council |
| NSAID | non-steroidal anti-inflammatory drug |
| NSP | non-starch polysaccharide |
| NST | nutrition support team |
| OGD | oesophageal gastroduodenoscopy |
| OGIB | obscure gastrointestinal bleeding |
| PABA | para-amino benzoic acid |
| PBC | primary biliary cirrhosis |

| | |
|---|---|
| PCA | patient-controlled anaesthesia |
| PCR | polymerase chain reaction |
| PCT | primary care trust |
| PE | push enteroscopy |
| PEC | percutaneous endoscopic colostomy |
| PEG | percutaneous endoscopic gastrostomy |
| PEG-J | percutaneous endoscopic gastro-jejunostomy |
| PEJ | percutaneous endoscopic jejunostomy |
| PG | pyoderma gangrenosum |
| PICC | peripherally inserted central catheter |
| PJS | Peutz–Jeghers syndrome |
| PME | partial mesorectal excision |
| PN | parenteral nutrition |
| PNE | peripheral nerve evaluation |
| PPC | prescription prepayment certificate |
| PPI | proton pump inhibitor |
| PR | per rectum |
| PTML | pudendal terminal motor latency |
| PV | per vagina |
| RAIR | recto-anal inhibitory reflex |
| RIG | radiologically inserted gastrostomy |
| RLQ | right lower quadrant |
| RN | registered nurse |
| RNI | reference nutrient intake |
| s | second(s) |
| SC | subcutaneous |
| SCFA | short-chain fatty acid |
| SCI | spinal cord injury |
| SCN | stoma care nurse |
| SG | surgical gastrostomy |
| SI | safe intake |
| SJ | surgical jejunostomy |
| SNS | sacral nerve stimulation |
| SPN | supplementary parenteral nutrition |
| SSRI | selective serotonin-reuptake inhibitor |
| STI | sexually transmitted infection |
| TENS | transcutaneous electrical nerve stimulation |
| TIPS | transjugular intrahepatic porto-systemic shunt |
| TME | total mesorectal excision |
| TPMT | thiopurine metyl transferase |
| TTS | through the scope |
| UC | ulcerative colitis |

| VC | virtual colonoscopy |
| vCJD | variant Creutzfeldt–Jakob disease |
| w/v | weight/volume |
| WBC | white cell count |
| WCRF | World Cancer Research Fund |

# Overview of the gut and its function

Gross anatomy  2
Structure and function  4
Normal gut flora  6

# Gross anatomy

The gastrointestinal tract is a continuous hollow tube that extends from the mouth to the anus (Fig. 1.1). The structure and function of each region of the gut is outlined at the start of the relevant sections of this handbook. This overview outlines the factors that are common to the whole gut.

## Layers
- Outer layer—serosa; except in the oesophagus.
- Longitudinal smooth muscle.
- Circular smooth muscle.
- Submucosa.
- Mucosa.

## Serosa
In the abdominal cavity, the serosa comprises the following:
- Largest serous membrane in body.
- Parietal peritoneum lines the abdominopelvic cavity.
- Visceral peritoneum over the gut and organs.
- Space between layers—peritoneal cavity.
- Folds—binds organs to each other and the abdominal wall.

In the oesophagus, the serosa comprises the adventitia only.

## Gastrointestinal smooth muscle
Involuntary muscle comprising a circular inner layer and a longitudinal outer layer (which are connected).

## Submucosa
- Connective tissue.
- Blood and lymphatic vessels.
- Submucosal neuron plexus (Meissner's plexus; enteric nervous system).

## Mucosa
- Epithelium—columnar epithelium; except in the mouth, oesophagus, and distal anus.
- Renewal rate—cells renew rapidly every 4–7 days.
- Exocrine cells—secrete mucus.
- Endocrine cells—secrete hormones directly into the lumen or bloodstream.
- Lamina propria—connective tissue that contains the following:
  - Blood (absorption) and lymphatic (immunity) vessels.
  - Muscularis mucosae—muscle that arranges the gut surface into folds and ensures that all mucosa is in contact with the lumenal contents by means of local contraction and relaxation.

## Enteric nervous system

- Myenteric (Auerbach's) plexus—arranged in a linear fashion between muscle layers. It is responsible for motility (peristalsis) and inhibits the sphincters.
- Submucosal (Meissner's) plexus—controls secretion and blood flow.
- >100 million nerves in the enteric nervous system—'little brain'.

## Embryology

Formation of a tube occurs during week 4 of gestation; the tube is closed at both ends. At week 5 of gestation, the tube opens to form the mouth and anus. Three embryological sections of the gut:

- Foregut—pharynx, oesophagus, stomach, proximal duodenum, pancreas, and liver.
- Midgut—distal duodenum, jejunum, ileum, caecum, appendix, and ascending colon. It herniates through the umbilicus at weeks 5–10 of gestation and then returns to the abdominal cavity.
- Hindgut—transverse colon to anus.

## Further reading

Montague SE, Watson R., Herbert RA (eds) (2005). Innate defences. In: *Physiology for Nursing Practice*. London: Baillière Tindall.

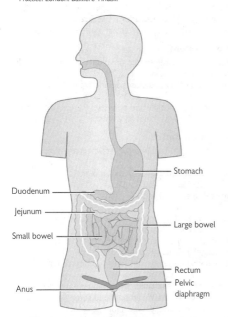

**Fig. 1.1** The gastrointestinal tract. Reproduced with kind permission © Burdett Institute 2008.

# Structure and function

The gut supplies fluid, nutrients, and electrolytes to the body for the following functions:
- Motility to propel food.
- Digestion—mechanical and chemical breakdown of food.
- Absorbs products of digestion.
- Blood supply to transport nutrients.
- Waste management.
- Barrier to ingestion of pathogens.
- Possible role in immunity—flora.
- Controlled by nerves and hormones.

### Enteric nervous system

Enteric nerves are mediators of movement and sensation in the gut. Chemical transmitters are shared with the brain.

Integrates extrinsic innervation (central nervous system) and local reflexes within the gut.

Gut motility is mostly controlled by the enteric nervous system, with stimulation or inhibition by the central autonomic nervous system. This is why the gut continues to work after complete spinal cord injury (albeit more slowly and commonly with constipation). Local reflexes are mostly in response to distension, modified by the luminal content of the gut.

### Autonomic nervous system

The gut is also supplied by the autonomic (involuntary) portion of the central nervous system:
- Sympathetic—slows gut motility and closes sphincters (gut activity is not useful for 'fight or flight').
- Parasympathetic—stimulates motility and opens sphincters (digestion is best conducted when the body is relatively at rest).

### Gastrointestinal smooth muscle

- Circular inner layer and longitudinal outer layer which are connected (Fig. 1.2).
- Fibres are 200–500 μm long and 2–10 μm in diameter.
- Arranged in large bundles (up to 1000 fibres).
- Large gap junctions between muscle cells—transmitters move easily between cells.
- Functional syncytium—the action potential travels easily, enabling smooth prolonged contractions that spread locally.
- Action potentials—calcium and (some) sodium ions enter muscle cells (calcium–sodium channels). Calcium causes contraction. The slow opening and closing of channels produces long-duration action potentials.
- Depolarize—more positive and excitable. Stretch in response to stimulation by acetylcholine (parasympathetic) and some hormones.
- Hyperpolarize—more negative and less excitable. In response to transmitters such as norepinephrine and epinephrine (sympathetic).

## Hormones in the gut

Hormones control secretion. There are many, including the following:

- Cholecystokinin—released in the duodenum and jejunum in response to the presence of fat. Inhibits stomach activity and stimulates the gall bladder to release bile.
- Secretin—released from the duodenum. Inhibits motility in response to acid from the stomach.
- Gastric inhibitory peptide—released in the small bowel. Produced in response to presence of fats, carbohydrate, and amino acids (a feedback mechanism to inhibit the stomach and allow time for digestion and absorption in the small bowel before more gastric contents are released).

## Secretion and absorption

- Food and fluids—2000 ml/day.
- Secretion—7000 ml/day. Occurs throughout the gastrointestinal tract, but more secretion occurs in the upper gut compared with the lower gut.
- Absorption—the small bowel absorbs nutrients, electrolytes, and water.
- The colon absorbs only electrolytes, water, and organic acids produced by luminal bacteria (except during starvation, when it can adapt and absorb some calories).

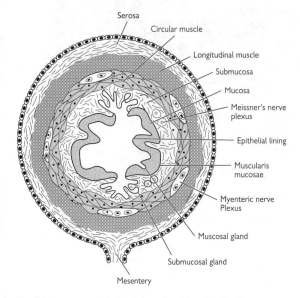

**Fig. 1.2** Typical cross-section of the gut. Reproduced with kind permission © Burdett Institute 2008.

# Normal gut flora

Microbes are present throughout the gastrointestinal tract, starting at the mouth.

## Mouth and pharynx

This contains a spectrum of flora including $\alpha$- and $\beta$-haemolytic streptococci, in addition to a number of anaerobes, staphylococci (including *Staphylococcus aureus*), *Neisseria* spp, diphtheroids, and yeasts.

## Stomach

The stomach harbours only transient organisms because the acidic environment is sterilizing. However, the gastric mucosa can be colonized by acid-tolerant lactobacilli and streptococci, in addition to *Helicobacter pylori*.

## Small intestine

Only lightly colonized by a floral population ($10^3$–$10^4$ organisms/ml; predominantly *E. coli*, streptococci, and lactobacilli) until just proximal to the ileocaecal valve. In this area of small bowel, bacterial concentrations $\uparrow$ to $10^6$–$10^7$ organisms/ml and consist of flora similar to that found in the colon.

## Colon

Here, bacterial counts are in the region of $10^9$–$10^{11}$ organisms/ml in the caecum, $\uparrow$ steadily to $10^{11}$ organisms/ml in the rectosigmoid. The flora consists of a large number of *Bacteroides* and spore formers, which significantly outnumber the aerobic and facultative anaerobic flora. Anaerobes, including *Bacteroides* spp, *Clostridium* spp, and anaerobic streptococci outnumber aerobic bacteria, such as coliforms, 1000-fold.

Density

Organisms

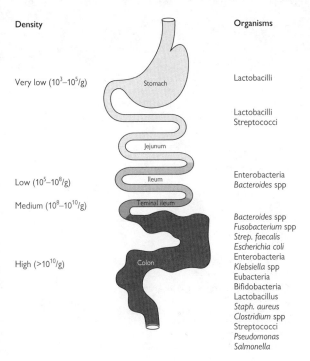

Very low ($10^3$–$10^5$/g)

Stomach

Lactobacilli

Lactobacilli
Streptococci

Jejunum

Low ($10^5$–$10^8$/g)

Ileum

Enterobacteria
*Bacteroides* spp

Medium ($10^8$–$10^{10}$/g)

Teminal ileum

*Bacteroides* spp
*Fusobacterium* spp
*Strep. faecalis*
*Escherichia coli*
Enterobacteria
*Klebsiella* spp
Eubacteria
Bifidobacteria
Lactobacillus
*Staph. aureus*
*Clostridium* spp
Streptococci
*Pseudomonas*
*Salmonella*

High (>$10^{10}$/g)

Colon

**Fig. 1.3** Densities and longitudinal distribution of the bacteria making up the normal flora of the human gastrointestinal tract. Reproduced with kind permission © Burdett Institute 2008.

# Nursing care of gastrointestinal (GI) patients

Clinical history-taking: general  10
Clinical history-taking: GI symptoms 1  12
Clinical history-taking: GI symptoms 2  14
Physical examination: environment, position, inspection  16
Physical examination: palpation, percussion, auscultation  18
Physical examination: per rectum (PR) examination  20
Stigma and taboos  22
Body image and sexuality  24
Presentation of psychological difficulties in GI patients  28
Management of psychological difficulties in GI patients  30

# Clinical history-taking: general

When nurses develop advanced practice skills and expertise in GI nursing, gaining the ability to undertake a thorough history and physical examination is essential because this process is the hub around which the patient's diagnosis and treatment revolve. The key factors are:

• Listening to what the patient volunteers.
• Taking time, not assuming a diagnosis.
• The nursing response to the information the patient provides.
• Recognizing whether the information is of high or low clinical value.
• Guiding the patient to reveal further possibly key symptoms.

The ability to interpret data obtained from a comprehensive history and physical examination will enable the nurse to initiate a comprehensive plan of care, which might include health promotion, treatment, follow-up, referral, or discharge.

## Scheme for history-taking

The SOAPIER format is most commonly used to structure the history-taking process (Subjective, Objective, Assessment (physical), Plan, Implementation, Evaluation, Review[1]). The format includes both subjective and objective data, and includes data assessment and planning, the components of which are outlined below.

### Subjective

• Present illness—presenting complaints; a short statement using the patients own words.
• History of present complaint—this should record details of each problem; let the patient tell the story and then ask specific questions to clarify or elicit further information.
• Past medical history—note all previous non-trivial illnesses, operations, and hospital admissions.
• Drugs and allergies—note all prescribed and over-the-counter drugs that the patient is taking.
• Social and personal history—including alcohol and smoking history, any use of recreational drugs, occupation, family history, recent exotic travel, whether the patient lives alone, and whether the patient uses social services.
• Family history—particularly any history of cancer, ulcerative colitis, or Crohn's disease.

### Objective

• Review of systems.
• Physical examination.
• Investigations.

### Assessment

• Formulation of a diagnosis.

---

1 Kettenbach G (1995). *Writing SOAP Notes* (2nd edn). FA Davis, Philadelphia, PA.

*Plan*
• Development of a plan of care.

Implementation, Evaluation, and Review then complete the SOAPIER process.

# Clinical history-taking: GI symptoms 1

▶ When taking a GI health history, ensure the following topics are fully explored within the SOAPIER history-taking format (negative findings should also be recorded).

- Nutrition—appetite, change in eating pattern, recent intentional or unintentional weight loss or gain, food preferences, food intolerances, special diets, lifestyle influences on dietary intake, and cultural influences on eating.
- Nausea, vomiting, difficulty in swallowing, and indigestion.
- Any jaundice, colour of urine, and colour of stools.
- Use of laxatives, stool softeners, anti-diarrhoeal agents, high doses of aspirin, non-steroidal anti-inflammatory agents, and steroids.
- Stool characteristics (frequency, consistency, colour, odour, and continence). Beware of terms such as 'diarrhoea' and 'constipation'; make sure you understand what the patient means by these terms.
- Bowel habit and the nature of a change in bowel habit.
- Travel history.
- Family history of diabetes, cancer, ulcerative colitis, or Crohn's disease.
- Previous surgery.
- Continence—post-defecation soiling, urge incontinence, or passive incontinence. A continence score is useful in quantifying the severity of the problem (Table 2.1).

The following are given as examples of key aspects of history-taking when patients describe specific symptoms.

▶ Ensure that all aspects of the history for the following specific symptoms are elicited.

## Bleeding

- Frequency and amount.
- Mixed with faeces.
- On the surface of faeces.
- Separate from faeces.
- On the toilet paper.
- Colour—bright red, dark, or melaena.

## Pain

- Site and radiation to other locations.
- Time and mode of onset—specific date, sudden or gradual, and persistent or intermittent.
- Severity—how bad is the pain on a scale of 1–10?; does it affect daily activities?
- Nature—cramping, aching, burning, or knife-like.
- Duration.
- Course—getting better or worse?
- Relieving factors—e.g. defecation.
- Exacerbating factors—e.g. defecation.
- Cause—what the patient feels is the cause.

**Table 2.1** St Mark's incontinence score[1]

|  | Never | Rarely <1x month | Sometimes <1x week | Usually <1x day | Always daily |
|---|---|---|---|---|---|
| Solid | 0 | 1 | 2 | 3 | 4 |
| Liquid | 0 | 1 | 2 | 3 | 4 |
| Gas | 0 | 1 | 2 | 3 | 4 |
| Lifestyle | 0 | 1 | 2 | 3 | 4 |

|  | No | Yes |
|---|---|---|
| Need to wear Plus or pad | 0 | 2 |
| Taking constipating medicines | 0 | 2 |
| Ability to defer for 15 minutes | 0 | 4 |

Total score: 0 = perfect continence; 24 = total incontinence

1 Vaizey CJ, Carapeti E, Cahill JA, and Kamm MA (1999). Prospective comparison of faecal incontinence grading systems. *Gut* **44**, 77–80.

# Clinical history-taking: GI symptoms 2

## Lump
- Location/description.
- Duration—when it was first noticed?
- First symptom—what brought it to the patient's notice?
- Other symptoms—what symptoms does it cause?
- Progression—how has it changed since it was first noticed?
- Persistence—has it ever disappeared (e.g. when lying flat)?
- Multiplicity—has the patient had other lumps?
- Cause—what does the patient think is the cause?

## Nausea and vomiting
- Onset and duration—relationship to food intake; odours.
- Vomiting preceded by nausea.
- Character of emesis—fresh blood, undigested food, bile, coffee grounds, fluid, solid or projectile.
- Associated symptoms—fever, headache, or abdominal pain.

## Indigestion
- Onset—relationship to meals, time of day or night, sudden or gradual.
- Character—bloated after eating, belching or flatulence, heartburn, loss of appetite, or severe pain.
- Location—generalized, or radiating to shoulders or arms.
- Alleviating or precipitating factors—type and quantity of food, and response to antacids, rest, and activity.

## Diarrhoea
- Onset and duration—gradual or sudden, frequency of stools, number per day, or change in usual bowel habit.
- Characteristics—watery, explosive, colour, mucous, blood, undigested food or fat, odour.
- Course—improving or getting worse.
- Associated symptoms—fever, chills, weight loss, abdominal pain, thirst, or recent antibiotics.
- Alleviating or precipitating factors.

## Constipation
- Onset and duration—recent occurrence or long-standing problem, sudden or gradual, last bowel movement.
- Characteristics—dry hard stool, number of bowel movements per week, change in size of stools, black or tarry, bright red blood, accompanied by abdominal or rectal pain, or alternating with diarrhoea.
- Feeling of incomplete evacuation—bulging towards vagina or post-defecation soiling.
- Course—continuous or intermittent.

- Associated symptoms—feeling of incomplete evacuation, feeling of a bulge, dragging sensation, prolapse, bloating, or abdominal pain.
- Alleviating or precipitating factors—diet, fluid intake, use of laxatives, enemas, suppositories, or manual evacuation.

## Further reading

Cox C (2004). *Physical Assessment for Nurses.* Blackwell, Oxford.

# Physical examination: environment, position, inspection

The history, no matter how comprehensive and accurate, is never complete without a physical examination.

## Environment
- Private, warm, and well-lit—if the patient is cold, they can't relax their abdominal muscles fully.
- Explanation.
- Is the patient comfortable—empty bladder.

## Position
- Recumbent at 15–20°.
- Arms by their sides—maintains lumbar lordosis and opens access to abdomen.
- If the abdominal wall is tense, ask the patient to bend their knees and draw their feet up slightly.

## Inspection
### General
Careful observation of the patient as a whole: do they look ill, in pain, distressed, alert, drowsy, obese, or wasted?
- Hand clubbing—ulcerative colitis, Crohn's disease, or cirrhosis (or non-GI causes).
- Palmar erythema—chronic liver failure.
- Dupuytren's contracture—alcohol excess.
- Liver flap—alcoholic liver disease.
- Spider naevi—liver disease.
- Koilonychia (spoon-shaped nails)—iron-deficiency anaemia.
- Leuconychia (white nails)—cirrhosis.
- Eyes—jaundice, liver disease, or excess circulation of bile pigments.
- Pallor—anaemia.
- Neck—supraclavicular nodes on the left (Virchow's node) or spread of a GI malignancy.
- Mouth—halitosis, fetor oris, or GI disease.
- Ketotic breath—fasting.
- Angular stomatitis/aphthous ulcers—Crohn's disease, ulcerative colitis, or iron deficiency.
- Glossitis (smooth, shiny tongue)—vitamin $B_{12}$ or folate deficiency.
- Lips—'freckle'-like pigmentation of lips is indicative of Peutz–Jeghers syndrome.
- Skin—erythema nodosum, pyoderma gangrenosum, soreness, or excoriation.

### Abdominal inspection
- Shape and symmetry—flat, scaphoid, or distended (flatus, faeces, fetus, fluid, fat, or fibroid).
- Scars.
- Straie—obesity, pregnancy, or Cushing's syndrome.

- Dilated veins—radiating from the navel (caput medusae) or portal hypertension.
- Visible peristalsis.
- Pulsations.
- Lumps/hernias—diversification of the rectus abdominus.
- Skin colour—erythema abigme (pigmentation from chronic use of a hot water bottle) and chronic pain.

## Further reading

Cox C (2004). *Physical Assessment for Nurses*. Blackwell, Oxford.

# Physical examination: palpation, percussion, auscultation

## Palpation

- Palpate all four quadrants.
- Always look at the patient's face, not your hand, to observe for any signs of pain.
- Light palpation—should begin opposite any area of pain. It is useful to ask the patient to pinpoint areas of pain themselves.
- Deep palpation.
- Liver—liver edge, firm, regular, irregular, or tender.
- Spleen—only possible to feel when it has doubled in size.
- Gall bladder—tenderness in the right hypochondrium on palpation (especially if asked to take a deep breath in—Murphy's sign) is indicative of cholecystitis.
- Guarding—voluntary tightening of abdominal muscles when you palpate.
- Rebound tenderness—sudden withdrawal of manual pressure causes sharp exacerbation of pain, which is indicative of peritonitis.
- Rigidity—board-like abdomen is indicative of peritonitis.

If a mass is noted on palpation, note the following:

- Position.
- Shape.
- Size.
- Surface—smooth or nodular.
- The colon can often be grossly distended with faeces, most commonly in left iliac fossa (LIF); faeces can feel firm but are indented by firm pressure with the fingers and this dent persists after releasing the pressure.

## Percussion

- Used to establish whether abdominal distension is caused by gas or fluid—tympani (normal sound caused by air) or dullness (organ or mass, fluid-filled loops or ascites).
- To assess the size of the liver and spleen.
- To detect ascites—lie patient on one side, mark the upper level of dullness, roll the patient flat, and percuss to see if the level of dullness shifts ('shifting dullness').
- To detect a distended bladder.
- To confirm a mass felt on palpation.

## Auscultation (using a stethoscope)

Listen in each of the four quadrants:

- Begin in the right lower quadrant (RLQ) over the ileocaecal valve.
- Listen for bowel sounds.
- Intermittent low-pitched gurgles are normal.
- Peritonitis—silent abdomen.
- Obstruction—excessive exaggerated high-pitched tinkles.
- Succession splash—paralytic ileus, small bowel obstruction, or pyloric stenosis.

## Further reading

Cox C (2004). *Physical Assessment for Nurses*. Blackwell, Oxford.

# Physical examination: per rectum (PR) examination

Anorectal examination includes inspection and palpation. Sigmoidoscopy and proctoscopy comprise an integral part of this examination. The issues of consent and chaperoning must not be forgotten. The procedure must be clearly explained to the patient, and either written or verbal consent recorded (📖 p. 34).

*Position*
- Left lateral, hips flexed to 90° but knees flexed >90° and buttocks to the edge of the couch.

*Inspection*
- Skin rashes—excoriation, skin disorders such as eczema or fungal or viral infections.
- Scars from previous surgery or infection.
- Skin tags—fissuring or haemorrhoids.
- Sinus—hidradenitis suppurativa.
- Faecal soiling—poor hygiene or incontinence.
- Lumps and bumps—polyps, warts, prolapsed piles, perianal haematoma, skin tags, sentinel pile, mucosal prolapse, rectal prolapse, or squamous cell carcinoma.
- External opening—fistula.
- Ask the patient to strain and observe for perineal descent (the position of the anus in relation to the ischial tuberosities at rest and on straining), rectal prolapse, mucosal prolapse, or prolapsing piles.

*Palpation*
Palpation includes feeling the skin around the perineum, in addition to digital examination of the anorectum.

*Perianal palpation*
- Tracks leading from the external openings of fistulae can be felt.
- Induration/fibrosis from sepsis.

*Digital examination of the anorectum*
Ensure that the examining finger is well lubricated. If patients have an acute fissure, they will often not tolerate a PR examination. This examination must be methodical and include the following:
- Assessment of resting tone.
- Squeeze pressures.
- Assessment of any thickening or masses in the anal canal and lower rectum.
- Prostate.
- Faeces—presence, volume, and consistency.
- Cervix.
- Abnormalities in the recto-vaginal septum (e.g. rectocele or weak perineal body). After examination, always check the withdrawn finger for blood and faeces.

► Record all findings in the multidisciplinary notes. Negative findings are often as important as positive findings.

## Further reading

Cox C (2004). *Physical Assessment for Nurses*. Blackwell, Oxford.

# Stigma and taboos

Patients with GI disorders are often disadvantaged because gut function is surrounded by stigma and taboos in Western cultures.

The term 'stigma' is derived from a Greek word referring to a tattoo mark that people who were devotees to a temple were branded with to show their affiliation. However, branding was later used to identify people, such as slaves or criminals, who were to be shunned, particularly in social arenas.

Stigmatization refers to a process whereby a person is not fully accepted by society because of their appearance or behaviour, which is not accepted as a cultural 'norm'. This can lead to them being discriminated against and socially excluded from everyday activities.

To avoid such exclusion, people might attempt to conceal their differences and impose self-exclusion, which can be detrimental to their physical and psychological health.

People with GI disease can feel stigmatized because their symptoms might relate to bowel function and faeces. Faeces provoke expressions of disgust. Faeces have been regarded as unclean for centuries, and are known to transmit disease if not disposed of appropriately. Defecation occurs in a specific private room and discussion of this activity is not deemed socially appropriate.

Bowel control is a learned but largely subconscious process, so when alterations in bowel habit occur, the person has difficulty understanding these symptoms and, because of the taboo nature of the subject, is reluctant to seek help. Not seeking assessment could lead to a worsening of symptoms, increased anxiety, and possibly death from the condition itself (e.g. bowel cancer).

▶ Therefore, during any assessment process, nurses should provide a supportive environment to facilitate discussion, allowing the person time to describe their symptoms using words or pictures, and respond in a calm non-judgemental manner.

## Further reading

Mason T, Carlisle C, Watkins C, *et al.* (2001). *Stigma and Social Exclusion in Healthcare*. Routledge, London.

Norton C (2004). Nurses, bowel continence, stigma and taboos. *Journal of Wound, Ostomy, and Continence Nursing* **27**, 279–91.

# Body image and sexuality

The entire experience of having a GI illness represents a major change in a patient's life. The patient is in a position where they might have to cope with a complex roller coaster of emotions, and social and physical problems resulting from continued drug therapy or surgical intervention. The anxieties faced will include feelings of alteration to their body image, function, and control of bowel function, in addition to restrictions on their current lifestyle and activity, all of which, in turn, have the potential to impinge on sexual function.

The way we see ourselves is an important part of our everyday lives. If there is a sudden alteration in this picture, it can have psychological implications for our behaviour. Illness tends to make us more self-aware of our bodies.

Factors that have been associated with poor body image include the following.
- Poor self-esteem.
- Social anxiety.
- Self-consciousness.
- Depressive features.

Beliefs, attitudes, and values towards the concepts of body image are developed from an early age and are swayed primarily by our upbringing, with influences from our parents, friends, families, and peers, in addition to attitudes within society.

Price[1] presents a useful triangular model of body reality, presentation, and ideal, which offers a framework for working towards improving body image (Fig. 2.1):
- Body reality—how the body really is: tall, short, fat or thin.
- Body ideal—how we feel the body should look.
- Body presentation—how the body is presented to the outside world.

An imbalance in any given area is likely to result in an alteration in body image, the severity of which will depend on the individual's support network and coping strategies.

## Sexuality

This complex issue has an important role in, and is an integral part of, our personality; sexuality is entwined in all aspects of our lives and influences everything we do. Sexuality is more than the act of sex; it is concerned with relationships and feelings about others, in addition to ourself. Major changes in sexual role and function are experienced by patients with GI illnesses because of the disease trajectory, surgical procedures, and long-term drug use (Tables 2.2 and 2.3).

**1** Price B (1990). *Body Image: Nursing Concepts and Care.* Prentice Hall, Hemel Hempstead.

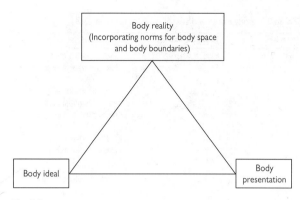

**Fig. 2.1** Body image framework (Reproduced from *Body Image: Nursing Concepts and Care*. Prentice Hall. Price B 1990, 📖 p. 4).

**Table 2.2** Body image and sexuality issues for men

| Problem | Probable cause | Treatment/solution |
|---|---|---|
| Impotence | Drugs | Stop or change medication |
| | Surgery | Sperm banking before surgery |
| | Progression of disease | Intercavernosal drugs |
| | Concurrent disease | Vacuum devices |
| | Psychological | Medication |
| | | Prosthetic implants |
| | | Pelvic floor exercises |
| | | Psychological support |
| Retrograde ejaculation/dry orgasm | Drugs | Counselling |
| | Surgery | Pelvic floor exercises |
| Sterility/inability to produce sperm | Drugs | Counselling |
| | Surgery | Sperm banking |
| Lack of libido | Change in body image | Counselling regarding sexual issues |
| | Lack of confidence | |
| | Unsure of partner's feelings | |
| | Surgery | |
| | Fear of intercourse | |
| | Fear of rejection | |

**Table 2.3** Body image and sexuality issues for women

| Problem | Probable cause | Treatment/solution |
| --- | --- | --- |
| Dyspareunia | Lack of oestrogen | Topical oestrogen creams |
| | Surgery | HRT (hormone replacement therapy) |
| | Infection | |
| | Stricture | Treat infection |
| | Psychological | KY Jelly/artificial saliva (unlicensed use) for lubrication |
| | | Vaginal dilators |
| | | Encourage intercourse |
| | | Psychological support |
| Vaginal dryness | Lack of oestrogen | Topical oestrogen creams |
| | Surgery | HRT |
| | | KY Jelly/artificial saliva (unlicensed use) for lubrication |
| | | Psychological support |
| Lack of libido | Change in body image | Counselling regarding sexual issues |
| | Lack of confidence | |
| | Unsure of partner's feelings | |
| | Surgery | |
| | Fear of intercourse | |
| | Fear of incontinence | |
| | Fear of rejection | |
| Infertility | Drugs | Counselling |
| | Surgery | *In vitro* fertilization (IVF) |
| | | Egg-sparing |

# Presentation of psychological difficulties in GI patients

It is well recognized that ~50% of patients presenting to gastroenterology outpatient clinics will be found to have a functional (non-organic) disorder. In many of these patients, a diagnosis of anxiety or depression can be made, and treatment thereafter will be in conjunction with psychological services, with good evidence for psychodynamic therapy, hypnotherapy, and/or cognitive–behavioural therapy. Such patients might resist a referral for psychological treatment, believing it to be stigmatizing or fearing it will uncover troubling memories or emotions. Pressure is placed on the general practitioner, primary care staff, and hospital staff to investigate further, sometimes even to operate, which should be resisted unless there are very good medical grounds for proceeding. Additional diagnoses, which might co-occur, include:

• An eating disorder (anorexia and/or bulimia).
• Obsessive–compulsive disorder.
• Other functional syndromes.

Patients with organic illnesses, such as inflammatory bowel disease (Crohn's disease or ulcerative colitis) present with a different set of psychological difficulties, often relating to the illness and its effects on their lives:

• Depression.
• Body-image disturbance.
• Problems of compliance with medication.
• Psychosexual difficulties.
• Problems associated with coping with (inter alia) a stoma, a fistula, parenteral nutrition, and/or periods of hospitalization.

In such cases, individual and/or family counselling or psychotherapy can be useful, helping the patient with his/her ability to cope with the illness. Similarly, patients with GI malignancy, hepato-biliary disease, or pancreatic disorders will present with disturbances pertaining to their particular condition, which are always coloured by their own past histories and their current family and personal situations, and these will be conveyed to staff members verbally and in their actions.

Patients might occasionally present to the gastroenterology service with a psychiatric disorder affecting the GI tract. Anorexia and/or bulimia are obvious examples, with complaints of constipation, bloating, and sometimes vomiting, but occasionally patients with severe depression develop delusions about their insides rotting. Patients might self-harm, injuring their bowel or harming their stoma or central line, and alcohol abuse can have severe consequences for the liver, pancreas, and entire GI tract.

Furthermore, many of the drugs used in psychiatry have effects on the GI tract (Box 2.1).

This is just a small fraction of the ways in which GI patients might present with psychological difficulties or psychiatric syndromes, and the effects of patient's psychological state on GI nursing cannot be underestimated. This emphasizes the importance of good clinical supervision when managing these patients.

### Box 2.1 Psychiatric drugs affecting the GI tract

- Selective serotonin-reuptake inhibitors (SSRIs) (antidepressants, such as fluoxetine)—nausea or altered bowel habit.
- Tricyclic antidepressants (e.g. amitriptyline)—constipation.
- Antipsychotic agents (e.g. olanzapine)—increased appetite.
- Antipsychotic agents (e.g. olanzapine)—nausea and vomiting, dyspepsia, or constipation.

# Management of psychological difficulties in GI patients

- Recognition of psychological morbidity—often this is recognized first by nurses who are often particularly closely involved in the ongoing hands-on care of the patient (especially in-patients) and their emotions.
- Discussion of the patient's psychological state with other team members.
- If possible, the provision of clinical supervision/case-discussion workshops for such cases; alternatively, a staff support group might be helpful in dealing with patients and the stresses of work.
- It is crucial that there is a pathway for referring such patients to professionals with the appropriate expertise. Not all GI units have access to in-house psychological services, but nurses must know that there is a link with local psychological services.
- Patients might be offered a number of different treatments after referral, but the options will tend to be one of two types—psychological therapy (e.g. counselling, hypnotherapy, group therapy, psychodynamic therapy, cognitive–behavioural therapy, etc.) and/or pharmacotherapy (i.e. drug treatment). In all cases, it is important for the GI team to get feedback from the mental health practitioner, because this could be crucial in therapeutic work with the patient.
- Ongoing education—GI nurses must remain well informed regarding psychiatry in general and the psychology of GI disorders in particular. This should be an important, and sometimes central, component of any continuing professional development (CPD).
- Clinical nurse specialists can often offer ongoing support to patients and their family/carers, but must recognize any limits to their scope and competence in this area.

### Further reading

Stern J (2003). Psychiatry, psychotherapy and gastroenterology: bringing it all together. *Alimentary Pharmacology and Therapeutics* **17**, 175–84.

# Nursing specialties in GI practice

Role of the nurse specialist in GI nursing  32
Training for advanced practice roles  33
Medico-legal issues and accountability in GI nursing  34
Nurse prescribing  36

# Role of the nurse specialist in GI nursing

In the past decade, there has been a huge expansion in the provision of specialist services for people with GI disorders. For example, the number of dedicated consultant gastroenterologists has doubled and virtually every district general hospital now has a colorectal surgeon. In parallel with this expansion, there has been a proliferation of nursing posts, roles, and the scope of practice, including the following.

• Stoma and pouch care.
• Endoscopist (upper or lower GI)—diagnostic or screening/surveillance.
• Inflammatory bowel disease (IBD) nurse specialist.
• Nutrition.
• Colorectal nurse practitioner.
• Biofeedback/benign disorders.

The nurse specialist's role might cover a single specialty or a combination of specialties, depending on the local needs and history of service. There is a limited evidence base for effectiveness of these roles, but they are often reported as popular with patients.

   However, there is a danger of fragmenting care and de-skilling 'generalist' ward, department, and community nurses. The nurse specialist's role might combine any of the following (and other roles locally).

• Specialist clinical care—but beware taking over routine care.
• Nurse-led clinics.
• Consultancy for professional colleagues.
• Development of protocols, guidelines, and care pathways.
• Coordination of patient pathways.
• Liaison with a multidisciplinary team—but beware administrative overload.
• Patient groups—education or support.
• Patient information.
• Patient advocacy.
• Telephone helpline or clinics.
• Teaching or mentoring clinical colleagues and clinical supervision.
• Formal teaching.
• Audit and research.

# Training for advanced practice roles

Training is poorly defined and often ad hoc locally,[1] with a few exceptions (e.g. the British Society of Gastroenterology endoscopist training guidelines).[2] The Nursing and Midwifery Council (NMC) advises 'competence', but this is poorly defined. It is increasingly accepted that MSc preparation should be the benchmark for nurse practitioner or advanced practice roles, but it can be difficult to access, fund, and find the time to study at this level.

1 Norton C and Kamm MA (2002). Specialist nurses in gastroenterology. *Journal of the Royal Society of Medicine* **95**, 331–5.

2 British Society of Gastroenterology (2006). *Care of Patients with Gastrointestinal Disorders in the United Kingdom*. BSG, London.

# Medico-legal issues and accountability in GI nursing

## Accountability

All registered nurses are governed by the NMC code of professional conduct (2002).[1] They must be trained and competent to provide care; there is an obligation to disclose any lack of competence and not to provide care in such circumstances. In law, they are required to practice with a level of skill and knowledge expected of own peer group.

## Negligence

If the nurse is working within their job description and competency, an employer will usually take vicarious liability for actions performed in good faith (but not those that are deliberately harmful). It is the employer, rather than the individual, who can be sued in a civil court for negligence. Vicarious liability does not cover deliberately criminal offences.

## Consent

Before any episode of care, consent must be obtained. This ensures permission for care and nurse–patient trust and cooperation.
- Valid informed consent—given by a competent adult who can weigh up the information provided, including benefits and significant (common or major) risks.
- Implied consent—the patient cooperates before the procedure, e.g. adopts the requested posture for examination. Consider the need for a chaperone.

A patient can withhold or withdraw consent at any time (without the need to give a reason). Care without consent can result in accusations of battery (a criminal offence) or trespass to the person (in civil law).
- Written consent—has no greater validity in law and is invalid if the patient did not understand the consent process.
- Legal capacity to consent—only needs to apply to proposed treatment (not an IQ test).
- <18 years of age—parents or legal guardians can consent (but note Gillick competence for teenagers who are considered capable of understanding the implications of their own consent).
- >18 years of age—no-one else (including parents or spouse) can give or withhold consent unless authorized by a court. A healthcare professional must give care in the patient's best interest if the patient is incapable.

---

1 Nursing and Midwifery Council (2002). *Code of Professional Conduct*. NMC, London.

# Nurse prescribing

## Introduction

In 1989, Dr June Crown proposed that qualified district nurses (DNS) or health visitors (HVS), who had completed an approved course, should be allowed to prescribe from a limited formulary. In addition, certain nurses should be able to supply and adjust the timing/dosage within a group protocol agreed for a particular situation. Since then, there has been an extension of the concept of 'nurse prescribing' to include other health-care professionals, a formalized course, and certain specified drugs from the *British National Formulary (BNF)*.[1]

In 2002, supplementary prescribing was introduced, which was defined as 'a voluntary partnership between an independent prescriber (doctor/dentist) and a supplementary prescriber (nurse/pharmacist) to implement an agreed patient-specific clinical management plan'. This led to an expansion of the Nurses Extended Formulary, allowing more drugs to be available. The types of nurse prescribing are shown in Box 3.1.

## Prescribing course

The content of the course includes the following.
- Consultation and decision-making.
- Safe and secure handling of medicines.
- Clinical pharmacology/pharmacokinetics/adverse drug reactions.
- Legal and ethical issues.
- Accountability.
- Patient assessment.

## Clinical governance

Clinical governance focuses on the patient's experience as the main indicator of quality. Nurse prescribing is a relatively new initiative that must be carefully monitored and evaluated to ensure that patients are receiving the best care possible. Healthcare establishments should always be considering and reviewing their strategic intent regarding any service offered and whether the patient's needs are being met.

Risk assessment protects patients and encourages healthcare professionals to examine what they do and how they can improve. Nurse prescribing is no exception. To date, there have been no legal 'test' cases for the issue of nurse prescribing and vicarious liability by health care trusts. It is the responsibility of the nurse prescriber to ensure that they feel confident and competent, after completing the course, in order to practice safely.

Appropriate training, education, reflective practice, and continuing professional development are imperative to support this exciting initiative and to ensure that the patient receives the highest quality of care.

---

**1** Courtenay M and Griffiths M (2004). *Independent and Supplementary Prescribing: an Essential Guide*. Cambridge University Press.

In May 2006 the Nurse Prescribers' Extended Formulary was discontinued and qualified nurse independent prescribers were authorized to prescribe any licensed medicine for any medical condition within their competence, including some controlled drugs.[2]

---

### Box 3.1 Types of nurse prescribing

*Patient group directions (formerly 'protocols')*
- Written instructions for the supply and administration of specified medicines for specified conditions.
- No limit on clinical focus.
- 'Condition/situation' focused—not 'patient-focused'.

*Nurse prescriber's formulary*
- Limited to a few 'prescription-only' medicines.
- Mainly consists of wound dressings and non-drug items designed to meet the needs of housebound patients.
- The DN/HV is eligible to prescribe after completion of a course.

*Nurse-prescribing extended formulary*
- List of 'prescription-only' drugs, plus licensed products for general and pharmacy sales (a list at the back of the *BNF*).
- Focusing on minor illness, health promotion, and palliative care.
- Extensive nurse-prescribing course to be completed.

*Supplementary prescribing*
- Legally allowed to prescribe from a wide range of medicines, except 'off-license' drugs.

Use of a clinical management plan for each patient to be agreed between doctor and prescriber. Permission must also be sought from the patient.

---

2 Beckwith S and Franklin P (2007.) *Oxford Handbook of Nurse Prescribing.* Oxford University Press.

# Imaging the GI tract

Radiological imaging  40
Barium swallow  42
Barium meal ('upper GI series')  43
Barium follow-through  44
Barium enema  45
Evacuating proctogram (defecography,
    defecating proctogram)  46
Abdominal ultrasound  47
Computed tomography (CT)  48
Virtual colonoscopy (VC) or CT colonography  50
Magnetic resonance imaging (MRI)  52
Scintigraphy (radionuclide imaging or nuclear
    medicine studies)  54

# Radiological imaging

All abdominal imaging that involves radiation (X-rays) is of potential harm to the patient in terms of a risk of inducing cancer. For example, an abdominal computed tomography (CT) scan has a risk of 1 in 1000 of inducing cancer. Furthermore, exposure during pregnancy, to even small amounts of radiation, has a risk of teratogenesis in the fetus. The use of X-rays should be kept to a minimum. If possible, good clinical history and examination findings, in addition to ultrasound, can help ↓ the need for radiation-based investigations.

## Plain abdominal X-ray (radiograph)

Shows an overview of the bony and soft tissue structures in the abdomen and can show gas within an obstructed or diseased bowel.

*Indications*
• Suspected bowel obstruction and abdominal distension accompanied by nausea and vomiting, with ↓ bowel output.
• Assessment of the extent of disease in acute colitis.

## Contrast studies of the gastrointestinal tract (GIT)

Heavy metal (barium or iodine) based solutions (which are both inert) are taken orally and travel through the stomach and small bowel in 1–2 h in a fasted patient. The metal shows up on radiographs because it stops the incident radiation in a similar way to bones, appearing white and providing a map of the bowel at the time at which the radiograph is taken.

Barium sulphate (which is not absorbed from the GIT) is a chalky solution of varying thickness, from watery to milkshake/yoghurt-type thickness. It can also be made up in the form of a paste and used to simulate a food bolus, for assessment of swallow function, or given as an enema, to enable assessment of evacuation. If taken orally, it is usually flavoured to make it more palatable. The barium sticks to the dry fasted mucosa of the gut lining as it travels through; the thicker the solution, the more sticky it is and the more detail is obtained of the mucosal surface.

## Iodine-based water-soluble and low-osmolar contrast media (LOCM)

If barium escapes from the bowel into the mediastinum or peritoneum, it can cause irritation and, in some cases, severe inflammation. For this reason, in the immediate post-operative period, or if perforation is sus-pected, an alternative iodine-based solution (gastrografin or other water-soluble agent) is given. This is a more watery solution, which is similar to the intravenous contrast media used in other imaging techniques. These cannot produce good mucosal detail of the bowel but are used commonly in the post-operative setting to exclude or confirm leaks at anastomoses or, in cases of small-bowel obstruction, if the effect of these agents can relieve the obstruction.

Spasmolytic agents, such as glucagon or hyoscine-*n*-butyl bromide (Buscopan®) can be used to induce hypotonicity of the GIT. A segment of spastic bowel, e.g. mimicking a benign stricture or malignancy, can be identified by watching the bowel segment regaining its normal appearance after the spasmolytic drug has been administered intravenously.

### Complications
- Leakage of barium from an unsuspected perforation.
- Aspiration.

Barium has a constipating effect and, in the presence of a colonic stricture, bowel obstruction owing to barium impaction is a rare complication. Water-soluble contrast agents should be used if aspiration is probable or a leak is suspected. Gastrografin is hypertonic, drawing water into the bowel, and can cause diarrhoea. It also results in pulmonary oedema if aspirated, so LOCM should be used in preference if aspiration is a risk.

### Aftercare
Patients are advised to ↑ their fluid intake for a few days after a barium study, to prevent constipation, and to take gentle laxatives if they usually need to.

# Barium swallow

### Indications
- Dysphagia—difficulty swallowing solids or liquids.
- Odynophagia—pain on swallowing.
- Globus sensation—lump in throat.
- Suspected pulmonary aspiration.
- Suspected oesophageal perforation—LOCM ± barium.

### Contraindications
- Suspected leak.
- Known colonic stricture.
- Severe dysphagia, with an obvious oropharyngeal component. The patient is unlikely to be able to take sufficient contrast for a complete study.
- Severe immobility and difficulty standing unaided.

### Preparation
- Fasting for 4 h before the procedure.

### Choice of contrast agent
- 100% weight/volume (w/v) barium for most patients.

### Procedure
- The patient should be in the standing position.
- The contrast agent is given orally and swallowed on instruction.
- The passage of the contrast agent down the oesophagus is visualized in real time and a series of images is taken from the upper to lower part of the oesophagus at different angles.

This study enables radiographic real-time visualization of moving anatomical structures; in particular, the swallowing process and contractions of the oesophagus can be evaluated and any obstruction or stricture can be identified.

### Average procedure time
- 10–15 min.

### Aftercare
- ↑ fluid intake.

# Barium meal ('upper GI series')

## Indications
- Dyspepsia.
- Weight loss.
- Upper abdominal mass.
- Assessment of a site of perforation or anastomosis (LOCM).
- Failure or contraindication to endoscopy oesophageal gastroduodenoscopy (OGD).

## Preparation
- Fasting for 4 h before examination.

## Choice of contrast agent
- Barium sulphate (250% w/v) and a gas-producing agent to create gaseous distension of the stomach.

## Contraindications
📖 Barium swallow, p. 43.

## Procedure
The barium meal is an extension of the barium swallow study, which visualizes the passage of orally ingested contrast agent into the duodenum. Because endoscopy has become more commonplace, the use of upper GI series has continued to diminish. OGD has a high sensitivity and ability to biopsy and/or treat, and has made OGD first-choice investigation. Nonetheless, a high-quality barium meal, using a double-contrast technique (barium-coated mucosa within a gas-distended stomach), can provide excellent diagnostic information of the gastro-oesophageal junction, and both gastric and duodenal mucosa, in particular. The patient should be in lying position and asked to turn several times into sideways, supine, and prone positions. These manoeuvres are necessary to test for gastro-oesophageal reflux disease (GORD) and for visualization of the entire gastric mucosa. Spasmolytic agents (e.g. hyoscine butyl bromide) are given to ↓ gastric motility.

## Average procedure time
- 15 min.

# Barium follow-through

This refers to the use of barium to outline the small bowel from the duodenum to the terminal ileum. A larger volume of more dilute barium is taken orally (~600 ml). Images are then taken at 20-min intervals, demonstrating a column of barium travelling along the small intestine. Strictures, inflammation, diverticula, and tumours are easily identifiable.

Alternatively, a 'small bowel enema' may be given via a nasogastric tube. This is a quicker examination than oral barium, with no difference in sensitivity. However, it can be more uncomfortable for the patient.

### Indications
• Intermittent small-bowel obstruction.
• Assessment of known small-bowel disease—Crohn's disease, coeliac disease, and polyposis syndromes.

### Contraindications
📖 Barium swallow, p. 42.

### Preparation
• Fasting for 6 h.

### Average procedure time
• 2.5 h.

# Barium enema

A double-contrast technique is used in a fully prepared colon to outline the mucosa of the colon while it is distended with air or carbon dioxide.

Note: A single-contrast enema can be given in an unprepared colon for rapid exclusion of colonic obstruction.

### Indications
• Altered bowel habit and suspected stricture/tumour.
• Rectal bleeding.

### Contraindications
📖 Barium swallow, p. 42.

### Preparation
• Low-residue diet for 48 h.
• Good oral fluid intake, in addition to two sachets of sodium picosulphate (Picolax®) during the 24 h before the procedure, to produce a cleansed colon with minimal fluid residue.

### Procedure
650 ml of 70% w/v barium sulphate is introduced per rectum through an enema bag and tube, starting with the patient in a left-lateral position. The patient is turned prone, to encourage the barium to travel along the colon into the splenic flexure. Barium coats the bowel wall after several more changes of the patient's position and, following insufflation of carbon dioxide or air, the entire colon is visualized in double contrast. Strictures, polyps, tumours, diverticula, and inflammatory changes are easily identified.

# Evacuating proctogram (defecography, defecating proctogram)

This examination is designed to study the dynamic processes in the pelvic floor that enable defecation. Defecation is not replicated, only simulated, because urgency is induced by insertion of a barium-paste enema into the rectum. Dilute barium solution is taken orally to delineate the small bowel so that any hernia (enterocele) can easily be demonstrated. Sometimes it can be useful to fill the bladder in more complex pelvic floor dysfunction, but this is not routine. Patient privacy and a relaxed reassuring environment is essential, and the test is usually only performed in centres at which this environment can be developed. Evacuation of the barium paste is recorded using fluoroscopy. Perineal descent, retention, or incomplete evacuation of the enema and abnormal herniation of the rectum, rectal wall, or other structures are definable.

## Indications
- Intractable constipation—to exclude obstructed defecation as the cause.
- Perineal herniation—to exclude anismus as a predisposing factor.
- Suspected rectal intussusception or prolapse.

## Contraindication
- Faecal incontinence.

## Complications/aftercare
- None.

# Abdominal ultrasound

Ultrasound uses high-frequency sound waves, in a similar way to radar, to map out different tissue interfaces and display the information in a two-dimensional real-time image that represents the internal tissues of the body being examined. Sound waves do not travel through air, so some detail is lost in looking at the abdomen, because bowel containing air or gas obstructs the view of deeper structures. It is best used for examining the solid or fluid-containing organs of the abdomen, and is the most sensitive examination for detecting gallstones because its spatial resolution, if optimally performed, is better than both CT and magnetic resonance imaging (MRI). Although loops of bowel can make examining the abdomen and pelvis difficult, good detail of the bowel wall makes it possible to identify bowel inflammation in colitis, thickened bowel loops suggestive of inflammatory bowel disease, diverticulitis, or other inflammatory conditions of the small bowel.

## Indications
- Abdominal pain.
- ↑ liver enzyme levels.
- Jaundice.
- Hepatomegaly.
- Symptoms of biliary-tract pathology.
- Renal insufficiency.
- Abdominal masses.
- Suspected abdominal sepsis.
- Inflammatory bowel disease (IBD).

## Contraindications
- None.
- Multiple abdominal dressings/stoma bags make access to the abdominal wall difficult and are a relative contraindication.
- Pancreatic imaging may be poor because of overlying bone and gas.

## Preparation
Patients should be nil by mouth for 4 h before the examination, to enable visualization of the gall bladder.

## Complications
- None.

## Aftercare
- None.

# Computed tomography (CT)

CT uses X-rays and high-powered computer reconstruction techniques to create a cross-sectional image through the body, showing all the different organs by virtue of their different water and fat contents, in addition to their vascularity.

## Indications

CT is indicated if ultrasound is technically difficult or non-diagnostic and for whole-body staging in malignancy. The main disadvantages are a relatively high radiation dose and the difficulty of transferring sick and unstable patients to the scanner.

## Procedure

The examination table advances at a constant rate through the CT scanner gantry, while the X-ray tube rotates continuously around the abdomen, emitting controlled beams of radiation. Each time the X-ray tube makes a 360° rotation, a digital image of a thin transverse section of the abdomen is acquired. The average procedure time is 20 min, with a scan time of between 20 s and 5 min, depending on the type of scan being performed. The patient must hold their breath, usually for 6–10 s at a time.

## Contrast administration for CT

Within the abdomen, the use of contrast materials is necessary to enhance the visibility of soft tissue, visceral organs, and blood vessels. The contrast material used can be swallowed, injected through a vein directly into the bloodstream, or administered by enema, depending on the type of examination. Most commonly, an abdominal CT scan requires the patient to drink some oral contrast agent, and an intravenous (IV) high-rate infusion is performed during the examination.

## Preparing the patient

Four aspects must always be considered:

*Renal function: are urea and creatinine levels within their normal ranges?*

Patients with kidney problems carry an ↑ risk of potential problems eliminating the contrast material from their system after the examination.

The degree of renal dysfunction, risk of causing renal failure, and type of contrast agent are important.

*Previous idiosyncratic reaction to contrast medium*

The risk of an anaphylactic reaction or inducing renal failure should be weighed against the risk of failing to find a diagnosis in a critically ill patient. Exploratory surgery might be a better option in some cases, and a multidisciplinary discussion is an essential component of the decision on how best to manage such patients.

*Scheduling of patients*
Patients who are considered for an abdominal CT scan using oral contrast medium must be scheduled 30–60 min earlier to enable sufficient time for the contrast agent to travel through the GIT before the procedure.

*Scheduling a CT scan and surgery*
- The right contrast medium should be chosen (no barium before surgery).
- Investigations should be carefully planned (previous barium studies cause severe artefacts in CT scans for the following ~3 days).

## Contraindications
- No absolute contraindications.

## Complications
- None.

## Aftercare
Occasionally, patients can experience a laxative effect from the oral contrast, so warning of this is useful.

# Virtual colonoscopy (VC) or CT colonography

### Indications

Suspected colorectal cancer or its precursor, the colonic polyp. VC can be performed with standard CT to provide a complete staging scan if an obstructing cancer cannot be traversed at colonsocopy. However, VC may not be as sensitive as colonoscopy for polyp detection. Additionally, any abnormalities detected cannot be biopsied or treated.

### Contraindications

- Previous surgery that has left an oversewn rectal stump or mucous fistula.
- The presence of IBD is a relative contraindication owing to the ↑ risk of perforation, particularly in active disease.

### Preparation

Similar to a barium enema, the bowel must be cleansed. Commonly, a formal full bowel preparation is given, but newer techniques are being developed that will use modified and less laxative regimens or no bowel cleansing at all.

### Choice of contrast agent

Usually, no contrast agent is used because this enables a more rapid examination time. An IV contrast agent is used if the patient is to have staging of malignancy at the same visit.

### Procedure

The patient lies on the CT scanner table top and is asked to assume a left-lateral position, for insertion of a soft thin rectal catheter. Carbon dioxide is introduced by a pressure-controlled pump to insufflate the colon. IV hyoscine butylbromide is used as an antispasmodic. Once insufflated, two scans are acquired: one with the patient in a supine position, and the other scan with the patient lying prone, supported by a pillow under their chest.

### Average procedure time

- 20 min.

### Complications

Perforation is a rare complication; the incidence is significantly less than that reported in conventional colonoscopy.

### Aftercare

- None.

# Magnetic resonance imaging (MRI)

MRI is similar to CT, in that it produces cross-sectional images of the body and internal organs. It has three main advantages.
- It does not use ionizing radiation.
- The contrast resolution between different tissue types is better, enabling better characterization of abnormal tissue.
- The computer software enables display of the information in any plane, which affords a better understanding of the relationships between different organs/structures and the abnormality—an advantage in surgical planning.

The technique uses a large-bore high-field-strength magnet, with a central tunnel. When the patient lies inside the tunnel, the magnet aligns the protons of all atoms of the patient's body in one direction. High-energy audible-frequency sound is used to transfer energy to these protons, which deflects their alignment. When they return to a normal relaxed state, energy is emitted, which is detected by the scanner, and the information is used to map the internal structure of the body in terms of tissue structure and characteristics.

## Indications
Primarily used for assessment of rectal and perineal disease caused by IBD or as part of staging of anorectal cancer. Increasingly used for exclusion of pancreatic and biliary pathology, if ultrasound is inconclusive. Specialist centres might use MRI to identify small and large bowel pathology.

## Contraindications
- Metallic implants, e.g. a cardiac pacemaker or other metallic mechanical/electrical device in the heart or brain.
- Metal in crucial or sensitive areas, e.g. shrapnel in the eyeball.
- Relative contraindications—claustrophobia and ventilated or monitored patients.

## Preparation
- None required.

## Choice of contrast agent
For some small bowel and pancreatic studies, injections of antispasmodic or antisecretory agents might be required. Some staging examinations might require an intravascular contrast agent.

## Procedure
The patient must be able to lie still on the scanner table, inside the magnet bore. It is noisy, with a fairly monotonous sound, similar to a road-worker's pneumatic tools. Despite this, with earplugs and a calmly lit environment, most patients manage to fall into a light sleep and remain comfortable throughout.

**Average procedure time**
• 15–45 min.

**Complications**
• None.

**Aftercare**
• None.

# Scintigraphy (radionuclide imaging or nuclear medicine studies)

The three main examinations used to look at the GI tract are as follows.
• White cell scan—to look for inflammation or abcesses.
• Hepatobiliary iminodiacetic acid (HIDA) scan—to examine hepatic excretory and gall bladder functions.
  Might be used to delineate bile leaks or congenital anomalies in infants with jaundice.
• Position emission tomography (PET) (or PET/CT) scan—excludes the spread of tumours to distant sites if major surgery is being considered. Can identify small areas of recurrence, if these cannot be identified by other imaging techniques.

### Contraindications and preparation
• Specific to the indication.

### Procedure
The patient receives an injection of a radiolabelled physiological protein, which is incorporated into the organs of the body and metabolized as normal. The low-level radiation emitted by the substance can be detected by a gamma camera, on which the patient lies for intervals of 20–30 min. The average procedure time is 3–4 h. The patient can return to the ward after injection of the radionuclide; instructions will be given to the ward staff regarding precautions, if appropriate. The radioactive material administered to the patient is not powerful enough to leave the patient and is absorbed into their body. In some cases, however, excretion occurs into faeces and urine, making minor precautions necessary.

### Complications
• None.

### Aftercare
• None.

# Nutrition

Introduction  56
Nutritional requirements in health  57
Balance of good health  58
Influence of diet on health  60
Obesity  62
Management of obesity  64
Diet and cancer  66
Functional foods and supplements  68
Nutrients  70
Fats  72
Carbohydrates  74
Fibre  76
Proteins  78
Vitamins  82
Minerals  88
Water  94

# Introduction

Nutrition, as a science, includes many disciplines. In addition to being the foundation of good health and disease prevention, the food we eat has important psychological and social roles in our lives.

Data from the National Food Survey[1] reported the average household expenditure on food and drink (excluding alcohol) for 2005–06 was 10% of gross income. Although we are spending more on food, there is ↑ concern that we make poor food choices. The consequences of our food choices and the eating behaviour of our children are influenced greatly by our knowledge and attitudes. Because we have ↓ individual involvement in the cultivation and preparation of food, it seems that we are abdicating the responsibility for making good food choices. Our daily routines and busy lifestyles have led us to turn to the convenience of processed food, with little concern for how the food is grown and pre-pared. This lack of interest has meant that we are less knowledgeable about food and how important nutrients are to health.

Nurses require a thorough knowledge of nutrition to understand how it influences health throughout an individual's lifespan. The gastrointestinal tract is the organ responsible for ingestion, digestion, and absorption; furthermore, a healthy gastrointestinal tract (GIT) is essential in maintaining nutritional health. The nurse working within this speciality must have a sound knowledge of how an altered GIT will affect an individual's health.

▶ The nurse should also understand how the function of the GIT is influenced by food and nutrients.

There is an ↑ amount of information regarding the health benefits of certain foods, in addition to an ↑ number of 'nutritionists' willing to advise the public. The nurse must be confident that the information his/her patients are receiving is correct and be able to identify and liaise with appropriately qualified professionals.

For the patient to benefit from the nurse's knowledge, the nurse must first make an assessment of the individual's needs and plan care. This will require the application of patient education and health promotion skills.

This chapter focuses on the importance of a balanced diet and provides an overview of nutrients.

## Further reading

British Nutrition Foundation. http://www.nutrition.org.uk (accessed 25.05.07).

**1** Dunn E and Gibbs C (2007). *Family Spending: 2006 Edition*. Office for National Statistics. Palgrave Macmillan London. http://www.palgrave.com/ONS/ (accessed 25.06.07).

# Nutritional requirements in health

Recommendations for nutrient intake were first published in 1969. The subsequent revision of this document reflects the ↑ knowledge of nutrients and aims to assess the adequacy of the diets of groups of people. The 1991 guidance produced by the Committee on Medical Aspects of Food and Nutrition Policy[1] adopted the term 'dietary reference values', which implied that it was a general point of 'reference' rather than an absolute or definitive recommendation. There is current agreement that guidance needs to ensure maximum health and function while ↓ the risk of degenerative illness, rather than just aiming to prevent symptoms of deficiency.

## Dietary reference values

People need many different nutrients to maintain good health. The amount of nutrients required is related to the difference between absorption and metabolism, in addition to age, gender, state of health, and level of activity. Dietary reference values include the following categories of estimates derived from the principle that the requirement for a nutrient is normally distributed.

- Estimated average requirement (EAR)—used to guide the average requirement for energy (no other value is used for energy requirements) or a nutrient. By definition, 50% of the population require more than the average and 50% require less. An EAR has been set for dietary fibre (adults), energy (fat and carbohydrate), nine vitamins (📖 p. 82), and 11 minerals (📖 p. 88).
- Reference nutrient intake (RNI)—an amount of nutrient that meets the needs of almost all individuals (97.5% of the population). Healthy individuals consuming this level of nutrients are unlikely to be deficient. An RNI has been set for nine vitamins and 11 minerals.
- Lower reference nutrient intake (LRNI)—an amount of nutrient that is enough for only a small number of the population (2.5% of the population). An LRNI has been set for nine vitamins and 11 minerals.
- Safe intake (SI)—the term used to refer to the intake of nutrient that does not have enough information to provide an EAR, RNI, or LRNI. It gives a value that is expected to avoid deficiency but set below a level that might cause toxic effects. An SI has been set for four vitamins (pantothenic acid, biotin, vitamin E, and vitamin K) and four minerals (manganese, molybdenum, chromium, and fluoride).

The Committee on Medical Aspects of Food has been superseded by the Scientific Advisory Committee on Nutrition.[2] This group of independent experts is supported by a joint secretariat of the Department of Health and Food Standards Agency.

1 Department of Health (1991). *Dietary Reference Values for Food Energy and Nutrition for the United Kingdom.* Committee on Medical Aspects of Food Policy Report. HMSO, London.

2 Scientific Advisory Committee on Nutrition. http://www.sacn.gov.uk (accessed 25.06.07).

# Balance of good health

The Food Standards Agency[1] has translated the recommendations of the Committee on Medical Aspects of Food Policy report[2] into a more user-friendly format. The 'balance of good health' depicts a range and amount of foods that are required to make up a balanced diet.

The pictorial guide represents a plate and is divided into the five following food groups.

• Bread, other cereals, and potatoes—should make up 33% of daily food intake. Include at least one portion of starchy food at each main meal. This food group provides carbohydrate, calcium, iron, B vitamins, and fibre.

• Fruit and vegetables—eat at least five portions per day (33% of food consumed). This food group provides water-soluble vitamins, carbohydrate, and fibre.

• Milk and dairy products—eat two to three portions per day (15% of food consumed). This food group provides calcium, protein, vitamin $B_{12}$, and fat-soluble vitamins.

• Meat, fish, and alternatives—eat two to three portions per day (12% of food consumed). This food group provides iron, protein, B vitamins, zinc, and magnesium.

• Foods containing fat and sugar—eat only zero to three portions per day (8% of food consumed). This food group provides fat, carbohydrate, fat-soluble vitamins, and salt.

A balanced diet includes a variety of foods which, if consumed in the above proportions for a period of time, will provide energy and nutrients for the majority of the population to remain healthy.

## Guidelines for a healthy diet

• Base your meals on starchy foods.
• Eat plenty of fruit and vegetables.
• Eat more fish.
• Limit the amount of foods containing saturated fat and sugars.
• Eat less salt—no more than 6 g/day.
• Get active and eat the right amount to maintain a healthy weight.
• Drink plenty of water.
• Don't skip breakfast.

Promoting a whole-diet approach to healthy eating is essential because it considers the consequences of the whole diet on health, rather than just individual nutrients or food groups.

1 Health Education Authority (1996). *The Balance of Good Health. Health Education Authority: Ministry of Agriculture, Fisheries, and Food, London;* or via Food Standards Agency. *Eat well, be well.* http://www.eatwell.gov.uk (accessed 25.06.07).

2 Department of Health (1991). *Dietary Reference Values for Food Energy and Nutrition for the United Kingdom.* Committee on Medical Aspects of Food Policy Report. HMSO. London.

## Food labelling

The Food Standards Agency is promoting the use of traffic-light labelling to identify for the consumer foods that contain high (red), medium (amber), or low (green) levels of saturated fat, salt, and added sugar.

# Influence of diet on health

There is ↑ evidence that an individual's diet is associated with the risk of chronic disease in adult life. Diet-related chronic diseases, also known as 'nutrition-related non-communicable diseases' (NCDs), are attributed to an unbalanced (not always excessive) intake, genetic predisposition, and ↓ levels of physical activity.

Diet-related chronic illnesses include the following.

- Alcoholism—alcohol provides 7.1 kcal/g. If consumed in moderation, alcohol has a protective effect against cardiovascular disease. If taken in excess, it can become addictive. Consequences of alcoholism include weight gain and, in extreme cases, malnutrition, which is associated with poor nutritional intake and malabsorbption, damage to the liver, brain, and heart, and an ↑ risk of cancer.

- Obesity (📖 p. 62)—a direct consequence of a diet with excess energy intake compared with activity. It is linked to a number of chronic diseases, including cardiovascular disease, cancer, type 2 diabetes, and osteoarthritis.

- The metabolic syndrome is associated with an ↑ risk of type 2 diabetes mellitus and cardiovascular disease. It is characterized by insulin resistance, dyslipidaemia, abdominal obesity, and hypertension. The disease process involves several metabolic pathways. Nutrition is thought to have a key role in the development of this syndrome because obesity is an underlying causative factor.

- Cardiovascular disease is the most common cause of death in the UK. Dietary factors contribute to the pathophysiology of atherosclerosis and thrombosis. To ↓ the risk of atherosclerosis and thrombosis, individuals are advised to reduce the total amount of fat consumed, in particular to change the ratio of saturated to mono- and poly-unsaturated fats, to regulate their cholesterol levels by ↓ the amount of saturated fat in the diet, ↑ the amount of mono-unsaturated and n-6 poly-unsaturated fats (sunflower and corn oil), and ↑ the amount of soluble fibre in the diet. Oil-rich (n-3 fatty acids) fish consumption can also ↓ the level of triglycerides and has anti-thrombotic properties (as precursors to prostaglandins), ∴ ↓ the risk of clot formation. A ↓ in high blood pressure is advised, which can be achieved through weight ↓, ↓ salt intake, ↑ level of exercise, and cessation of smoking.

- Type 2 diabetes mellitus is associated with obesity, characteristically central abdominal obesity. This results in a partial or complete lack of insulin production, which directly affects glucose and fat metabolism. Health advice emphasizes weight loss, maintenance of a normal blood sugar level, and ↑ physical activity. Some patients with type 2 diabetes will require insulin therapy if drug and diet therapies are unsuccessful. Uncontrolled diabetes leads to an ↑ risk of heart disease, renal failure, neuropathy, and blindness.

- Cancer (📖 p. 66).

## Food intolerance

▶ Although food intolerance (unless untreated) does not lead to chronic disease, it has direct health consequences. Food intolerance is associated with an adverse reaction to a specific food or ingredient, which will produce the same reaction if exposure occurs again. This definition does not include reactions to foods that have a psychological basis. There is a wide interpretation as to what constitutes an adverse reaction because individuals vary in their tolerance. Food intolerance includes the following.

• Food allergy—requires an immunological reaction. The scope of reaction includes urticaria, angio-oedema, rhinitis, worsening of atopic eczema, respiratory symptoms (e.g. wheezing, coughing, and dyspnoea), gastrointestinal symptoms (e.g. vomiting, diarrhoea, and abdominal pain), and anaphylactic shock (an extreme reaction).
  ▶ A sound diagnosis of food allergy is important, especially in children who are on exclusion diets who should be managed by an immunologist and specialist dietitian.

• Enzyme defects—inborn errors of metabolism might affect digestion, absorption, and storage of carbohydrate, fat, or protein. Whereas several enzyme deficiencies are limited to the GIT (e.g. lactase deficiency, which generally causes the loose stools and bloating associated with the consumption of milk), other enzyme deficiencies (e.g. fructose intolerance) have more immediate life-threatening consequences. If an enzyme in the process responsible for the breakdown of fructose is missing, it causes a build-up of fructose-1-phosphate, which, in turn, inhibits the enzyme converting glycogen to glucose in hepatic cells and results in hypoglycaemia, shock, convulsions, and sometimes liver disease.

• Pharmacological reactions—several components of food are known to have pharmacological effects. Caffeine has stimulant effects that are usually dose dependent. Reactions include a fast heart rate, an irregular heartbeat, tremor, anxiety, sleeplessness, heartburn, diarrhoea, and colic.

• Drug–food interactions—the most common intolerance/interaction is associated with tyramine-containing food (e.g. cheese, yeast, and fermented soya products) and a class of antidepressant drugs (monoamine oxidase inhibitors).

• Toxic products—several plants are toxic and must be processed before consumption. Plant proteins (phytohaemagglutinins or lectins) are present in legumes, and can, in extreme circumstances, agglutinate red blood cells. Inadequate cooking of red kidney beans can cause severe gastrointestinal symptoms.

• Food contamination—during storage, chemical changes can occur that cause toxic reactions. Poor storage of mackerel, with bacterial spoilage, can ↑ the level of histamine in the fish. Reactions can also occur through contamination by antigens, such as mites, bacterial spores, and fungi.

# Obesity

Obesity is defined as a body mass index (BMI) of 30 kg/m$^2$ or more (Table 5.1). In the UK in 2002, ~22 % of ♂ and ~23 % of ♀ were classed as clinically obese. An ↑ waist circumference also enables an assessment of the individual's risk of being overweight and associated risk of cardiovascular disease.[1]

Obesity occurs if more energy is consumed than used. The reasons for this include the following.

- Lack of regular exercise.
- Sedentary occupation.
- Irregular eating activity and snacking behaviour.
- Availability of high-calorie convenience foods.
- ↑ alcohol intake.
- Genetics/ethnicity.

## Impact on health

An ↑ in body fat is associated with changes in physiological function. Many of these changes are linked to the distribution of adipose tissue, as follows.

- Generalized obesity—↑ total blood volume and cardiac function.
- Thoracic and abdominal adipose deposition—↓ respiratory function.
- Intra-abdominal visceral deposition—hypertension, ↑ level of insulin, and associated insulin resistance and hyperglycaemia. People of Asian origin have a tendency to more visceral fat and associated health risks than Caucasians, although they might have a lower BMI.

Obesity-associated conditions affect the cardiovascular, respiratory, gastrointestinal (e.g. cirrhosis, gallstones, colorectal cancer, hiatus hernia, and gastro-oesophageal reflux), renal, reproductive, musculoskeletal, genitourinary, and endocrine systems, and the skin.

**Table 5.1** Classification of obesity[1]

| Classification | Body mass index (kg/m$^2$) |
| --- | --- |
| Underweight | <18.5 |
| Normal | 18.5–24.9 |
| Overweight | 25.0–29.9 |
| Obese (I) | 30.0–34.9 |
| Obese (II) | 35.0–39.9 |
| Obese (III) | ≥40 |

1 National Institute for Health and Clinical Excellence (2006). Obesity: the prevention, identification, assessment and management of overweight and obesity in adults and children. *Clinical Guidelines* **43**. http://www.nice.gov.uk (accessed 25.06.07).

# Management of obesity

## Aims

By ↓ the amount and distribution of body fat, the potential benefits include:

- Improving health and well-being.
- ↓ the risk of chronic illness.

A ↓ in weight of 5–10% is associated with improved clinical outcome (e.g. blood pressure, serum cholesterol, and improved blood glucose control). Successful weight regulation should be focused on ↓ risk, rather than a return to a normal weight.

## Treatment

Obesity is a chronic relapsing condition that requires long-term treatment strategies, such as those described below.

### Diet

Defined as 'low-calorie' (800–1500 kcal/day) or 'very-low-calorie' (800 kcal/day) diets. They include a variety of diets that restrict calories according to the quantity of macronutrients, amount of supervision provided, and need for the purchase of commercially produced replacement meals. Some diets have more scientific underpinning than others. The long-term maintenance of weight is also dependent on activity levels and long-term changes in food behaviour.

### Physical activity

Lack of exercise is a contributory factor for the development of obesity. Similarly, it is an important component of the management of obesity, in combination with dietary interventions. In individuals who are exercising, loss of weight is associated with the preservation of fat-free mass. Additionally, regular exercise contributes to a ↓ in blood pressure and improved insulin sensitivity.

### Behavioural therapy

A variety of techniques that require the individual to explore the reasons for their abnormal eating behaviours and participate in techniques to unlearn established eating patterns. Participants are required to take responsibility for their behaviour, both diet-related and exercise.

These programmes characteristically involve self-monitoring, goal-setting, stimulus control, problem-solving, and cognitive adaptation (challenging beliefs about weight control, exploring thoughts and emotions, and using positive-thinking techniques).

### Drug therapy

Only considered following an evaluation of diet, exercise, and behavioural interventions. Pharmacological agents include orlistat (a gastric and pancreatic lipase inhibitor that ↓ absorption of dietary fat) and sibutramine (↑ the sense of satiety by its action as a serotonin-reuptake inhibitor). Patients who have a priority for treatment include those with comorbidities (e.g. type 2 diabetes, hypertension, and dyslipidaemia), whose activity is (directly or indirectly) limited by weight, or who are thought to be high risk (e.g. with a family history). These drugs are not without their risks and require pre-assessment and ongoing monitoring.

### Surgical intervention

The criteria for selecting patients for surgery include a BMI $\geq 40$ kg/m$^2$ or $\geq 35$ kg/m$^2$ with a serious comorbidity. Assessment includes consideration of operative morbidity and long-term adverse effects. Surgical techniques include the following.

- Jaw wiring—no longer advocated because of a lack of long-term efficacy.
- Gastric restriction (gastric banding or gastroplasty)—these techniques involve restricting the gastric volume to ~20–30 ml. Dietary compliance is still required.
- Gastric bypass—involves ↓ stomach capacity (~20–30 ml); the stomach is connected to the jejunum. In addition to an inability to tolerate normal volumes of food, gastric bypass promotes malabsorption. Although it achieves ↑ weight loss than just gastric restriction, it causes dumping syndrome (📖 p. 368) and nutritional deficiencies.

Surgical intervention should be undertaken as part of a multidisciplinary approach to treatment; ongoing dietetic and primary healthcare management is essential.

## Further reading

Colquitt J, Clegg A, Loveman E, et al. (2003). Surgery for morbid obesity. *Cochrane Database of Systematic Reviews* 2. http://www.cochrane.org/reviews/en/ab003641.html (accessed 07.11.07).

*International Obesity Task Force.* http://www.iotf.org (accessed 25.06.07).

National Institute for Health and Clinical Excellence (2006). Obesity: the prevention, identification, assessment and management of overweight and obesity in adults and children. *Clinical Guidelines* 43. http://www.nice.gov.uk (accessed 25.06.07).

Shaw K, O' Rourke P, and Del Mar C (2005). Psychological intervention for overweight or obesity. *Cochrane Database of Systematic Reviews* 3. http://www.cochrane.org/reviews/en/ab003818.html (accessed 07.11.07).

# Diet and cancer

The World Cancer Research Fund (WCRF) reported that approximately 33% of all cancers are preventable.[1] However, the evidence linking diet to cancer is complex because cancer is a complicated disease to study. The reasons for this include the following.
- Cancer takes many years to develop.
- There are several different forms.
- There are multiple risk factors—genetic predisposition, environmental factors, and hormonal factors.
- Some substances can initiate the cancer process, whereas others can affect its progression.

Diet is considered to be an environmental factor. Our diet is made up of many different foods and nutrients. Some diets (containing many different combinations of nutrients) influence the risk of developing cancers (Table 5.2), either directly (e.g. red and processed meat and bowel cancer) or indirectly (e.g. maintaining a healthy body weight ↓ the risk of bowel, breast, kidney, oesophageal, and uterine cancers).

## General advice
- Eat five different portions of fruit and vegetables per day—provide a range of vitamins and minerals, in addition to ↑ dietary fibre.
- Choose whole-grain varieties of starchy food.
- Avoid energy-dense foods and drinks.
- Eat smaller and fewer portions of red and processed meats.
- Use low-temperature methods of cooking—avoid eating meat that has been burnt.
- ↓ the amount of saturated fat in the diet, including processed foods.
- Consume more oily fish, e.g. salmon, mackerel, or sardines.
- Maintain a healthy body weight/be physically active.
- Limit the intake of salt.
- If you drink alcohol, stay within safe limits—♀ should consume no more than 1 drink /day (2 units alcohol=16 g) and ♂ should consume less than 2 drinks /day (max 30 g alcohol).

## Further reading
Cancer Research UK. http://www.cancerresearchuk.org (accessed 25.06.07).
Scientific Advisory Committee on Nutrition. http://www.sacn.gov.uk (accessed 25.06.07).

**1** World Cancer Research Fund and American Institute for Cancer Research (2007). Food, nutrition, physical activity and the prevention of cancer. American Institute for Cancer Research. Washington, DC. http://www.dietandcancerreport/downloads/ (accessed 8.11.07)

**Table 5.2** Effect of diet/nutrients on cancer risk

| Food group | Effects on cancer risk |
| --- | --- |
| Fruit and vegetables | ↓ the risk of mouth, oesophageal, pharynx, larynx, stomach, and colorectal cancers |
| Bread, cereals and starchy roots, pulses, nuts, seeds | Fibre-rich foods ↓ the risk of colorectal cancer |
| Meat, fish, and eggs | |
| Red and processed meat | ↑ the risk of colorectal and, possibly, stomach cancers |
| Fish | Might ↓ the risk of colorectal cancer |
| Foods containing fat | |
| Diets high in saturated fat | ↑ the risk of breast cancer, possibly lung and colorectal cancers |
| Milk and dairy food | High intakes of milk and cheese are known to ↓ the risk of colorectal cancer and diets high in calcium increase prostate cancer |
| High-salt foods | Might ↑ the risk of stomach cancer and cancer of the nasopharynx |
| Alcohol | ↑ the risk of mouth, pharynx, larynx, oesophageal, liver, colorectal, and breast cancers |
| | Micronutrient deficiencies are common in chronic alcoholics |

# Functional foods and supplements

## Functional foods

These foods are either promoted as improving health or ↓ the risk of disease. The food industry also use the term 'superfoods' in marketing these foods. Although there is no standard definition of a 'functional food', the implication is that a constituent within the food is physiologically active beyond its accepted nutritional role. Evidence for how frequently, and in what quantities, these foods must be consumed to demonstrate a benefit is limited.

Functional foods include the following.

• Conventional foods, e.g. broccoli (which contains sulphoraphane, an anticarcinogenic) and tomatoes (which contain lycopene, an antioxidant with an anticarcinogenic effect).

• Enriched or enhanced foods, e.g. spreads with added phytosterols to ↓ serum cholesterol and foods containing prebiotics and probiotics to promote gut health.

## Food supplements

This term is confusing as there are different definitions. The 2002 European Union Directive for the regulation of food supplements (2002/46/EC)[1] defines supplements as 'foodstuffs the purpose of which are to supplement the normal diet and which are a concentrated source of nutrients or other substances with a nutritional or physiological effect, alone or in combination marketed in dose form.'

Evidence supporting the routine use of supplements is lacking. Recommendations for the use of vitamin supplements include folic acid supplementation[2], as part of preconception and early pregnancy care to ↓ the risk of neural tube defects, and supplementation of vitamin D for breastfeeding mothers, children <2 years, and the institutionalized elderly. However, routine dietary supplementation is not recommended. Consuming a 'whole-food' diet is ideal, because there are many beneficial substances in food (not conventionally identified as nutrients) that offer protection against cancer and other chronic diseases. Manufactured supplements cannot reproduce the range of substances naturally present in food. Combining vitamin and mineral preparations can be potentially harmful because some vitamins are toxic. Excessively high intake of one nutrient can affect the absorption of other vitamins and minerals. Some studies have shown that high doses of antioxidant vitamins for the prevention of gastrointestinal cancers actually ↑ mortality.[3]

1 European Parliament and Council of the European Union (2002). Directive 2002/46/EC of the European Parliament and of the Council of 10 June 2002 on the approximation of the laws of the Member States relating to food supplements. *Official Journal of the European Communities* L183/51–L183/57.

2 Scientific Advisory Committee on Nutrition. http://www.sacn.gov.uk (accessed 25.06.07).

3 Bjjelakovic G, Nikolova P, Simonetti R, *et al.* (2004). Antioxidant supplements for preventing gastrointestinal cancers. *The Cochrane Database of Systematic Reviews* 4: CD004183. http://www.cochrane.org/reviews/en/ab004183.html (accessed 07.11.07).

## Regulation and legislation

Claims made about the health properties of foods fall under the Trade Descriptions Act 1968[4], Food Safety Act 1990[5], and Food Labelling Regulations Act 1996. The development and marketing of functional foods might also be affected by the European Union Directive on Medicinal Products for Human Use (2004/27/EC).[6] This regulation is specifically related to substances presented as having properties for treating or preventing disease or aiming to restore, correct, or modify physiological function through a pharmacological, immunological, or metabolic action.

Regulation is concerned with ensuring that claims made about foods or supplements are truthful and help the consumer to make informed choices.

4 UK Parliament (1968). *Trades Description Act 1968*. HMSO, London.

5 UK Parliament (1990). *Food Safety Act 1990 (C. 16)*. http://www.opsi.gov.uk/acts1990/ukpga_199000/6_eni.ntm

6 European Commission (2004). Directive 200/27/EC of the European Parliament and of the council of 31 March 2004, on the community code relating to medical products for human use. *Official Journal* **EU LI35**. 35–57.

# Nutrients

Nutrients are required for growth, maintenance of body tissue, storage of energy for physiological functions, and control of metabolic processes. Nutrients are generally classified into two types:
- Macronutrients—include fats, carbohydrates (starches, sugars, and dietary fibre), and proteins.
- Micronutrients, also defined as 'regulatory nutrients'—include water-soluble vitamins, fat-soluble vitamins, macrominerals, and microminerals.

Alcohol is not considered a nutrient. The Department of Health guidelines for the intake of alcohol are that it should not provide >5% of the energy in the diet.[1]

## Non-essential nutrients

Some nutrients can be made by the body from other nutrients (e.g. vitamin D, some fatty acids, and amino acids) or micro-organisms found in food (e.g. vitamin $B_{12}$) or the large intestine (e.g. vitamin K). Do not assume that these non-essential nutrients can be left out of the diet, because their manufacture is dependent on optimal health and normal metabolic processes.

Foods are ingested and broken down mechanically and chemically. The efficiency of digestion and absorption is dependent on a healthy functioning GIT, in addition to the bioavailability of the nutrient. Absorption requires the transport of the nutrient into the blood and lymphatic system. The term 'metabolism' is used to describe the mechanisms by which nutrients are processed in the body (i.e. how they are assimilated and incorporated into tissue or detoxified and excreted). Metabolism includes:
- Catabolism—broadly, the breakdown of complex substances.
- Anabolism—the synthesis of complex substances from simple substances.
- Basal metabolic rate (BMR)—the rate at which the body uses energy at rest. This measurement is dependent on age, sex, and body weight.
- Physical activity level—used to estimate an individual's daily activity level as a multiple of BMR, which varies from 1.4 (light energy expenditure in work, with non-active leisure pursuits) to 1.9 (energy-demanding work and leisure-time activity).
- Energy—the kilocalorie (kcal) is the unit of energy used to measure the energy value of food. Guidelines for the intake of energy are based on activity levels of the UK population. Fat, protein, carbohydrate, and alcohol provide energy.

## Further reading

British Nutrition Foundation. http://www.nutrtion.org.uk (accessed 25.06.07).

**1** Department of Health (1991). *Dietary Reference Values for Food Energy and Nutrition for the United Kingdom*. Committee on Medical Aspects of Food Policy Report. HMSO. London.

# Fats

Fat is obtained from dietary sources in either solid or liquid (oil) form and is also known as 'lipid'.

## Functions

- Source of energy—1 g of fat provides 9 kcal.
- Constituent of all cell membranes and steroid hormones.
- Essential fatty acids are precursors to eicosanoids (fatty acids 20 carbon atoms in length), which include the physiologically potent groups of substances called prostaglandins and thromboxanes (intracellular messengers regulating blood pressure, diuresis, immune function, and platelet aggregation), in addition to leukotrienes (chemical mediators of hypersensitivity and inflammatory reactions).
- Subcutaneous insulating layer.
- Transport of fat-soluble vitamins.

## Classification

Dietary fats are usually consumed in the form of triglycerides, which are composed of a glycerol molecule attached to three fatty acid molecules. Fatty acids are made up of a hydrocarbon chain, which varies in length. The physical properties of fats are influenced by the combination of fatty acids that comprise the triglyceride. Fatty acids are classified by their chemical make-up. Naturally occurring fatty acids are either 'saturated' or 'unsaturated' (see Table 5.3 for reference values).

### Saturated fatty acids

Each carbon atom is bound to two hydrogen atoms. The bonding capability of the carbon atoms is 'saturated' with hydrogen. Characteristically, these fats are solid at room temperature and associated with adverse health consequences if consumed in excess.

### Unsaturated fatty acids

Unsaturated fatty acids contain double carbon bonds where there is no hydrogen. Unsaturated fatty acids are further classified according to how many double bonds exist in the hydrocarbon chain. If there is only one double bond, it is known as a 'mono-unsaturated' fatty acid. Oleic acid is the most commonly consumed fatty acid of this type.

### Poly-unsaturated fatty acids

This type of fatty acid has two or more double bonds between carbon atoms. This group of fatty acids contains two subgroups:

- $n$-6 (omega-6).
- $n$-3 (omega-3).

'Omega' or '$n$' is a designation that refers to the position of the carbon atom of the first double bond within the fatty acid chain. This group contains the two essential fatty acids linoleic acid ($n$-6; found in sunflower oil) and α-linolenic acid (found in some vegetable and seed oils). These fatty acids must be obtained from dietary sources because they cannot be synthesized by the body.

*Cholesterol*
A component of every living cell wall. Although it can be obtained from food, most cholesterol is made by the body. The synthesis of vitamin D requires cholesterol.

*Trans-fatty acids*
The process whereby oil is changed into solid is known as 'hydrogenation'. This process, despite extending the shelf-life of processed food, alters the structure of the lipid. Fats that are altered to a 'trans' configuration are known to contribute to an ↑ in low-density lipoprotein cholesterol, ↑ the risk of coronary heart disease.

## Metabolism

Short- and medium-chain fatty acids are directly absorbed. Long-chain fatty acids are packed into chylomicrons which travel through enterocytes into the lymphatic system, entering the circulation via the thoracic duct. Triglycerides in chylomicrons are broken down into glycerol and fatty acids by lipoprotein lipase, which is found on the surface of cells. This enables the fatty acids and glycerol to enter the cells. Fat metabolism is regulated by catabolic hormones (epinephrine, glucagon, glucocorticoids, and thryroxine) and the anabolic hormone insulin.

Fatty acids and glycerol have the following functions:
• Broken down for energy (oxidation).
• Rebuilt into triglycerides for storage (anabolism) within adipose tissue.

## Health implications

A diet high in mono-unsaturated fatty acids is thought to be protective, because people from Mediterranean countries, who characteristically consume large amounts of oleic acid, have a low incidence of heart disease. Note that there are other factors in the Mediterranean diet (↓ overall consumption of fat and saturated fat and ↑ intake of fruit and vegetables) that might also contribute to the overall health outcomes. Linoleic acid is known to help ↓ blood cholesterol.

**Table 5.3** Dietary reference values for fat intake[1]

| Fat | Average for the population (% of total daily energy intake) |
| --- | --- |
| Saturated fatty acids | 10 |
| Poly-unsaturated fatty acids | 6 |
| Mono-unsaturated fatty acids | 12 |
| Trans-fatty acids | 2 |
| **Total fatty acids** | **30** |

1 Department of Health (1991). *Dietary Reference Values for Food Energy and Nutrition for the United Kingdom*. Committee on Medical Aspects of Food Policy Report. HMSO. London.

# Carbohydrates

Carbohydrates are constructed from carbon, oxygen, and hydrogen atoms. Table 5.4 gives dietary sources and Table 5.5 reference values.

## Functions
- Source of energy—1 g of carbohydrate provides 3.75 kcal.
- Protein-sparing—an adequate level of carbohydrate in the body enables proteins to be used for growth and repair, rather than as an energy source.
- Stored as glycogen in the liver and muscle.
- Dietary fibre (📖 p. 76) has a number of physiological effects—preventing constipation and regulation of blood cholesterol and glucose levels.

## Classification
Carbohydrates can be classified as follows.
- Monosaccharides or simple sugars—cannot be hydrolysed to smaller units.
- Disaccharides—two parts of monosaccharides.
- Oligosaccharides—short chains of varying monosaccharides joined by covalent bonds.
- Polysaccharides—long chains of monosaccharide units (from several to 100 repeating units of glucose or different types of monosaccharide).

## Metabolism
Metabolic pathways are regulated according to the need for energy. Pathways of carbohydrate use and storage include the following.
- Glycogenesis—conversion of glucose to glycogen (e.g. in liver and skeletal muscle).
- Glycogenolysis—conversion or breakdown of stored glycogen to glucose.
- Glycolysis—breakdown of glucose (intercellular) to the metabolic intermediate pyruvate. Under anaerobic conditions, pyruvate is used to provide energy by production of lactate; under aerobic conditions, pyruvate enters the Krebs cycle (within mitochondria) and is oxidized to release energy.
- Gluconeogenesis—reversible reaction of glycolysis, resulting in the synthesis of glucose from non-carbohydrate sources (usually occurs in the liver but, during starvation, the kidney contributes to glucose production). Non-carbohydrate sources include lactate, pyruvate, glycerol (from the breakdown of triglycerides), and specific amino acids.

## Health implications
- Intrinsic sugars (sugars that are naturally incorporated into the cellular structure of foods) and lactose do not have harmful effects on health (they can cause ↑ gut transit if consumed in large quantities).
- Non-milk extrinsic sugars contribute to dental caries.

- Consumption of non-milk extrinsic sugars is energy dense (although less so than fats and alcohol) and often associated with excess calorie intake, and ∴ is associated with weight gain.
- Intake of sucrose >200 g/day can be associated with ↑ cholesterol and blood glucose.
- Starches should be consumed in preference to other energy-producing foods (fat and alcohol).

**Table 5.4** Classification and dietary sources of carbohydrates

| Classification | Example | Food source |
|---|---|---|
| Monosaccharides | Glucose, fructose, galactose | Fruit, honey |
| Disaccharides | Maltose (two units of glucose) | Barley, wheat |
| | Lactose (galactose and glucose) | Milk |
| | Sucrose (glucose and fructose) | Cane and beet sugar, honey, fruit |
| Polysaccharides | Glycogen (repeating glucose units) | Meat |
| | Starch (repeating glucose units) | Cereals, potatoes, legumes |
| | Cellulose/non-starch polysaccharide or dietary fibre | Plant cell walls, e.g. wholegrain cereals and vegetables |

**Table 5.5** Dietary reference values for carbohydrate intake[1]

| Carbohydrate | % of total daily energy intake |
|---|---|
| Non-milk extrinsic sugars | 10 |
| Intrinsic sugars, milk sugars, and starch | 37 |
| Total | 47 |

1 Department of Health (1991). *Dietary Reference Values for Food Energy and Nutrition for the United Kingdom.* Committee on Medical Aspects of Food Policy Report. HMSO. London.

# Fibre

Dietary fibre is found in fruit, vegetables, and wholegrain cereal foods. If eaten, it reaches the caecum unchanged. Although there is no universally accepted definition of 'dietary fibre', it includes polysaccharides (non-starch polysaccharide (NSP)) and lignin. Plants are made up of a variety of chemically different NSPs.

## Functions

Although dietary fibre cannot be broken down by human digestive enzymes, it has important physiological effects and can be broken down by bacteria in the large bowel. Fibre has the following properties.
- Bulking—delayed gastric emptying, enhanced satiety, reduced intestinal transit time, ↓ intraluminal pressure, and ↑ frequency of defecation.
- Cholesterol ↓.
- Delays glucose absorption.
- ↑ bile acid excretion.
- Fermentation provides energy (in colon).

## Classification

There are two main categories of non-starch polysaccharide.
- Soluble—some hemicellulose (found in the cell walls of plants, e.g. bran and whole grains), pectin (found in the cell walls of plants, e.g. apples and citrus fruits), gum (also known as 'hydrocolloid'; found in oatmeal, barley, and legumes), and mucilages and algae (hydrocolloids obtained from plant secretory cells—mucilages, algae, and seaweed).
- Insoluble—some hemicellulose (found in the cell walls of plants, e.g. bran and whole grains), lignin (non-carbohydrate component of root vegetables, wheat, and fruit), and cellulose (found in the cell walls of bran, legumes, peas, apples, and root vegetables).

## Digestion, absorption, and metabolism

Anaerobic bacteria in the large bowel ferment pectins, gums, mucilages, algal polysaccharides, cellulose, and hemicellulose. The products are short-chain fatty acids (butyric, acetic, and propionic acids). Gases produced (methane, carbon dioxide, and hydrogen) are excreted as flatus or expired during respiration.

The short-chain fatty acids (SCFAs) are absorbed by colonocytes and promote water and sodium absorption. Some SCFAs (e.g. butyric acid) are used as an energy source for cells in the colon. Others (e.g. propionic and acetic acids) travel through the portal vein to the liver, where they are metabolized, or to the peripheral circulation, from where they are taken up by the muscle and used.

## Dietary reference values[1]

- Non-starch polysaccharide—population average 18 g/day (equates to 24 g/day dietary fibre).

---

1 Department of Health (1991). *Dietary Reference Values for Food Energy and Nutrition for the United Kingdom*. Committee on Medical Aspects of Food Policy Report. HMSO. London.

**Health implications**
Low-fibre diets are associated with diverticular disease and an ↑ risk of colon cancer.

▶ Advice to ↑ daily fibre intake should also include advice on ↑ daily fluid intake.

Excessively high intake of fibre can impair the absorption of minerals (cations, e.g. calcium, zinc, and iron). These minerals are released for absorption in the colon if they undergo fermentation.

# Proteins

Proteins are found in every living cell. They are large complex molecules made up of many different amino acids, which, in turn, comprise carbon, hydrogen, oxygen, and nitrogen atoms. All amino acids, in addition to their carbon structure, have four side groups:

- An acid (COOH) group.
- An amino ($NH_2$) group.
- A hydrogen site.
- The fourth side group varies among amino acids—∴ this chemical structure makes the amino acid unique.

Amino acids are joined by a peptide link between the acid group of one amino acid and the amino group of another: these are described 'dipeptide' bonds. Longer-chain amino acids are polypeptides, which are joined in a more complex manner than just a peptide bond. Proteins typically contain many hundreds of amino acid combinations; specific proteins are produced (synthesized) from a genetic blueprint. Dietary reference values are given in Table 5.6.

## Functions

- Growth, development, and repair of body structures and tissues.
- Source of energy, (recommendations 10–15% food intake[1]). 1 g protein = 4 kcal.
- Dietary protein is used for growth and repair, rather than as an energy source. However, it will be used as a source of energy if no other is available. The functional role of proteins is determined by their structure and organization.

Categories of proteins include the following.

- Enzymes—responsible for catalysing chemical reactions required for normal physiological processes, e.g. digestion, cellular energy production, coagulation, and neuromuscular activity.
- Peptide hormones—responsible for the regulation of body functions by directing the production or activity of enzymes, e.g. insulin, glucagon, thyroid hormones, and many other hormones.
- Transport proteins—these proteins can combine with substances so that the substances can be carried in the bloodstream, e.g. haemaglobin, transferrin, and retinol-binding protein.
- Immunoproteins—produced by white blood cells (B lymphocytes). They bind to antigens, to recognize and inactivate them.
- Structural proteins—including the fibrous proteins (elastin, keratin, and collagen) found in connective tissue, skin, hair, and nails, in addition to the contractile proteins of muscle (actin and myosin).

## Classification

This is determined by the quality of amino acids contained in the protein source (Table 5.7). The body makes some amino acids through a process of transamination, which is possible if the diet contains 'essential' (also

**1** Department of Health (1991). *Dietary Reference Values for Food Energy and Nutrition for the United Kingdom.* Committee on Medical Aspects of Food Policy Report. HMSO. London.

known as 'indispensable') amino acids. These amino acids contain an amino group that, if broken down, can be transferred to form other types of amino acid. Some non-essential amino acids become essential under specific physiological conditions and are classed as conditionally essential (Table 5.7).

### High-biological-value proteins

Foods that contain proteins comprise essential amino acids in adequate amounts. They are generally derived from animal sources (e.g. meat, milk, and eggs), and soya.

### Low-biological-value proteins

Foods lacking one or more of the essential amino acids. This group includes all plant proteins, excluding soya.

Consuming a range of foods containing complementary low-biological-value amino acids will ↑ the quality of the amino acids consumed.

## Metabolism

Unlike glucose and fat, excess protein in the diet cannot be stored by the body. Free amino acids are available within cells, providing a 'metabolic pool' for protein synthesis. These amino acids come from both dietary sources (exogenous amino acids) and the breakdown of tissue proteins (endogenous amino acids). To ensure that a balance is achieved, protein metabolism is a continuous process of catabolism (breakdown) and anabolism (synthesis). A balance is achieved if the amount of protein made is equal to the amount used. A positive nitrogen balance occurs if the protein synthesized exceeds the amount broken down (e.g. in tissue repair and muscle building/growth). During starvation and the associated loss of fat-free mass, the body has a negative nitrogen balance.

## Health implications

A poor intake of protein will contribute to malnutrition. However, excessive amounts of protein in the diet can cause an ↑ loss of calcium, which ↑ the risk of bone disease. Additionally, high intake of protein over a period of time is thought to contribute to impaired renal function in vulnerable individuals, particularly diabetics.

**Table 5.6** Dietary reference values for protein[1]

|  | Weight (kg) | EAR (g/day) | RNI (g/day) |
|---|---|---|---|
| ♂ 19–50 years | 74 | 44.4 | 55.5 |
| ≥50 years | 71 | 42.6 | 53.3 |
| ♀* 19–50 years | 60 | 36 | 45 |
| ≥50 years | 62 | 37.2 | 46.5 |

* Additional requirement in pregnancy and for breastfeeding.

**Table 5.7** Classification of amino acids

| Non-essential | Essential |
|---|---|
| Asparagine | Histidine |
| Aspartate | Isoleucine |
| Cysteine* | Leucine |
| Glycine* | Methionine |
| Glutamate | Phenylalanine |
| Glutamine* | Threonine |
| Proline* | Tryptophan |
| Serine | Lysine |
| Tyrosine* | Valine |
| Arganine* | |
| Alanine | |

* Conditionally essential.

1 Department of Health (1991). *Dietry Reference Values for Food Energy and Nutrition for the United Kingdom.* Committee on Medical Aspects of Food Policy Report. HMSO, London.

# Vitamins

This group of nutrients includes a diverse range of compounds that are required for normal growth and the maintenance of health. To prevent vitamin-deficiency diseases, these organic compounds are required in very small quantities (i.e. milligrams (mg) or micrograms (mcg) per day). Generally, provision of vitamins in the diet is 'essential' because they cannot be synthesized by the body; however, exceptions include vitamin D (synthesized in the skin if it is exposed to sunlight) and niacin (synthesized from the essential amino acid tryptophan).

## Functions

Vitamins contribute to the following fundamental processes:
- Growth.
- Metabolism.
- Maintenance of health.

## Classification

Vitamins are classified as either water soluble (e.g. A, D, E, and K; see Table 5.8) or fat soluble ($B_1$, $B_2$, niacin, $B_6$, folic acid, $B_{12}$, biotin, and C; see Table 5.9). In addition, vitamins are chemically related compounds that share the same biological activity.
- Vitamin A—retinol and β-carotene.
- Vitamin E—tocopherols and tocotrienols.
- Vitamin K—phylloquinone and menaquinones.
- Niacin—nicotinic acid and nicotinamide.
- Vitamin $B_6$—pyridoxal and pyridoxamine.

## Dietary recommendations[1]

- Water-soluble vitamins—see Table 5.8.
- Fat-soluble vitamins—see Table 5.9.

Safe intake (SI) levels of intake have been set for the following vitamins.
- Pantothenic acid—3–7 mg/day.
- Biotin—10–200 mcg/day.
- Vitamin E—>4 mg/day for ♂ and >3 mg/day for ♀.
- Vitamin K—1 mcg/kg body weight/day.

## Metabolism

The two groups of vitamins are processed differently by the body.

### Water-soluble vitamins
- Absorbed into the portal bloodstream.
- Carried in the blood by transport proteins.
- Cellular uptake facilitated by vitamin-specific enzymes.
- Storage in the body tissues is limited—except vitamin $B_{12}$ and biotin.
- Toxicity is rare because these vitamins are excreted if the plasma level reaches the renal threshold.

1 Department of Health (1991). *Dietary Reference Values for Food Energy and Nutrition for the United Kingdom*. Committee on Medical Aspects of Food Policy Report. HMSO. London.

*Fat-soluble vitamins*
- Transport requires chylomicrons in the lymphatic system and then the general circulation.
- Stored in body fat.
- If taken in large doses over long periods toxicity can develop as they are excreted more slowly than water-soluble vitamins.

## Further reading

British Nutrition Foundation. http://www.nutrition.org.uk (accessed 24.06.07).

**Table 5.8** Water-soluble vitamins[1,2]

| Vitamin and reference value | Source | Function | Deficiency | Groups at risk |
|---|---|---|---|---|
| **Vitamin C** (ascorbic acid)<br>RNI (mg/day)<br>♂ >18 yrs—40<br>♀ >18 yrs—40 | Citrus fruit<br>Soft fruits/berries<br>Potatoes | Connective, vascular, and cartilage tissue formation<br>Promotes the absorption of non-haem iron<br>Antioxidant | Scurvy, poor wound healing | Critically ill<br>Smokers |
| **Vitamin B₁** (thiamine)<br>RNI (mg/day)<br>♂ 19–50 yrs—1<br>♂ >50 yrs—0.9<br>♀ >18 yrs—0.8 | Wheatgerm<br>Wholegrain cereals<br>Nuts, pulses,<br>Pork<br>Eggs<br>Fortified cereals and flour | Metabolism (energy release) of carbohydrates, fat, and alcohol<br>Normal functioning of nervous system | Beriberi<br>Wernicke–Korsakoff syndrome | Chronic alcoholics |
| **Vitamin B₂** (Riboflavin)<br>RNI (mg/day)<br>♂ >18 yrs—1.3<br>♀ >18 yrs—1.1 | Liver, dairy products, eggs<br>Green vegetables<br>Fortified cereals<br>Meat | Metabolism (energy release)<br>Integrity of mucus membranes | Lesions of mucous membranes<br>Glossitis<br>Seborrhoeic skin lesions | Chronic dieters |

**Table 5.8** (Contd.)

| Vitamin and reference value | Source | Function | Deficiency | Groups at risk |
|---|---|---|---|---|
| **Niacin** (nicotinic acid equivalent) **RNI** (mg/day) ♂ 19–50 yrs—17 ♂ > 50 yrs—16 ♀ 19–50 yrs—13 ♀ > 50 yrs—2 | Meat, liver, fish Yeast extract Fortified breakfast cereals (can be synthesized from the amino acid tryptophan) | Part of the nicotinamide nucleo-tide coenzymes Energy metabolism | Pellagra (skin lesions, diarr-hoea, dementia) | |
| **Vitamin B₆** (pyridoxine) **RNI** (mg/day) ♂ >18 yrs—1.4 ♀ >18 yrs—1.2 | Beef, fish, poultry Wholegrains Bananas Nuts | Cofactor in protein, glycogen, and lipid metabolism Iron metabolism and transport Conversion of tryptophan to niacin | Unknown | |
| **Vitamin B₁₂** (cyancobalamin) **RNI** (mcg/day) ♂ >18 yrs—1.5 ♀ >18 yrs—1.5 | Milk, meat, eggs Fortified breakfast cereals Oily fish | Cell division, cell formation and function Maintenance of blood homocysteine levels Cofactor in amino acid metabo-lism | Megaloblastic anaemia and neurological damage | Vegetarians Those with ileal resection and those lacking instrinsic factor |

**Table 5.8** (Contd.)

| Folate (folic acid) RNI (mcg/day) ♂ >18 yrs—200 ♀ >18 yrs—200 | Liver, yeast extract Green leafy vegetables Pulses Breakfast cereal | Cell division Formation of blood cells Formation of the nervous system | Megloblastic anaemia | Malabsorption Alcoholics, Developing fetus Some drug therapy (methotrexate and anticonvulsants) |
|---|---|---|---|---|
| Panthothenic acid SI (mg/day) ♂ >18 yrs—3–7 ♀ >18 yrs—3–7 | Liver, meat Yeast extract Eggs, mushrooms Green leafy vegetables | Part of coenzyme A molecule required energy metabolism | Unknown | Unknown |
| Biotin SI (mcg/day) ♂ >18 yrs—10–200 ♀ >18 yrs—10–200 | Liver Soya bean, pulses Egg yolk Nuts, wholegrains Synthesized by intestinal flora | Fatty acid synthesis Metabolic pathway of gluconeogenesis and the catabolism of branched-chain amino acids | Dermatitis, hair loss, glossitis, anorexia, nausea, hallucinations and depression | Those with ↑ intake of raw egg white |

1 Department of Health (1991). *Dietary Reference Values for Food Energy and Nutrition for the United Kingdom.* Committee on Medical Aspects of Food Policy Report. HMSO. London.

2 Thomas B and Bishop J (eds) (2007) *Manual of Dietetic Practice,* 4th edn. Blackwell, Oxford.

Table 5.9 Fat-soluble vitamins [1,2]

| Vitamin and reference value | Source | Function | Deficiency | Groups at risk |
|---|---|---|---|---|
| **Vitamin A** (retinol and carotenoids) RNI (mcg/day) ♂ >18 yrs—700 ♀ >18 yrs—600 | Liver Oily fish Egg yolk, dairy products Yellow and orange fruit. Green, yellow, and orange vegetables | Growth and normal development Differentiation of tissues Vision | Dry conjunctiva and cornea leading to loss of vision Night blindness Fatigue | Excessive laxative use Fat malabsorption Chronic low-fat dieters |
| **Vitamin D** (cholecalciferol and ergocalciferol) RNI (mcg/day) ♂ 18–65 yrs* ♂ >65 yrs—10 ♀ 18–65 yrs* ♀ >65 yrs—10 | Sunlight Fortified fat spreads and margarine Oily fish Eggs Dairy products Meat | Regulation of calcium and phosphorus absorption Bone mineralization and structure Cell division | Rickets Osteomalacia and osteoporosis | Asian ethnicity, Housebound/ institutionalized Fat malabsorption Breast feeding |
| **Vitamin E** (tocopherals) SI (mg/day) ♂ >18 yrs—3–4 ♀ >18 yrs—3–4 | Vegetable oils Nuts Cereals Meat | Protects cells and cell membranes from oxidation damage | Low intakes associated with increased risk of cardiovascular disease and some cancers | Fat malabsorption High intake of n-6 PUFA |
| **Vitamin K** (phylloquinone) SI (mcg/kg/day) ♂ >18 yrs—1 ♀ > 18 yrs—1 | Dark green leafy vegetables Rapeseed, soya, and olive oils Menaquinone synthesized by intestinal bacteria | Synthesis of coagulation proteins Bone structure | Haemorrhagic disease of newborn Increased clotting time | Newborn babies Drugs affecting the intestinal flora Fat malabsorption |

* No recommendation. Safe Intake (SI), Reference Nutrient Intake RNI. No RNI for Tocopherals equivalents (requirement related to intake of PUFA intake) or Vitamin K (not enough evidence to establish a range of adult requirements).

1 Department of Health (1991). *Dietary Reference Values for Food Energy and Nutrition for the United Kingdom*. Committee on Medical Aspects of Food Policy Report. HMSO. London.

2 Thomas B and Bishop J (eds) (2007) *Manual of Dietetic Practice*, 4th edn. Blackwell, Oxford.

# Minerals

Essential minerals and trace elements are inorganic elements with important physiological functions required in small amounts from the diet.

## Functions

Each essential mineral and trace element has one or more physiological functions. The quantity needed of each element varies; the body has different requirements for each essential element. For optimal function, the concentration of the element falls within a range. Levels outside this range lead to deficiencies or toxicities that impair physiological functioning and might result in death. Minerals have the following functions.

- Structural component of bones, teeth, and other body tissues.
- Constituents of body fluids.
- Nerve function.
- Enzyme function.
- Cell membrane stability and transport.

## Classification

Minerals can be classified as follows.

- Minerals—required from the diet in quantities of milligrams per day, including sodium, potassium, calcium, magnesium, phosphorus, iron, zinc, and chloride.
- Trace elements—required from the diet in quantities of micrograms per day, including copper, selenium, iodine, manganese, molybdenum, nickel, silicon, vanadium, arsenic, boron, and cobalt.

## Dietary requirements

Values have been set for minerals (Table 5.10) and trace elements (Table 5.11).[1,2]

## Digestion, absorption, and metabolism

The digestion of food releases many of the minerals so that they can be absorbed in inorganic form. The uptake of these nutrients from both small and large bowel is regulated by the need for the nutrient. The absorption of minerals is also affected by foods consumed (e.g. phytate and oxalate ↓ the absorption of calcium, iron, and zinc, whereas vitamin C promotes the absorption of non-haem iron) and normal gastrointestinal functioning (e.g. steatorrhoea ↓ calcium absorption). Plasma concentrations of the elements are finely regulated by absorption and renal excretion, which makes toxicity rare in healthy individuals.

## Health implications

In the healthy population, a varied diet means that the use of mineral supplements is not required. Some minerals have protective effects against cancer and heart disease, whereas others have antioxidant properties.

## Futrther reading

British Nutrition Foundation. http://www.nutrition.org.uk (accessed 26.06.07).

1 Department of Health (1991). *Dietary Reference Values for Food Energy and Nutrition for the United Kingdom*. Committee on medical aspects of food policy report. HMSO. London.
2 Thomas B and Bishop J (2007) (eds) *Manual of Dietetic Practice*, 4th edn. Blackwell Publishing. Oxford.

Table 5.10 Dietary reference values for minerals[3]

| Mineral and reference value | Source | Function | Comment |
|---|---|---|---|
| Calcium<br>RNI (mg/day)<br>Adults >18 yrs—700 | Dairy products<br>Fish with soft bones<br>Leafy green vegetables<br>White and brown fortified flour<br>Pulses | Growth and development of bone<br>Maintenance of bone mass, cell structure, metabolic function, signal transmission | Calcium is absorbed more efficiently from dairy foods than from plant sources<br>Phytates, oxylates, and supplementation of zinc inhibit calcium absorption<br>Absorption is promoted if serum calcium or phosphorus levels are low, during pregnancy and lactation, and when vitamin D status is adequate |
| Magnesium<br>RNI (mg/day)<br>♂ >19 yrs—300<br>♀ >19 yrs—270 | Green vegetables<br>Wholegrain, cereals<br>Nuts and tofu<br>Meat | Bone development and maintenance<br>Nerve and muscle membrane electrical potential, cofactor for enzymes needing ATP (adenosine triphosphate)<br>Replication of DNA and the formation of RNA | Homeostasis achieved by regulating the efficiency of magnesium absorbed from the intestine and renal losses<br>Fibre ↓ bioavailability<br>Protein ↑ absorption |
| Phosphorus<br>RNI (mg/day)<br>Adults >18 yrs—550 | Meat<br>Fish<br>Eggs, cereals<br>Dairy products<br>Nuts | Component of bone, cell membranes, nucleotides, and nucleic acid, buffer, storage and transfer of energy, activation of catalytic enzymes | Increased intakes in fizzy drinks and food additives affect calcium metabolism and bone health |

**Table 5.10** (Contd.)

| Mineral and reference value | Source | Function | Comment |
|---|---|---|---|
| **Sodium**<br>RNI (mg/day)<br>Adults<br>>18 yrs—1600<br>**Salt**[4]<br>6 g/day | Processed foods: bread, ham, bacon, cheese, smoked fish<br>Cereals | Major extracellular electrolyte<br>Maintenance of extracellular fluid volume, acid–base balance, plasma membrane sodium/potassium pump (required for nerve cell signal transmission, muscle contraction, and active transport of nutrients) | Absorption increased by glucose, citrate and bicarbonate; regulated by hormone system; excreted in urine<br>High intakes associated with cardiovascular risk[4] |
| **Potassium**<br>RNI (mg/day)<br>Adults >18 yrs<br>—3500 | Fruit: bananas, apricots, blackcurrants, citrus<br>Vegetables including potatoes | Main intracellular electrolyte, plasma membrane sodium/potassium pump (required for nerve cell signal transmission, muscle contraction)<br>Cofactor in energy metabolism cell growth and division | Absorbed by passive diffusion<br>Excess potassium excreted in urine |
| **Iron**<br>RNI (mg/day)<br>♂ >18 yrs—8.7<br>♀ 19–50 yrs—14.8<br>♀50+—8.7 | Red meat, fish, offal, eggs, wholegrain food, fortified cereals, nuts, pulses, dried fruit, dark green vegetables | Component of haemoglobin, myoglobin (oxygen transport)<br>Enzymes required in energy metabolism | Iron absorption is inhibited by the consumption of tea (containing tannin) and ↑ with high intakes of ascorbic acid<br>↑ intakes required during growth and women with high menstrual losses<br>Stored in reticulo-endothelial system as ferritin; deficiency—range of functional impairments which may present before hypochromic anaemia<br>Toxicity can be fatal |

| | | |
|---|---|---|
| **Zinc**<br>**RNI** (mg/day)<br>♂ > 18 yrs—9.5<br>♀ > 18 yrs—7.0 | Red meat, liver<br>Seafood<br>Eggs<br>Milk | Structural, regulatory, and catalytic role for a number of enzymes, e.g. protein and nucleic acids synthesis, energy metabolism, bone formation, membrane integrity, and immunity | Homeostatic mechanism results in ↑ absorption when intake of zinc is low and reduced excretion when intake of zinc is low<br>Absorption is impaired with high phytate diets and low animal protein diets |
| **Fluoride**<br>**SI** (mg/kg/day)<br>Infants —0.05 | Tap water | Prevention of dental caries | Not an essential mineral as no known deficiency<br>Toxicity—Flurosis (discoloration of teeth) |

3 British Nutrition Foundation http://www.nutrition.org.uk.

4 Department of Health (1994). *Nutritional Aspects of Cardiovascular Disease*. Report of the Cardiovascular Review Group of the Committee of Medical Aspects of Food Policy. HMSO. London.

**Table 5.11** Trace elements[5]

| Trace element | Source | Function | Comment |
|---|---|---|---|
| **Copper** RNI (mg/day) Adults >18 yrs—1.2 | Nuts, shell fish Liver Cereals | Component of enzymes, cofactors, and proteins in the functioning of the nervous, cardiovascular, immune, and skeletal systems as well as the formation of red blood cells and the regulation of energy metabolism | Absorption regulated by dietary intake (less efficient with high intakes) Absorption impaired with high intakes of zinc, iron, and ascorbic acid Absorption promoted with high-protein diets |
| **Selenium** RNI (mcg/day) ♂ >18 yrs—75 ♀ >18 yrs—60 | Brazil nuts Meat Fish, offal Bread, eggs | Component of a large number of proteins including enzymes with a range of functions: antioxidant systems, production and regulation of thyroid hormone, muscle function, and immunity | Selenium content of wheat is dependent on the soil content; mercury in seafood may inhibit selenium absorption Diets high in selenium impair zinc absorption and deplete iron stores Toxicity with high intakes |
| **Molybdenum** SI (mcg/day) Adults—50–400 | Legumes, nuts, grains Leafy vegetables | Cofactor for iron and flavin containing enzymes in hydroxylation reactions | Readily absorbed, excreted in urine and bile, high levels of molybdenum in the body deplete copper stores |
| **Manganese** SI (mg/day) Adults >1.4 | Wholegrains, cereals nuts, dried fruit, leafy vegetables | Activator and cofactor of a number of enzymes; glycoprotein synthesis, carbohydrate and fat metabolism, sex hormone production, and skeletal development | Absorption inhibited by iron and phytate; regulation of manganese levels by hepatobiliary excretion and by the kidney Deficiency unknown |

| | | | |
|---|---|---|---|
| **Chromium** SI (mcg/day) Adults > 25 | Meat, offal, wholegrains, potatoes | Promotes the effectiveness of insulin, structural role in the integrity of of nuclear strands and gene expression | Deficiency causes carbohydrate intolerance |
| **Iodine** RNI (mcg/day) Adults 18+ yrs —140 | Seafood, milk, sea salt | Component of thyroid hormones | Thyroid hormone metabolism is also dependent on adequate selenium status |

5 Scientific Advisory Committee on Nutrition. http://www.sacn.gov.uk (accessed 25.06.07).

# Water

Although water is not formally recognized as a nutrient, it is the most abundant constituent of the human body. Estimates of water content range from 60% to 72% (42–45 L) of fat-free weight for an average 70 kg man. The water content of an adult remains relatively constant. Men generally have a higher composition of water, which is related to the greater fat-free mass. Total body water is divided into two main reservoirs.

- Intracellular compartment (water contained within cell membranes— 30 L).
- Extracellular compartment (water found outside cell membranes—15 L, 3 L of which is from the intravascular space, the remainder is fluid surrounding the cells or interstitial fluid).

Electrolytes contribute to the osmolality of body fluids and help to maintain body fluid in the appropriate compartment. Monovalent electrolytes— sodium, potassium, and chloride—are found mainly in the extracellular compartment, while potassium, magnesium, and phosphate are found in the intracellular fluid.

## Function

The vital functions of water include:
- Regulation of body temperature
- Lubricant
- Solvent and transport medium for nutrients ions and molecules
- Medium for chemical (metabolic) reactions
- Transport medium for the excretion of osmotically active solutes (e.g. urea, sodium ($Na^+$), chloride ($Cl^-$), and potassium ($K^+$).

## Requirements

In health, the need for fluid is approximately 30–35 ml/kg. Dietary intake of water includes liquid sources (beverages, fruit juice and squash, carbonated drinks, and milk); in addition about a third of our liquid intake is from the food we eat (fruit and vegetables have high water content). A small amount of water is produced as the result of the metabolism of food (see Table 5.12). In health, fluid intake is influenced by factors (social influences/habit, consumption of food) in addition to thirst. Fluid losses include fluid required for:
- Regulation of body temperature (sweating)
- Respiration (as water vapour)
- The elimination of waste products (the kidneys remove solute from the blood for elimination as urine; water is also lost from the GIT in faeces; see Table 5.13).

## Regulation

Thirst is experienced as the result of a water deficit and is a mechanism for the regulation of fluid intake. This water deficit (dehydration) will cause an increase in osmolality of all body fluids. Increased osmolality of plasma circulating through the hypothalamus will cause the sensation of thirst (prompting an increase in fluid intake) and the release of the antidiuretic hormone vasopressin. Vasopressin acts on the area for water absorption (renal tubule), increasing the water-absorbing capacity and therefore conserving body water and concentrating the urine.

## Absorption and elimination

In addition to the dietary intake of fluids, up to 8 L of fluid are secreted into the GIT each day. Most water is absorbed before entering the colon. Water movement across the gastrointestinal lumen is a passive process influenced by the (ionic) electrolyte movement. The colon has an absorptive capacity of about 4 L/day. Fluid lost in the stool is determined by the fibre content of the diet.

## Health implications

Fluid imbalance is not a problem in healthy individuals with unregulated access to water. Unusual episodes of hot weather put vulnerable groups such as frail older people at risk of dehydration. Loss of as little as 1% of body water can cause physiological impairment. An increase in fluid consumption is needed during periods of exercise or manual labour to avoid dehydration. The consumption of large amounts of caffeine in fluids has a diuretic effect. The consumption of large amounts of carbonated drinks (especially in the young) should be reduced as they may contain high levels of sugar and are known to affect bone metabolism.

**Table 5.12** Fluid intake (24 h)[1]

| Source | Volume (ml) |
| --- | --- |
| Liquids | 1500 |
| Food | 1000 |
| Metabolism | 300 |
| Total | 2800 |

**Table 5.13** Fluid losses (24 h)[1]

| Source | Volume (ml) |
| --- | --- |
| Urine | 1500 |
| Faeces | 150 |
| Lungs | 400 |
| Skin | 750 |
| Total | 2800 |

1 Thomas B and Bishop J (eds) (2007) *Manual of Dietetic Practice*, 4th edn. Blackwell, Oxford.

# Clinical nutrition

Organization of nutrition support  98
Roles of nutrition support team members  100
Undernutrition  102
Nutrition screening  104
Nutrition assessment  106
Estimating requirements  108
Nutrition support  110
Withholding and withdrawing nutrition support  112
Refeeding problems  114
Enteral nutrition  116
Short-term feeding  118
Long-term feeding  120
Nasogastric tube placement  122
Nasogastric tube management  124
Gastrostomy tube placement  126
Gastrostomy tube management  128
Replacement of gastrostomy tubes  130
Percutaneous intestinal feeding  132
Enteral feed preparations  134
Complications of enteral feeding  136
Mechanical complications of enteral feeding  138
Infective complications of enteral feeding  139
GI disturbances in enteral feeding  140
Monitoring enteral nutrition  142
Home enteral nutrition  144
Drug administration and enteral nutrition  146
Parenteral nutrition  148
Parenteral nutrition: central venous catheter access  150
Parenteral nutrition: peripheral vein catheter access  152
Parenteral nutrition: catheter insertion  154
Parenteral nutrition: catheter care  156
Parenteral nutrition: formulation  158
Parenteral nutrition: administration  160
Parenteral nutrition: monitoring  162
Home parenteral nutrition  164
Nutrition and the surgical patient  166
Nutritional management of gastrointestinal disease  168

# Organization of nutrition support

The use of artificial nutrition support for patients who cannot take sufficient nutrition orally has gained widespread acceptance, resulting in the development of both new techniques for insertion of feeding tubes and catheters, and a wider variety of feeds and access devices. The ↑ complexity of nutrition support means that practitioners require an expert knowledge of its risks, benefits, and complications. It can, therefore, be difficult for individual practitioners, who are not trained in nutrition support, to make appropriate choices for ensuring they provide optimal nutritional management for their patients. Even if practitioners do have a nutritional background (e.g. dietitians and nutrition nurses), it is unlikely that, as an individual, they would have sufficient knowledge, skill, or experience in all aspects of nutrition support to provide optimum patient care. Nutrition support teams (NSTs) bring the relevant expertise together and have been recognized as essential in providing safe and effective care.[1]

## Nutrition support teams

The composition of NSTs varies according to local needs and resources, but the following personnel are essential.
• Dietitian.
• Nutrition nurse.
• Pharmacist.
• Consultant clinician.

The grades of the above personnel and number of hours allocated to the NST might depend on local circumstances and needs, but the recent NICE guidelines[1] recommend that all acute hospital trusts should employ at least one nutrition nurse specialist. Funding of this post, in particular, has often proved a stumbling block for trusts trying to set up such a team. Trusts must consider the potential cost-savings that such a team might achieve.

In addition to the above personnel, the NST should be supported by a microbiologist, speech and language therapist, and biochemist.

NSTs can function in either an advisory or a consultancy capacity, whereby responsibility for the overall management of the patient remains with the senior consultant. Alternatively, responsibility for the management of the patient is transferred to the NST. Both these approaches have their advantages and disadvantages. The approach chosen will depend on local resources and clinical management systems. In either case, to ensure cooperation, the NST should appreciate the benefits of tact and diplomacy in dealing with their colleagues.

1 National Collaborating Centre for Acute Care (2006). *Nutrition Support in Adults: Oral Nutrition Support, Enteral Tube Feeding and Parenteral Nutrition. Clinical Guideline 32.* National Institute for Health and Clinical Excellence, London. http://www.nice.org.uk/CG32 (accessed 25.06.07).

# Roles of nutrition support team members

Although it is possible to outline the roles of individual members of the team, remember that there will often be overlaps (Table 6.1). View this in a positive light because it is vital that the team can continue to function effectively in the absence of one or more of its members.

All members of the team should participate in audit activities, teaching, and research.

The potential benefits of NSTs include the following.
- ↓ in unnecessary or inappropriate treatment.
- Prevention of complications in both enteral and parenteral nutrition.
- Optimizing drug therapy in patients receiving enteral and parenteral nutrition.
- Development of guidelines.
- Education and training of staff, patients, and carers.
- Cost-savings.

NICE recognized that the scale of these benefits was open to debate and conducted a review of this issue,[1] concluding that, although many of the studies were limited in quality, small, and heterogeneous, the evidence suggested that these teams ↓ complications through ↓ unnecessary treatments and preventing complications. NICE recommends that all acute hospital trusts should have a multidisciplinary nutrition support team.

### Alternative team configurations

Although the above is the most usual form a NST will take, it might not be suitable, or indeed necessary, for all areas. Smaller hospitals, care homes, and community-based teams might wish to consider a more informal set-up, whereby a group of individuals come together to discuss individual patients, as required. At the opposite end of the scale, several large acute trusts might require separate teams for adults, paediatrics, and neonates.

### Conclusion

Within our changing NHS, we are ↑ asked to provide evidence of the provision of high-quality patient care to the purchasers of our services. Within the field of nutrition support, a NST that is functioning well and auditing its practice should be able to provide evidence of this level of care being provided.

---

1 National Collaborating Centre for Acute Care (2006). *Nutrition Support in Adults: Oral Nutrition Support, Enteral Tube Feeding and Parenteral Nutrition. Clinical Guideline 32.* National Institute for Health and Clinical Excellence, London. http://www.nice.org.uk/CG32 (accessed 25.06.07).

**Table 6.1** The nutrition support team

| Team member | Key roles |
| --- | --- |
| Dietitian | Assessing nutritional intake and status |
| | Estimating nutritional requirements |
| | Monitoring patients receiving nutrition support (in collaboration with other NST members) |
| | Advising on, and monitoring, the transition from artificial nutrition support to eating and drinking |
| | Discharge planning and follow-up for patients being discharged into the community on enteral nutrition (in collaboration with other NST members) |
| Nutrition nurse specialist | Functioning as the patient's advocate |
| | Placing enteral and parenteral access devices |
| | Estimating nutritional requirements (in collaboration with other members of the NST) |
| | Monitoring patients receiving nutrition support (in collaboration with other members of the NST) |
| | Training healthcare professionals in the practical management of patients' enteral and parenteral feeding tubes and catheters, to minimize complications |
| | Training, supporting, and counselling all patients receiving nutrition support in the hospital or community |
| | Ensure adherence to nutrition support protocols |
| Pharmacist | Formulation of parenteral nutrition regimens (in consultation with other members of the NST) |
| | Advising on problems relating to drug therapy and enteral/parenteral nutrition |
| | Monitoring patients receiving parenteral nutrition and advising on changes to the regimen, as necessary |
| Consultant clinician | Link between the NST and his/her consultant colleagues, to ensure that the team's work has their support |
| | To plan, with the patient's senior consultant, an overall treatment plan that includes appropriate nutrition support |
| | Might place enteral/parenteral access devices, depending on specialty |
| | Advise on the prevention and management of complications related to nutrition support |

# Undernutrition

Although the terms 'malnutrition' and 'undernutrition' are often used interchangeably, they are not the same. Malnutrition or 'bad' nutrition refers to states of both under- and overnutrition. Although undernutrition is often unrecognized, it is a significant public health issue, with an economic cost that is greater than the cost of treating obesity.

## Incidence
Undernutrition affects ~10% of the population[1] and 40% of people admitted to hospital.[2]

## Definition
'Undernutrition' describes a state of insufficient dietary intake that is not enough to maintain a balance between energy intake and the amount of energy required for growth, maintenance of normal body function, and physical activity. In adults, chronic malnutrition characteristically results in an inability to maintain a healthy body weight and changes in body composition and function. The International Dietary Energy Consultancy Group[3] defines 'chronic undernutrition' as an individual with a body mass index (BMI) <18.5 kg/m$^2$. This condition is often referred to as protein–energy malnutrition (low protein and energy status).

Acute undernutrition, demonstrated by unintentional weight loss, reflects an acute change in protein–energy status. An individual with a normal BMI who has experienced unintentional weight loss of >5% over period of 3–6 months can be categorized as acutely malnourished.[4]

## Causes
Undernutrition in the UK is more likely to be the result of disease than poverty, although social and economic factors have been found to contribute. Causes might include:
• Poor nutritional intake—physical problems affecting the individual's ability to purchase, cook, and feed themselves, mastication and swallowing difficulties, ↓ appetite (e.g. anxiety, depression, or taste changes associated with medication or malignancy), eating disorders such as anorexia nervosa, and impaired mental function.

1 Elia M, Stratton T, Russell C, *et al.* (2005). *The Cost of Disease Related Malnutrition in the UK and Economic Considerations for the Use of Oral Nutritional Supplements in Adults.* Report by the Health Economic Group of the British Association for Parenteral and Enteral Nutrition (BAPEN), Redditch.

2 McWhirter JP and Pennington CR (1994). Incidence and recognition of malnutrition in hospital. *British Medical Journal* **308**, 945–8.

3 James WPT, Farro-Luzzi A, and Waterlow JC (1988). Definition of chronic energy deficiency in adults. A report of the working party of IDECG. *European Journal of Clinical Nutrition* **42**, 969–81.

4 Elia M (ed.) (2000). *Detection and Management of Under Nutrition in the Community.* Report by the Malnutrition Advisory Group. Maidenhead.

- ↑ metabolism and nutrient requirements—associated with surgery, trauma, and sepsis and pathology affecting energy expenditure (e.g. malignancy).
- Nutrient losses—poor gut absorption (e.g. active Crohn's disease, enteropathy, gut atrophy, or ↓ bowel length) and loss of protein from wound exudates, fistula, or dialysis.

## Consequences

The following complications associated with malnutrition are due to impairment of vital physiological protein-dependent functions.
- Muscle weakness—↓ mobility and associated complications, fatigue, ↑ risk of respiratory infection, and impaired cardiac function.
- Impaired immune function—↑ susceptibility to infection.
- Impaired wound healing.
- ↓ tolerance to cytotoxic drugs and chemotherapy.

Malnutrition is also associated with depression, anxiety, a ↓ ability to concentrate, and an ↑ perception of pain (requiring ↑ analgesia). These factors significantly affect the individual's perception of their quality of life. Additionally, ↑ morbidity results in a prolonged hospital stay and an associated economic burden.

## Treatment

The first step in managing a patient who is malnourished or at risk of malnutrition is identification of the problem through a process of screening (📖 p. 104). A range of possible interventions, from improving the quality of food taken by mouth to artificial nutrition support, will be considered by the dietitian or NST (📖 p. 110).

# Nutrition screening

Assessment of patients is essential in effective planning and implementation of individualized patient care. Nutritional screening has been incorporated into the nursing assessment process. Nutritional screening differs from a nutritional assessment ([ ] p. 106) in that it is a brief evaluation of factors that could indicate an individual is malnourished or at risk of malnutrition. These screening tools characteristically give a score to each of the indicators, which, added together, give an overall risk category. In addition to identifying risk, good screening tools also indicate the type of intervention required and need for ongoing assessment.

## Why use a screening tool?

A great number of screening tools have been developed in response to the ↑ awareness that malnutrition and those at risk of malnutrition are not effectively identified. This means that the patient's need for treatment is unrecognized and their condition continues to deteriorate.[1] Best practice guidelines published by NICE[2] advocate nutritional screening for all patients.

## Which screening tool?

In considering which screening tool should be used, it is essential to establish that the instrument is evidence based, validated, and simple to use. The Malnutrition Advisory Group of the British Association of Parenteral and Enteral Nutrition published the Malnutrition Universal Screening Tool (MUST),[3] which was researched and developed by a multidisciplinary group (Fig. 6.1). One of the strengths of this nationally recognized tool is that it is designed to be used in the adult population in both acute and community settings. Continuity of care is promoted because patients screened in the community can be reviewed using the same criteria if they are admitted to hospital. This tool provides management guidelines relating to monitoring and interventions. The document also provides useful information, including how to establish a BMI using surrogate measurements for height for those who cannot be measured.

## When to screen?

National best practice guidelines[2] recommend that all patients should be screened on admission to hospital or a care home and at the first out-patient appointment. Nutrition screening should be repeated at weekly intervals for in-patients. Nutrition screening is not intended as a substitute for clinical assessment. Any change in the patient's clinical condition or treatment plan warrants repeated nutrition screening and review of the care plan.

1 McWhirter JP and Pennington CR (1994). Incidence and recognition of malnutrition in hospital. *British Medical Journal* **308**, 945–8.

2 National Collaborating Centre for Acute Care (2006). *Nutrition Support in Adults: Oral Nutrition Support, Enteral Tube Feeding and Parenteral Nutrition. Clinical Guideline 32.* National Institute for Health and Clinical Excellence, London. http://www.nice.org.uk/CG32 (accessed 25.06.07).

3 BAPEN (2003). *Malnutrition Universal Screening Tool (MUST).* British Association of Enteral and Parenteral Nutrition. http://www.bapen.org.uk/must_tool.html (accessed 25.06.07).

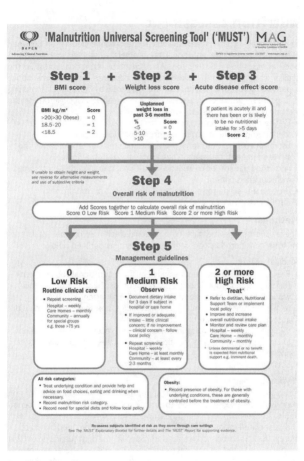

**Fig. 6.1** Malnutrition universal screening tool (MUST). Reproduced with kind permission of BAPEN.

# Nutrition assessment

The nutritional status of an individual is the dynamic association between nutritional intake and nutritional requirements, resulting in changes to body composition and function. Assessment of nutritional status in the clinical setting is usually undertaken in response to concerns about a patient's nutritional health that are triggered by nutritional screening (📖 p. 104). Nutritional assessment is a detailed investigation of the individual's nutritional health, which aims to:

- Define nutritional status.
- Identify those who might benefit from nutrition support.
- Establish goals of nutritional therapy to minimize deterioration in the stressed patient, to maintain nutritional status in the normally nourished patient, or to improve nutritional status in the non-stressed malnourished patient.
- Provide a baseline for planning and assessment of (monitoring) nutrition support.

## Methods

There is no single measure of nutritional health. A number of factors must be considered as part of the assessment, as outlined below.

### Medical history

- Previous and current illness—which might ↑ nutritional requirements (e.g. sepsis and wound healing), ↑ nutrient loss (e.g. vomiting, fistula/wound exudates, and haemorrhage), or limit nutrient ingestion (e.g. early satiety or vomiting), impaired digestion (e.g. pancreatitis), or absorption (e.g. coeliac disease).
- Weight history—including intentionality and recent changes in weight.
- Drug therapy—which might affect dietary intake, nutrient absorption, and metabolism.
- Socio-economic factors.

### Physical examination

Observing the patient's physical appearance will identify signs of the underlying disease, in addition to nutritional status, e.g. loss of subcutaneous fat stores, poor wound healing/pressure sores, ↓ muscle strength and associated poor mobility, dyspnoea, dehydration, oedema, and ↓ mental function/poor concentration. Specific nutrient deficiencies that might be suspected on physical examination include peripheral neuropathy in Wernicke–Korsakoff syndrome, which is associated with thiamine deficiency, and lesions of the lips and tongue, which are found in riboflavin deficiency.

### Dietary assessment

To determine whether dietary intake is sufficient to meet the patient's normal nutritional requirements and any additional requirements associated with illness. Recent and current dietary intakes should be assessed to establish any change in appetite, meal pattern, and food choice or consistency. A number of factors can influence dietary intake.

Factors affecting the individual's ability to buy and prepare food include socio-economic, psychological, and cognitive factors, and physical disability. Actual diet and fluid intakes can be estimated from patient recall and food records. An estimation of energy requirements (📖 p. 108) will be made to assess the adequacy of the diet.

### Body composition

Sequential body measurements or a comparison with standard population tables can be used to assess nutritional status. Anthropometric measurements can estimate adiposity (BMI and triceps skin-fold thickness), muscle mass (mid-arm muscle circumference), electrolyte and water composition, and total body weight. Accuracy depends on well-maintained equipment, training of clinical staff in the use of the technique, and interpretation of the results. Population standards are only available for healthy populations.

### Biochemical and haematological indices

Although nutritional compromise can affect the biochemistry of the body, biochemical and haematological measurements do not give clear indications of nutritional status. For instance, serum protein levels can vary owing to non-nutritional factors, e.g. posture, hydration, inflammatory response, and metabolic stress. These laboratory results should be interpreted in the light of the patient's changing clinical condition. Biochemical indices are of importance in monitoring artificial nutrition support and must be expertly interpreted if managing patients at risk of refeeding syndrome (📖 p. 114).

### Functional tests

Unsurprisingly, nutritional depletion impairs muscle function. Function can be measured by hand-grip and respiratory muscle strengths. On repletion, improvement in muscle function occurs before changes in body composition are detected.

## Further reading

Deurenberg P and Roubenoff R (2002). Body composition. In: Gibney MJ, Vorster HH, Kok F (eds). *Human Nutrition. The Nutrition Society Textbook Series.* Balckwell, Oxford, pp. 12–29.
Jeejeebhoy KN and Keith ME (2005). Nutritional assessment. In: Gibney MJ, Elia M, Lijungvist O *et al.* (eds). *Clinical Nutrition. The Nutrition Society Textbook Series.* Blackwell, Oxford, pp. 15–29.

# Estimating requirements

Establishing the patient's nutritional requirements is necessary to assess the adequacy of their dietary intake and advise on the provision of nutrition support. An accurate measurement of the patient's body weight is required because nutritional requirements are related to body composition. The goal of nutrition therapy depends on the patient's clinical/metabolic condition. In the management of a stressed patient, the nutritional goal is to minimize depletion. As the patient's condition improves, the goals of nutrition therapy will change in order to improve nutritional status.

## Energy requirements

Dietary sources of energy (kilocalories) are required to prevent the metabolism of body fat and protein. During periods of inadequate energy intake, catabolism occurs, with the breakdown of body protein. Exogenous sources of fat and carbohydrate are required. In clinical practice, energy requirements are calculated using the two methods outlined below.

### Predictive equations

A variety of equations are available. The British Dietetic Association[1] advocates the use of the Schofield equation for estimating basal metabolic requirements. Adjustments to the equation are needed to take into account the increased energy expenditure (stress factors) associated with the patient's illness and physical activity level.

### Indirect calorimetry

Energy expenditure can be determined from measurements of the oxygen consumed and carbon dioxide produced. Food consumed is burnt, i.e. combusted in the presence of oxygen, which releases carbon dioxide, water, and heat (energy).

Occasionally, it will be the intention to underfeed the patient. Adjustments to predictive equations are made to account for feeding an obese patient (using the patient's actual body weight will overestimate their basal energy requirements). Feeding the malnourished patient to meet their predicted energy requirement might cause cardiac, respiratory, renal, metabolic, and neuromuscular complications ( p. 114).

## Protein requirements

Protein is the only macronutrient containing nitrogen and therefore protein requirements are often referred to in terms of nitrogen requirements. Protein is not stored within the body; loss of protein has an effect on function. Proteins are continuously synthesized and degraded within a 'pool' that enables the formation of new proteins to meet the changing needs of the body. If the rate of protein synthesis is greater than the rate of protein breakdown, the body is said to be in an 'anabolic' state, with a positive nitrogen balance. If the rate of protein breakdown is greater than the rate of protein synthesis, this is a 'catabolic' state or negative nitrogen balance. To maintain the body in balance in the healthy individual, 0.75 g

---

1 Todoravic V, Micklewright A (2004). *A Pocket Guide to Clinical Nutrition* (3rd edn). British Dietetic Association, Birmingham.

of protein/kg body weight/day is required.[2] An ↑ protein/nitrogen intake is required in the metabolically stressed patient (e.g. owing to surgery, trauma, or sepsis),[1] although a positive nitrogen balance cannot be achieved in this altered metabolic state.

The aim is to limit protein loss. High protein intakes should be carefully monitored and avoided in those with liver and renal impairment.

## Fluid and electrolytes

Normal fluid requirements for adults between 18 and 60 years and >60 years are 35 ml/kg body weight/day and 30 ml/kg body weight/day, respectively.[1] Fluid balance can become disturbed during illness. In addition to estimating the fluid requirement on the basis of age and body weight, it is essential to make adjustments according to fluid loss (e.g. diarrhoea, fistula, vomiting, or pyrexia) to prevent dehydration. Overloading of fluids must also be avoided. In addition to impairing cardiac and respiratory function, fluid and electrolyte excess can slow gastric motility. Fluid-balance records, if kept accurately, are a useful tool. A positive fluid-balance chart of ~500 ml/day is desirable because this will account for insensible fluid loss that cannot be measured.

Electrolyte requirements for artificial nutrition support must be calculated on an individual basis.[1] Baseline serum levels should be measured to establish whether requirements are for maintenance or repletion. The National Institute for Health and Clinical Excellence have made recommendations for monitoring electrolytes during artificial feeding.[3]

2 Department of Health (1991). *Dietary Reference Values for Food Energy and Nutrition for the United Kingdom.* HMSO, London.

3 National Collaborating Centre for Acute Care (2006). *Nutrition Support in Adults: Oral Nutrition Support, Enteral Tube Feeding and Parenteral Nutrition. Clinical Guideline* 32. National Institute for Health and Clinical Excellence, London. http://www.nice.org.uk/CG32 (accessed 25.06.07).

# Nutrition support

The phrase 'food as treatment' is used to emphasize the importance of nutrition in the recovery of all patients. Without good nutrition, other therapeutic interventions are less effective. Nutrition support is concerned with the prevention and treatment of malnutrition.

Nutrition support includes a range of interventions, including:

- Improve food intake (oral diet).
- Fortification (energy and nutrient content) and modification (consistency) of the diet.
- Sip-feeds can provide a complete oral liquid diet if consumed in sufficient quantity (nutritionally complete preparations) or supplement an inadequate dietary intake.
- Artificial nutrition support is the provision of nutrients by artificial means—enteral or parenteral.

## Enteral nutrition (EN)

Delivery of feed via the gastrointestinal tract (GIT). It is used to supplement an inadequate dietary intake or provide the patient's total nutritional needs (📖 p. 116). EN can be used to introduce nutrients to the GIT following a period of intestinal failure while weaning from parenteral nutrition (PN).

## Parenteral nutrition (intravenous nutrition support)

Used to provide nutrients and fluid to patients with intestinal failure or if enteral tube access cannot be obtained (📖 p. 112). Supplemental PN might be used if enteral tube feeding is being introduced but is not meeting the patient's nutritional requirements. EN is generally considered to be more physiological and poses less risk to the patient.

## Artificial nutrition support

All patients who are malnourished and those at risk of becoming malnourished should be referred to nutrition and dietetic services. Patients requiring artificial nutrition support should be managed by a multidisciplinary NST.[1] Following an individual nutritional assessment (📖 p. 106), which will include an estimation of the patient's nutritional requirements (📖 p. 108), the route of nutrition support will be advised. The level of intervention depends on the patient's clinical condition (cause of nutritional depletion and disease process), function of the GIT, and potential accessibility for artificial feeding. Whenever possible, the patient should be involved in decision-making relating to artificial feeding (📖 p. 112: withholding and withdrawing nutrition support). Careful delivery and monitoring is essential as normal regulatory mechanisms are bypassed and complications associated with overfeeding (e.g. hyperglycaemia, hyperlipidaemia, fatty liver, and fluid and electrolyte disturbances) can be fatal.

**1** National Collaborating Centre for Acute Care (2006). *Nutrition Support in Adults: Oral Nutrition Support, Enteral Tube Feeding and Parenteral Nutrition. Clinical Guideline 32.* National Institute for Health and Clinical Excellence, London. http://www.nice.org.uk/CG32 (accessed 25.06.07).

# Withholding and withdrawing nutrition support

The principles surrounding the decision-making process for withholding or withdrawal of nutrition are derived from ethical (autonomy, beneficence, non-maleficence, and justice) and legal principles.

## Treatment or care

The provision of fluid and diet by mouth, and assistance that might be needed, are considered 'basic care'. Enteral tube feeding (☐ p. 116) and PN (☐ p. 148) are methods of artificial nutrition support and ∴ considered to be medical treatments.[1] The consultant responsible for the patient's care will need to decide if artificial nutrition is appropriate. On initiating artificial nutrition support, treatment goals should be clearly stated.[2] The provision of nutrition support might be intended to do the following:
- Impact on the disease process.
- Prolong life by allowing time for recovery.
- Improve quality of life.
- Provide compassionate care for the relief of symptoms.

## Autonomy

If a patient's nutritional intake is inadequate despite measures to improve the quality and quantity of dietary intake, or they cannot take diet by mouth, they must be consulted about the options for providing nutrition by artificial means. The rationale, risks, and benefits of treatment must be explained in terms that the patient will understand. Competent patients have the right to refuse treatment. Doctors are required to make treatment decisions in the 'best interest' of patients who lack the capacity to make their own decisions. Guidelines to assess competence have been produced jointly by the British Medical Association and the Law Society.[3]

Whereas the medical team is required to consult the family and carers of patients who lack the capacity to make decisions, family members do not have the right to demand treatment. Patients can make their wishes known regarding the advanced refusal of life-sustaining treatment; this might be done in anticipation of losing the ability to make treatment choices. Advance decisions, also known as 'advanced directives' or 'living wills', must fulfil specific criteria to be legally valid.[4]

1 *Airedale NHS Trust* v. *Bland* (1993), 1 All ER 821 (House of Lords).

2 Lennard-Jones J (1999). *Ethical and Legal Aspects of Clinical Hydration and Nutrition Support.* British Association of Parenteral and Enteral Nutrition, Maidenhead.

3 British Medical Association and the Law Society (2004). *Assessment of Mental Capacity: Guidance for Doctors and Lawyers* (2nd edn). BMJ Books, London.

4 Mental Capacity Act 2005. Stationery Office. London. http://www.opsi.gov.uk/acts/acts2005/20050009.htm (accessed 31. 10.07).

## Beneficence

Lack of adequate nourishment will cause the physical decline associated with malnutrition. Methods of artificial nutrition support should be considered in those who cannot take enough food by mouth, but also take into account the potential net benefits. The provision of artificial nutrition support might be beneficial in terms of maintaining the body's systems, but, in conditions such as persistent vegetative state, it will not contribute to a recovery. Doctors are not expected to provide treatment if it is deemed to be futile and against their clinical judgement. If the futility of treatment is unknown, the following is expected:

• A second opinion is sought,[5] perhaps from a clinical ethics team.
• A time-limited trial of nutrition should be provided.

## Non-maleficence

It is the medical team's responsibility to discuss the risks and burdens (including discomfort) of treatment, in addition to the potential benefits, with the patient and, if relevant, the patient's family. To avoid harm to the patient receiving nutrition support, care should be provided by competent practitioners.

## Justice

There is no legal or ethical basis for withholding or withdrawing nutrition support on the grounds of limited resources (equipment or appropriately trained personal). If care cannot be safely provided, the patient's care should be transferred.

## Nursing considerations

• Nurses should be aware that the authority to artificially feed, withhold, or withdraw nutrition lies with the consultant.
• Discussions regarding the provision, withdrawal, or withholding of artificial nutrition support should include the patient and their family, in addition to the nursing team.
• The nurse has a significant role in helping the patient to understand the need for the therapy, its potential risks and benefits, and the alternatives (including the consequences of not accepting the treatment), and in functioning as a patient advocate.
• Hospital nutrition support policy and procedure documents should contain guidelines on withholding and withdrawing nutrition support.

5 British Medical Association (2005). *Withholding and Withdrawing Life-Prolonging Treatment: Good Practice in Decision Making*. BMA, London.

# Refeeding problems

Life-threatening complications are associated with feeding patients who are malnourished or have had a poor dietary intake. Extreme care should be taken in initiating nutrition support. Micronutrient deficiencies, and fluid and electrolyte shifts, occur if too much feed is given, feed is given too quickly, or the feed is unbalanced. This might cause cardiac, respiratory, neurological, neuromuscular, renal, haematological, hepatic, and metabolic problems.

## Wernike–Korsakoff syndrome

The ↑ demand for thiamine, as the body reverts to carbohydrate metabolism, causes acute thiamine deficiency. Neurological symptoms of this syndrome include apathy, depression, ataxia, eye movement disorders, and short-term memory impairment.

Alcoholics and those with chronic vomiting disorders are at risk.

## Refeeding syndrome

During starvation, insulin production is ↓ because the intake of carbohydrate is ↓. Catabolism of protein and fat stores provides energy, with the loss of intracellular electrolytes. On feeding, carbohydrate becomes the main energy source, resulting in ↑ secretion of insulin. This, in turn, causes a metabolic shift, with the cellular uptake of electrolytes (phosphate, potassium, and magnesium) causing a rapid ↓ in serum electrolyte levels. There is ↑ demand for electrolytes and micronutrients.

Patients are at risk if they have two or more of the following.[1]

- BMI <18.5 kg/m$^2$.
- Unintentional weight loss of >10% of body weight in the previous 3–6 months.
- Little or no intake for >5 days.
- History of alcohol abuse, chemotherapy, antacids, or diuretics.

The following patients are at high risk.[1]

- BMI <16 kg/m$^2$.
- Unintentional weight loss of >15% of body weight in the previous 3–6 months.
- Little or no intake for >10 days.
- Low serum potassium, phosphate, or magnesium before feeding.

### Management

National guidelines[1] recommend that:

- All patients must be screened on admission, to identify their nutritional risk, and referred to the nutrition and dietetic services.
- Seriously ill patients, and those who have eaten little for >5 days, should have their artificial nutrition support started at no greater than 50% of their estimated need, ↑ gradually.
- All patients at risk should have baseline biochemical monitoring, with frequent monitoring while the feed is introduced.

---

1 National Collaborating Centre for Acute Care (2006). *Nutrition Support in Adults: Oral Nutrition Support, Enteral Tube Feeding and Parenteral Nutrition. Clinical Guideline 32.* National Institute for Health and Clinical Excellence, London. http://www.nice.uk/CG32 (accessed 25.06.07).

- Those at high risk of refeeding syndrome, and those at risk of Wernike–Korsakoff syndrome, should receive a high dose of thiamine and vitamin B complex supplementation before and during the first 10 days of feeding.
- Those at high risk should have feed introduced at a rate of 5–10 kcal/kg body weight/day, ↑ slowly over a period of 7 days.
- Prefeeding serum electrolyte levels are usually within the normal range; correction of low levels can only be successfully achieved once feeding has commenced.
- Daily requirements for potassium, phosphate, and magnesium are ↑.
- Off-the-shelf PN formulations must not be used without appropriate additions.

# Enteral nutrition

EN can be used as the sole route for nutritional therapy or to supplement inadequate oral intake.

## Indications

Patients requiring enteral tube feeding are those who are:
- Unable to take diet safely by mouth, e.g. the unconscious patient, those at risk of aspiration owing to dysphagia, or those who have an upper gastrointestinal pathology.
- Unable to take enough diet by mouth to maintain their body weight and nutritional status and ∴ need supplementary enteral tube feeding.
- Already underweight and/or malnourished and cannot take enough diet by mouth to meet their ↑ nutritional requirements.

## Assessment of risk

The benefits of starting EN should outweigh any potential risks and follow the ethical principles of benefit, non-harm, justice, and autonomy (📖 p. 112). A risk assessment should be carried out and documented according to local guidelines.

## Routes of access to the GIT

The GIT can be accessed through the mouth, nose, or skin (percutaneously) (Fig. 6.2). The choice of access depends on the proposed period of feeding, clinical condition of the patient, anatomy of the patient, patient choice, and expertise of the personnel available to insert the tube.

### Selecting enteral routes and feeding tubes

Routes for enteral feeding tube access are primarily chosen according to the anticipated duration of feeding (Table 6.2). The material from which the tube is made will indicate how long the tube can be kept in place (📖 short-term feeding p. 118; (📖 long-term feeding p. 120).

**Table 6.2** Routes and duration of enteral feeding

| Distal tip | Route | Tube description | Duration |
|---|---|---|---|
| Stomach | Mouth | Orogastric | Short term |
| | Oesophagus | Oesophagostomy /oesophogastric, pharyngostomy | Short term |
| | Nose | Nasogastric | Short term* |
| | Abdominal wall | Percutaneous gastrostomy | Long term |
| Intestine | Mouth | Nasoduodenal/jejunal | Short term |
| | Stomach | Percutaneous gastrojejunostomy | Long term |
| | Abdominal wall | Percutaneous duodenostomy/ jejunostomy | Long term |

* Might be long term, according to patient preference.

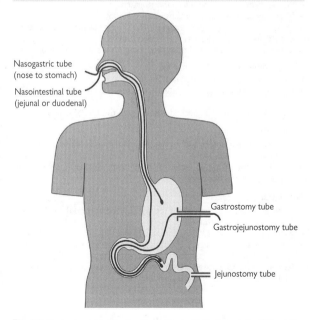

**Fig. 6.2** Routes for enteral feeding. Reproduced with kind permission © Burdett Institute 2008.

# Short-term feeding

This is usually defined as an anticipated period of feeding up to 4 weeks. Possible reasons for short-term feeding of stroke patients include:

- A short trial (1–2 weeks) of nasogastric feeding to maintain the patient's nutritional state and hydration during a period used to establish the possibility of recovery and assess the benefits of feeding, with the option of withdrawing tube feeding.
- Nasogastric tube feeding for a patient with oropharyngeal dysphagia, while awaiting the recovery of swallow function. The patient might progress to a modified-consistency diet, with supplemental nasogastric feeding, or require alternative long-term enteral access if there is little or no improvement.

Other reasons for short-term feeding include nasogastric or nasointestinal feeding in malnourished patients in preparation for surgery or the post-operative period.

## Short-term feeding routes

### Orogastric

- Placed through the mouth into the stomach.
- Placed by direct vision in the critical care setting.
- Used for patients in whom nasogastric (NG) tube placement is contra-indicated, e.g. basal skull fracture or facial fractures.
- Tube position should be checked according to the NG tube protocol.

### Pharyngostomy and oesophagostomy

- May be placed at the time of laryngectomy.
- It is now more common for patients to be referred for gastrostomy tube placement.
- Tube position must be checked according to the NG tube protocol.

### Nasogastric

- Most common and appropriate route for short-term enteral nutrition (<4 weeks).
- Long-term enteral option if alternative methods are unsafe, not possible, or not pursued by the patient.

### Nasointestinal

- Also referred to as post-pyloric feeding (placed beyond the pylorus of the stomach) (see Table 6.2).
- Includes nasoduodenal (ND) and nasojejunal (NJ) tubes.
- Selected if there is concern about gastro-oesophageal reflux causing aspiration into the lungs, delayed gastric emptying, or if intragastric feeding is contraindicated. Feeding beyond the ligament of Triez (NJ) is required for patients with pancreatitis.

## Short-term feeding tubes

These tubes are usually described according to how they are inserted into the GIT and the distal tip location where the feed is delivered (e.g. nasogastric) (see Table 6.2)

### *Ryles tubes: polyvinylchloride tubes*

- These large-bore tubes are mainly used for gastric decompression, but they can be used for short episodes of orogastric or NG feeding.
- Because of acid hardening, these tubes should be replaced within 10 days.

### *Fine-bore feeding tubes: polyvinylchloride (6–8FG)*

- Usually non-guide-wire assisted.
- Used for short periods of feeding or if the patient is self-intubating on a daily basis.

# Long-term feeding

This term is generally used for any patient requiring enteral feeding for >6 weeks. By this time, the benefits of continuing to feed are clearly established according to the goals of nutritional therapy. Although the use of gastrostomy tubes is advocated for the majority of patients requiring long-term feeding, do not assume that this is the patient's preference. If the patient wishes to continue NG feeding or gastrostomy tube placement is not thought to be in the patient's best interest, arrangements for long-term care of the patient in the community should include an assessment of the patient and/or carer's learning needs to safely prepare them for replacing the tube and managing the enteral feed-associated care (📖 p. 144).

## Long-term feeding tubes

These tubes are generally made from material that is more pliable (polyurethane and silicone) and therefore more comfortable for the patient.

### Fine-bore feeding tubes: polyurethane (6–8FG)

- Nasoenteric tubes.
- These tubes are resistant to acid hardening and ∴ can stay in place for >4 weeks—refer to the manufacturer's guidelines.
- Usually guidewire assisted.
- Might have a double lumen for those at risk of aspiration of gastric contents. This is to enable aspiration of stomach contents (see Fig. 6.3) through one port and permit feeding into the duodenum or intestine through a distal port (nasointestinal route). These can be placed at the bedside but may need endoscopic or radiological placement.

### Needle catheter jejunostomy

- Placed at the time of upper gastrointestinal surgery in patients who are malnourished, where post-pyloric feeding is indicated.
- Secured with sutures or with a Dacron® cuff.
- Usually <12 FG; avoid drug administration and take care with flushing; blocked tubes will need to be removed.

### Gastrostomy tubes and gastrojejunal tubes

- Most common method for long-term enteral feeding (📖 p. 126).
- Variable durability; some deteriorate more quickly due to interaction with some anti-epilepsy drugs and micro-organisms (e.g. Candida).

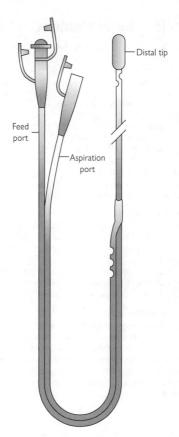

**Fig. 6.3** Double-lumen feeding tube. Reproduced with kind permission © Burdett Institute 2008.

# Nasogastric tube placement

The reasons for medical staff requesting NG tube insertion should be clearly documented in the patient's notes. Referral to the dietetic team should be timely to ensure that the patient has a nutritional assessment, with an estimation of nutritional and fluid requirements. This is to ensure that a feeding schedule or prescription is immediately available. NG tube insertion can be undertaken by a competent registered nurse (RN) or student nurse under direct supervision of a competent RN. A programme of education and supervision will be required if NG tube insertion was not included in the basic training for the register.

The successful placement of NG tubes will depend not only on your experience and attitude (if you are a novice at this procedure or have not placed a tube for some time, seek out a colleague whom you know to have a good success rate and learn the finer points of insertion), but also on how well you have prepared the patient.

## Placement procedure

Before undertaking this procedure, the RN should refer to their hospital policy and be knowledgeable about the type and characteristics of the available tubes. Insertion policies should be up to date and make reference to national guidelines.[1,2]

Details of the insertion (type of tube, length of tube inserted, method used to confirm tube position, planned replacement date, and any difficulties encountered during the insertion) must be clearly documented.

## Cautions and contraindications

NG is not always possible or carries ↑ risks associated with insertion or feeding. Careful assessment of the risks and benefits is necessary (Table 6.3).

If bedside placement of the feeding tube is not possible, alternative routes of tube placement (e.g. orogastric for those with a history of basal skull fracture) or NG placement using fluoroscopic methods should be considered. If the risks are associated with feeding, a plan of care should reflect actions to ↓ these risks.

1 National Collaborating Centre for Acute Care (2006). *Nutrition Support in Adults: Oral Nutrition Support, Enteral Tube Feeding and Parenteral Nutrition. Clinical Guideline 32.* National Institute for Health and Clinical Excellence, London. http://www.nice.org.uk/CG32 (accessed 25.06.07).

2 National Patient Safety Agency (2005). *Patient Safety Alert 05: Reducing the Harm Caused by Misplaced Nasogastric Feeding Tubes.* http://www.npsa.nhs.uk (accessed 25.06.07)

**Table 6.3** Contraindications for NG tube placement or feeding

| Condition | Risk |
| --- | --- |
| Basal skull fracture | Intracranial placement |
| Altered mental state | Misplaced tubes |
| Severe gastro-oesophageal reflux | Aspiration pneumonia |
| Oesophageal perforation | Misplaced tube |
| Pathology of the nasopharyx, oropharnyx, or oesophagus | Trauma/misplaced tube |
| Gastroparesis/poor gastric motility (high gastric aspirates) | Regurgitation/aspiration pneumonia |
| Severe acute pancreatitis | Exacerbation of pancreatitis |

# Nasogastric tube management

The focus of care is to reduce the risk of complications (some life threatening), ensure the liquid feed is administered and to promote comfort.

## Verifying tube tip placement

There is a risk that NG tubes can be misplaced on insertion or during use. It is, therefore, necessary to verify where the distal tip is before each use. Regardless of the type of NG tube used, verification of the position should be made using pH-grade indicator paper, using advice from the National Patient Safety Agency.[1] A pH of <5.5 is consistent with gastric placement. The routine use of radiography is not recommended because this delays feeding and exposes the patient to unnecessary radioactivity.

## Patient comfort

- NG tubes should be secured to the patient's cheek, not their nose, to prevent pressure necrosis.
- Regular inspection of the nostril should be undertaken.
- Patients should be assisted with oral hygiene.

## Maintaining tube patency

- Once the position of the tube has been confirmed the tube should be flushed with water,[2] before administering feed. This is important as the acid secretions of the stomach drawn up into the feeding tube will cause the administered feed to curdle.
- Feeding tubes must also be flushed prior to the administration of drugs, between drug administration, and to complete drug administration. This is to prevent drug–drug and drug–feed interactions that could block the tube (📖 p. 146).

## Preventing accidental removal

Most tubes are accidentally removed by either the patient or healthcare staff. To minimize the risk of accidental removal:

- Carefully plan the mobilization/repositioning of the patient to ↓ the incidence of accidental removal.
- Regularly remind the patient of the need for tube feeding and its benefits.
- Consider the use of a nasal bridle.[3]

## Tube removal

Care should be taken when removing NG tubes. The feeding tube should be flushed and capped. If the patient reports pain during tube removal, this procedure should be abandoned and investigated for possible knotting. It should be clearly documented that the tube has been removed and noted if the tube is intact.

1 National Patient Safety Association (2005). *Patient Safety Alert 05. Reducing the Harm Caused by Misplaced Nasogastric Feeding Tubes.* http://www.npsa.nhs.uk (accessed 12.07.07).

2 National Collaborating Centre for Nursing and Supportive Care (2003). *Prevention of Healthcare Associated Infection in Primary and Community Care.* National Institute for Clinical Excellence, London.

3 Anderson MR, O'Connor M, Mayer P, O'Mahoney D, Woodward J, Kane K (2004). The nasal loop provides an alternative to percutaneous endoscopic gastrostomy in high risk dysphagic stroke patients. *Clinical Nutrition* **23**, 501–6.

# Gastrostomy tube placement

Gastrostomy tubes (Fig. 6.4) are inserted through the abdominal wall into the stomach. Gastrostomy tube feeding should be considered if EN is needed for >4 weeks.[1] The decision to start gastrostomy feeding should be made by a multidisciplinary NST.[2] Occasionally, gastrostomy tubes are placed to facilitate gastric drainage, as a long-term alternative to NG tube placement. The principles of tube and site care are the same.

Gastrostomy tubes can be placed endoscopically, radiologically, or surgically. Endoscopic and radiological gastrostomy tubes are associated with fewer complications than surgically placed tubes. Gastrostomy tubes are generally placed with concomitant antibiotic prophylaxis.

## Percutaneous endoscopic gastrostomy (PEG)
- Requires sedation—local anaesthetic to abdominal wound.
- Disc or flange retained (Fig 6.5)—lifespan of months to years.
- (📖 p. 199 for indications and contraindications).

## Surgical gastrostomy (SG)
- Requires mini-laparotomy.
- Balloon or Malecot retained (Fig. 6.4).
- Requires deep abdominal sutures (T fasteners) to secure the stomach to the abdominal wall.

## Radiologically inserted gastrostomy (RIG)
- Requires sedation and local anaesthetic to abdominal wound.
- Malecot, pigtail, or balloon retained (Fig. 6.4).
- Long-term tube—Dacron cuff; lifespan of months to years.
- Requires deep abdominal sutures (T fasteners) to secure the stomach to the abdominal wall.
- Can be a one- or two-stage procedure, with a long-term tube placed through the tract once it has formed (2–4 weeks).

## Assessment
In preparation for gastrostomy tube insertion, a patient assessment should be carried out, with the following aims.
- Review of the appropriateness of artificial nutrition—this can only be answered if the goals of artificial nutrition were clearly stated.
- Assessment of the risks of the procedure.
- To inform the patient and relevant carers of the procedure, risks, and aftercare.

1 National Collaborating Centre for Acute Care (2006). *Nutrition Support in Adults: Clinical Guideline 32.* National Institute for Health and Clinical Excellence. London. http://www.nice.org.uk/CG32 (accessed 25.06.07).

2 NCEPOD (2004). *Scoping our Practice. National Confidential Enquiry into Patient Outcome and Death.* http://www.ncepod.org.uk (accessed 12.07.07).

## Pre-insertion management

Collaborative protocols between endoscopy units and NSTs aim to minimize potential complications associated with tube insertion (📖 p. 198).

## Post-procedure care

Local guidelines must include monitoring the patient for procedure-related complications, gastrostomy site (stoma) care, and the introduction of the enteral feed preparation (📖 p. 134).

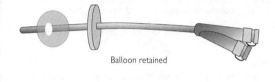

Balloon retained

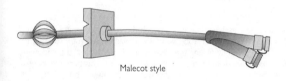

Malecot style

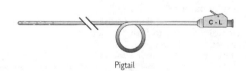

Pigtail

**Fig. 6.4** Gastrostomy tubes. Reproduced with kind permission © Burdett Institute 2008.

# Gastrostomy tube management

The correct repositioning of the external retention plate (Fig. 6.5) is extremely important during the first few weeks while the tract is forming and the abdominal wall and the stomach are fibrosing.

## Stoma site

Gastrostomy stomas should be cleaned daily as part of daily hygiene. In the days following insertion the site should be cleaned with saline and gauze. Dressings are only indicated if the site is oozing or infected. Dressings limit access to the stoma for observation and if placed under the external retention disc may cause pressure damage. Once healed the site can be cleaned with soap and water (refer to local policy) to reduce the risk of infection.

## Granuloma

A granuloma at the gastrostomy site is associated with excessive movement of the tube. Treated with steroid-based ointments or silver nitrate. Prevention is preferable.

## Buried bumper

As a general rule, gastrostomy tubes should be rotated through 360° daily. This is done by pushing the tube ventrally (inwards) 3–5 mm, rotating the tube, and then carefully pulling the tube until it is felt against the abdominal wall. The external retention plate should be secured. This prevents internal tissue necrosis and internal over-granulation causing a buried bumper. Intragastric granulation may occlude the feeding tube and may need surgical removal.

## Maintaining tube patency

Enteral feeding tubes should be flushed regularly, even if not in use. A minimal standard would be to flush the tube before, between, and after any medicines or feed. Syringes (50 ml enteral feeding syringes or oral syringes) that are not IV compatible should be used, thus preventing wrong route administrations of medicines or feed. In hospital, sterile water tends to be used for flushing for practical reasons, but at home freshly drawn tap water or cooled boiled water is more practical and not associated with any ↑ infective complications.[1]

---

1 National Collaborating Centre for Nursing and Supportive Care (2003). *Prevention of Healthcare Associated Infection in Primary and Community Care.* National Institute for Clinical Excellence. London.

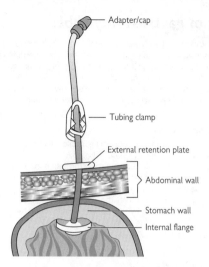

**Fig. 6.5** Cross-section showing an internal flange gastrostomy tube in the stomach. Reproduced with kind permission © Burdett Institute 2008.

# Replacement of gastrostomy tubes

A tract (fistula) develops over time (2–6 weeks), in addition to the adhesion of the anterior abdominal wall to the stomach. This is an important consideration in planning to replace the tube or if the tube falls out prematurely. An established tract enables tubes to be changed safely without loss of the tract. PEG tubes should be replaced using the manufacturer's advice. Balloon and Malecot tubes (Fig. 6.4) can be replaced through the tract by competent trained personnel.

## Low-profile gastrostomy tube

Use of low-profile replacement tubes is becoming more favoured in young adults and patients with active lifestyles (Fig. 6.6). These gastrostomy tubes are also referred to as button gastrostomies. A balloon retained device is commonly used. Other tubes of a Malecot style are available and have the advantage that they have a longer durability. The replacement tubes are usually funded through the patient's primary care trust (PCT). The procedure is undertaken by appropriately trained members of the NST, the district nursing team, or the patient.

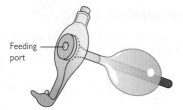

Feeding port

**Fig. 6.6** Low-profile balloon gastrostomy. Reproduced with kind permission © Burdett Institute 2008.

# Percutaneous intestinal feeding

Intestinal feeding tubes are becoming more common as they are useful in the management of post-operative patients and those with a GIT that is difficult to access.

### Indications

- Upper GIT dysfunction (e.g. delayed gastric emptying, reflux, and aspiration).
- Inaccessible upper GIT (e.g. oesophageal fistula, stricture, gastrectomy).

### Placement methods

- Surgical jejunostomy (SJ)—a stoma is created to facilitate intubation with an enteral tube.[1]
- Needle catheter jejunostomy (NCJ)—at the time of laparotomy/ surgical procedure a feeding tube is placed through the abdominal wall into the jejunum. The abdominal wall must be anchored to the intestine.[1]
- Percutaneous endoscopic jejunostomy (PEJ) based on the PEG procedure allows the jejunal extension tube to be placed directly into the jejunum.[2]
- Percutaneous endoscopic gastro-jejunostomy (PEG-J) refers to a tube which is placed percutaneously though the abdominal wall into the stomach (gastrostomy), with an intestinal extension placed beyond the pylorus into the jejunum (Fig. 6.7).
- Fistuloclysis is an uncommon method of feeding patients with small intestinal fistulation. This involves the insertion of a feeding tube (usually a balloon tube designed for gastrostomy placement) into the distal segment of the fistulated bowel.[3]

1 Payne-James J (2001). Enteral nutrition: tubes and techniques of delivery. In: Payne-James J, Grimble G, and Silk D (eds.) *Artificial Nutrition Support in Clinical Practice*. Greenwich Medical Media, London, pp. 281–302.

2 Maple JT, Peterson BT, and Baron TH (2005). Direct percutaneous endoscopic jejunostomy; outcomes of 307 consecutive attempts. *American Journal of Gastroenterology* **100**: 2681–88.

3 Farrer K and Teubner A (2003). *Fistuloclysis: Distal Feeding*. Salford Royal Hospital.

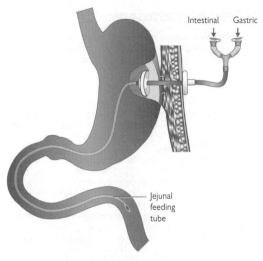

Intestinal    Gastric

Jejunal
feeding
tube

**Fig. 6.7** Percutaneous endoscopic gastro-jejunostomy. Reproduced with kind permission © Burdett Institute 2008.

# Enteral feed preparations

Most enteral feeds come as a ready-to-use prepackaged sterile liquid. They are usually nutritionally complete. A standard feed contains 1 kcal/ml, with or without fibre, and is suitable for the majority of patients, but there are preparations available with different compositions (Table 6.4).

## Prescribing

Enteral feed regimens are usually prescribed by a registered dietitian once the patient's nutritional requirements have been calculated (&#x1F4D6; p. 108).[1] Registered nurses have undertaken this role in accordance local need and supported by the local drugs and therapeutic committee after the introduction of non-medical prescribing.

Several hospitals have a policy whereby a feed can be started in the absence of a dietitian (during weekends). The nurse following these instructions should be aware of the consequences of commencing a feed for a patient who is malnourished and at risk of refeeding syndrome (&#x1F4D6; p. 114). All patients who are fed in the absence of a dietitcian, should have their baseline blood biochemistry reviewed and both weight and weight history recorded. An assessment of the risks of refeeding should be undertaken and, if there is any concern, the feed should be delayed until expert advice is available.

## Administration of enteral tube feeds

Feeds should be administered, and the regimen tailored to meet the individual needs of the patient, after consideration of any clinical constraints (e.g. medication delivery, nursing schedules, and rehabilitation programmes). Feeds can be delivered into the stomach or small intestine by syringe (a bolus feed), continuous pump delivery, or an intermittent pump (high rate), or any combination of these methods. Continuous pump delivery is the method of choice for acutely unwell hospital patients, in whom glycaemic control and fluid balance are important. Feeding into the stomach facilitates higher delivery rates, because it is better tolerated than feeding into the small intestine.

The majority of adult enteral feeds are commercially prepared, with consideration of the convenience of the feeding system and ↓ of the risks of microbiological contamination.

1 *British National Formulary* (2007). http://www.bnf.org. (accessed 05.07.07).

**Table 6.4** Summary of enteral feeds

| Type of feed | Indications |
| --- | --- |
| **Standard** (whole protein/polymeric) 1 kcal/ml, with or without fibre | Suitable for most patients Fibre—a mixture of soluble and insoluble forms |
| **High energy** (whole protein/polymeric) 1.2–2.0 kcal/ml, with or without fibre | ↑ nutritional requirements or fluid restrictions |
| **Low energy** (whole protein/polymeric) 0.5–1.0 kcal/ml | Contains complete mineral and vitamin profiles in lower volumes Suitable for long-term feeding in patients with low energy requirements |
| **Elemental/peptide** | Proteins are in the form of amino acids or peptides, to aid absorption |
| **Therapeutic feeds** For example, renal, respiratory, low-sodium, or immune-modulation feeds | Specific feeds targeted to meet the requirements of clinical conditions Should be used under the supervision of a dietitian or other clinical nutrition expert/healthcare professional |

# Complications of enteral feeding

Complications associated with enteral feeding can be categorized as metabolic, mechanical, infective, or gastrointestinal; several examples are summarized in Table 6.5.

## Metabolic complications

Can sometimes be predicted and require specific monitoring (📖 p. 142).

### Hyperglycaemia

Usually related to insulin resistance and might necessitate the initiation of hyperglycaemic medication or insulin regimens.

### Refeeding syndrome

(📖 p. 114)

Can develop if food is reintroduced too rapidly after a period of starvation or minimal oral intake. The syndrome is characterized by life-threatening micronutrient deficiencies, fluid and electrolyte imbalance, and organ and metabolic dysfunctions. Nurses are ideally placed to identify this group of patients.

### Electrolyte imbalance

Can result from over- or under-hydration, refeeding syndrome, medicine administration, or critical illness. Regular daily biochemical testing is required if electrolyte levels are abnormal or unstable. Intravenous (IV) or enteral correction might be necessary, depending on local policy (check with the pharmacist for clarification of local policy).

### Drugs nutrient interaction

Medicines and feed can each affect the absorption of one another, which can, in turn, alter physiological processes and sometimes cause toxicity or deficiency of either therapeutic medicine levels or nutrients. Interactions are usually predictable, and the pharmacist can advise on all medicine preparations and administration through feeding tubes (📖 p. 146).

**Table 6.5** Summary of enteral nutrition complications[1]

| Complication | Examples of specific complications |
|---|---|
| Metabolic | Hyperglycaemia, hypoglycaemia |
| | Over-hydration, under-hydration |
| | Electrolyte imbalance |
| | Refeeding syndrome |
| | Drug–nutrient interactions |
| Mechanical | Pulmonary aspiration |
| | Rhinitis, otitis, pharyngitis, oesophagitis (NG) |
| | Oesophageal erosions |
| | Tube blockage |
| | Tube displacement |
| | Colon perforation (PEG) |
| | Buried bumper syndrome (PEG, PEG-J, PEJ) |
| Infective | Diarrhoea |
| | Colonization of stoma site |
| | Aspiration pneumonitis |
| Gastrointestinal | Abdominal cramping |
| | Abdominal distension |
| | Nausea and vomiting |
| | Oesophageal reflux |
| | Malabsorption |
| | Diarrhoea |
| | Constipation |

1 National Collaborating Centre for Acute Care (2006). *Nutrition Support in Adults: Clinical Guideline 32*. National Institute for Health and Clinical Excellence, London. http://www.nice.org.uk/CG32 (accessed 25.06.07).

# Mechanical complications of enteral feeding

Contact between a tube and the mucosa of the GI tract can lead to ulceration, pressure necrosis, and infection. Assess the site of the tube daily, e.g. the nares for NG/NJ tubes and abdomen site for other tubes. If red, sore, indurated, or discharging, the site must be assessed by a member of the NST or doctor.

## Aspiration

Can occur in any patient with dysphagia or compromised swallow function, regardless of the route of feeding. Minimizing risk includes:
- Careful assessment of gastric residual volumes in patients with upper GI dysmotility or delayed gastric emptying.
- Careful use of prokinetic agents.
- Ensuring the patient is sitting up at an angle of at least 30°.
- Not letting the patient become constipated.

## Blockages

Tube blockages are a common occurrence in enterally fed patients. Prevention is the best cure and ∴ flushing the tubes, administering medicines in the correct form, and never leaving feed in the tube at the end of a feeding session is paramount. If blockage is apparent:
- Check the tube is not coiled or kinked under the dressing.
- Flushing with warm water is at least as effective as any other solution[1] and should be the first line of treatment.
- Use a 30 ml syringe and the push–stop technique—smaller syringes might rupture fine-bore feeding tubes.
- Other unblocking agents include sodium bicarbonate solution or pancreatic enzymes.
- Further advice should be sought from local healthcare professionals or policy.

## Displacement

Ensuring that feeding tubes are securely fixed to the skin will prevent most displacements. Daily checks should be encouraged. The use of nasal loops to prevent accidental NG/NJ tube removal has been successful[2] and is becoming more widely used.

**1** Colagiovanni L (2000). Preventing and clearing blocked feeding tubes. *NTPlus* **96**, 3–4.

**2** Anderson MR, O'Connor M, Mayer P, O'Mahoney D, Woodward J, and Kane K (2004). The nasal loop provides an alternative to percutaneous endoscopic gastrostomy in high risk dysphagic stroke patients. *Clinical Nutrition* **23**, 501–6.

# Infective complications of enteral feeding

Patients who are malnourished have an increased vulnerability to infection.

## Diarrhoea

Diarrhoea can occur in 30–68% of people who are enterally fed[1] (📖 p. 140). Stools of patients being enterally fed are abnormal and can sometimes be falsely diagnosed as diarrhoea, which would account for differences in reported numbers. Infective causes include bacteria, viruses, or, less frequently, protozoa.

- *Clostridium difficile* is one of the most common hospital-acquired infections—occurs after alteration of gut flora by antibiotic therapy and can be life threatening.
- Other bacteria include *Campylobacter* spp, *Salmonella* spp, *Shigella* spp, and *Escherischia coli*.

Using ready-made sterile feeds, changing administration sets daily, and paying attention to hand-washing before accessing the feeding tube will minimize contamination.

## Infected stoma site

Stoma sites can become colonized without being infected. Check the site daily and take action if it is red, hot, sore, indurated, or exuding pus; if positive for infection, the doctor should be informed.

### Treatment

- Topical cleansing antiseptics—the pharmacist or infection-control team can advise. Alcohol-based cleansers should only be used if compatible with the feeding tube.
- Systemic antibiotics must be given in severe cases.
- Topical antibiotics should generally be avoided because the preparations can cause damage to the feeding tube.
- Silver dressings—there is ↑ evidence for the topical use of silver-impregnated charcoal dressings, with encouraging results that show a ↓ of PEG-site colonization and ↓ in the incidence of clinically infected PEG sites.[2]

1 Duncan H, and Silk DBA (2001.) Enteral nutrition. In: Nightingale J (ed.) *Intestinal Failure*. Greenwich Medical Media, London, pp. 477–97.

2 Leak K (2002). PEG site infections: a novel use for Actisorb Silver 220. *British Journal of Community Nursing* **7**, 321–25.

# GI disturbances in enteral feeding

Abdominal cramping, abdominal distension, nausea, and vomiting are not uncommon in the early stages of EN. Monitoring for, and identification of, the causes of GI disturbances are within the remit of the NST. ↓ the rate of feeds and review of medicines might be necessary.

## Diarrhoea

In most circumstances, diarrhoea is unlikely to be caused by EN and other causes should be investigated. Inform the dietitian, pharmacist, nutrition nurse specialist, or healthcare professional because unresolved diarrhoea can ↑ requirements, lead to malabsorption of certain nutrients or vitamins/minerals, and affect fluid balance. In addition to infective causes diarrhoea can be caused by:

- Lactose intolerance—most feeds now are lactose free. The dietitian can advise.
- Medicines: e.g. antibiotics—alter gut flora and may increase gut motility.
- As a side effect of medicines:
  - Inert substances in medicines, e.g. magnesium stearate.
  - Any pharmacological concerns should be discussed with the local pharmacist.
- Feed—unlikely to be the cause, but the dietitian or other healthcare professional can advise you or change the feed if there are concerns with its content or osmolarity, or if there is a malabsorption syndrome.

## Constipation

Patients receiving EN might develop constipation—bowel activity should be monitored daily and recorded on the observation chart, according to local policy. Constipation can occur as a result of dehydration, a lack of fibre in the diet, certain medical conditions, or medicines. Regular assessment of fluid requirements is necessary, especially in hot weather.

# Monitoring enteral nutrition

Monitoring should be undertaken by healthcare professionals with the relevant skills and knowledge and is best conducted within the auspices of a multi-disciplinary NST because of the varying nature of the skills and knowledge needed. Patients receiving EN, either in hospital or in the community, need monitoring for the following reasons:

• To ensure they are meeting their nutritional goals.
• To ensure they are not developing complications.
• To ensure that the EN access device is patent and in working order.
• To enable evaluation of the type of nutrition support, content of the nutritional regimen, and efficacy of the nutritional plan.

The frequency at which monitoring takes place will depend on the condition of the patient and local policy, and should reflect recent guidelines (Table 6.6).

Local policy will determine the protocol for monitoring patients receiving EN. Generally, the frequency at which the patient is monitored will be ↓ when their clinical condition stabilizes and ↓ further once they become established on EN or transferred from secondary to primary care.

**Table 6.6** Summary of EN monitoring[1]

| Monitoring | Frequency | Rationale |
|---|---|---|
| Nutritional intake | Daily, ↓ to weekly, monthly, and then every 3 months, as established | Ensure the provision meets requirements Allow for changes to be made Ensure correct feed and volume is being administered |
| Biochemical monitoring | See NICE recommendations for further advice[1] | |
| Weight | At least weekly and then ↓, as established | Provide baseline measurements to inform ongoing assessment of nutritional status |
| BMI, anthropometry | On commencement and then at formal reviews | |
| GI function (nausea, vomiting, constipation, diarrhoea) | Daily until EN is established without complications and then on each review | To establish whether feed is tolerated because any dysfunction will affect intake or absorption |
| **Nasogastric tube** | | |
| Position | Before each use using pH-graded indicator paper | To ensure the tube is in the correct position for feeding |
| Fixation | Daily | Avoid accidental removal |
| Patency/condition | Before each use | To ensure the tube is in working order and ↓ risk of tube malfunction |
| **Gastrostomy/ jejunostomy** | | |
| Stoma site | Daily | To ensure the tube is in working order and to detect signs of infection or complications |
| Tube position | Daily | |
| Patency/condition | At each use | |
| Balloon volume | Weekly, if indicated | |
| **Nasojejunal tube** | At each use | |
| Tube position | | |
| Tube patency | | |

1 National Collaborating Centre for Acute Care (2006). *Nutrition Support in Adults: Clinical Guideline 32*. National Institute for Health and Clinical Excellence, London. http://www.nice.org.uk/ CG32 (accessed 25.06.07).

# Home enteral nutrition

There are >18 680 adults in the UK who have made the transition from hospital to receiving their tube feed in the community.[1] Swallowing disorders were reported as the main indication for home enteral tube feeding (HETF) in the British Artificial Nutrition survey. In 2005, >50% of patients were discharged from hospital with conditions of the central nervous system (e.g. cerebrovascular accident, motor neuron disease, and multiple sclerosis) and ~24% of these patients were discharged with disorders of the GIT. Gastrostomy tube feeding accounts for >80% of all EN; some patients have NG tubes (12%) and might self-intubate in preference to gastrostomy tube feeding or because gastrostomy tube placement is not possible.

## Funding and organization

GPs are responsible for the care of their patients in the community. Enteral feed formulations are only available on prescription (FP10 endorsed by Advisory Committee on Borderline Substances (ACBS)). HETF packages vary throughout the country. Often, PCTs have a contract with an enteral feeding company which can provide the feed, giving sets, syringes, and feeding pumps, in addition to community-based specialized nursing services. The cost of the care package might be the responsibility of the PCT, devolved to the district nursing service, or incorporated into the nursing home costs. Those involved in the discharge include the dietitian, speech and language therapist (for those with dysphagia), nutrition nurse, pharmacist, district nurse, and GP. All patients need access to community dietetic services.

## Discharge planning

Most patients will have their enteral feed commenced in hospital, although it might be possible for a GP to initiate tube feeding in the community. Access to good clinical nutrition services is required. For gastrostomy tube placement, a minimum overnight stay will be required; the stay will be longer if problems tolerating the feed are encountered. Those caring for patients with enteral feeding tubes should refer to their PCT's nutrition support policy documents. Guidance and standards for the preparation, discharge, and monitoring of patients requiring HETF is available in the National Institute for Clinical Excellence guidelines on preventing infection[2] and artificial nutrition support.[3] Although the majority of patients are cared for in their own homes, altered care needs might mean that

1 Jones B, Holden C, Dalzell M et al. (2006). *Artificial Nutrition Support in the UK 2005*. A report by the British Artificial Nutrition survey. http://www.bapen.org.uk (accessed 30 May 2007).

2 National Collaborating Centre for Nursing and Supportive Care (2003). *Prevention of healthcare associated infection in primary and community care*. National Institute for Clinical Excellence, London.

3 National Collaborating Centre for Acute Care (2006). *Nutrition Support in Adults: Clinical Guideline 32*. National Institute for Health and Clinical Excellence, London. http://www.nice.org.uk/CG32 (accessed 25.06.07).

patients require nursing-home care. Those responsible for the discharge of these patients should ensure that those caring for them in the community are adequately prepared and competent in the care of the feeding tube and system.

▶ Consider the support available for families. Non-professional carers responsible for patients receiving HETF report significant emotional and psychological stress.

The organization of HETF takes ~5 days. It is the ward nurse's responsibility to prepare the patient/carer for the safe administration of the feed (including good hygiene), maintenance and care of the feeding tube and tube site, how to deal with tube-related problems, use of the enteral feeding pump and drug administration. The dietitian will ensure that the feeding schedule is appropriate for the patient and contact the GP to request the prescription, arrange the home-delivery service, complete the British Artificial Nutrition Survey form, and provide information about the patient support group (Patients on Intravenous and Nasogastric Nutrition Therapy (PINNT)). The pharmacist will ensure that the medication is in the appropriate preparation to take home. Follow-up services and contact details should also be provided.

# Drug administration and enteral nutrition

Patients requiring artificial nutrition support through enteral feeding tubes will often require administration of medication through the feeding tube. The nurse must be aware of the professional and legal issues relating to this aspect of care.

## Professional and legal issues

Licensed drugs become 'unlicensed' if not prepared and administered in accordance with the manufacturers' specifications.[1]

▶ This has particular relevance to crushing tablets, opening capsules, or delivering the drugs (e.g. through the enteral tube) at a site other than that intended by the manufacturer.

Doctors have the authority to prescribe drugs for 'unlicensed' use and must state on the prescription how they should be prepared and administered. The nurse administering the drug must use his/her professional judgement according to his/her knowledge and skill in administration or omission of medication. In addition to the principles of drug administration, he/she must ensure he/she has sufficient knowledge of how to prepare and administer the drug safely. It is reasonable for the nurse to seek further advice from the pharmacist (drug information) regarding the suitability of the drug for enteral-tube administration, preparation, and dosage. The nurse must ensure that, if the patient cannot receive their usual medication in situations whereby the feeding tube is blocked, damaged, or unintentionally removed, the prescribing doctor is notified and alternative routes of administration are considered. It is unacceptable to simply omit the drug without acting in the patient's best interest to ensure that they receive their treatment.

## Practice guidelines

The enteral feeding guidelines of individual hospital trusts should contain up-to-date information about the administration of drugs through enteral feeding tubes.[2,3] The following should be considered.
- If safe to do so, drugs should be taken orally.
- Drugs might need to be given during a break in the continuous infusion if the drug is known to interact with the feed and ↓ the efficacy of the drug (e.g. antacids) or drug absorption (e.g. carbamazepine, theophylline, or phenytoin).
- Certain drugs might not be absorbed at the site of delivery.
- Enteric-coated tablets, hormones, cytotoxic drugs, and sustained-release capsules should never be crushed.

---

**1** Nursing and Midwifery Council (2004). *Guidelines for the Administration of Medicines*. NMC, London.

**2** National Patient Safety Agency (2007). *Patient Safety Alert* (19): *Promoting Safer Measurement and Administration of Liquid Medicines via Oral and Other Enteral Routes*. NPSA, London.

**3** British Association of Parenteral and Enteral Nutrition. *Administering Drugs via Enteral Feeding Tubes: A Practical Guide*. http://www.bapen.org.uk (accessed 26.06.07).

- Liquid suspensions should be used in preference to crushing tablets or administering syrups.
- A 50 ml enteric or catheter-tip syringe should be used—small syringes exert greater pressure and might damage the tube.
- Ensure that the drug is prepared in a syringe that is incompatible with IV systems.
- Drugs should never be added to the feed solution.
- Measures to ↓ the risk of microbiological contamination should be adhered to.
- Before administration, ensure that the tube is correctly positioned.
- The tube should be flushed with 30 ml of water (to remove residual feed and ↓ the risks of drug–feed interactions) before drug administration, 10 ml of water between drugs, and 30 ml to flush the tube after drug administration.

# Parenteral nutrition

Parenteral nutrition (PN) refers to the administration of nutrients into the circulatory system, bypassing the GIT. The terms 'parenteral nutrition' and 'IV' are used in preference to the term 'total parenteral nutrition'. This term is no longer promoted because the complete range of nutrients cannot always be safely administered in the parenteral nutrition solution. Additionally, nutritional therapy is likely to include some oral or enteral intake. In this instance, the term 'supplemental parenteral nutrition' (SPN) might be used. Although the terms 'intravenous hyperalimentation' (IVH) and 'hyperalimentation' are not commonly used in the UK, they are terms used in the North American literature. This term is now synonymous with IV nutrition.

PN is an expensive complex therapy. Inappropriate selection of patients and delivery of PN by those lacking expertise will put the patient at risk of potentially life-threatening complications. National guidelines emphasize the importance of managing patients requiring PN within a multidisciplinary NST.[1] The NST will generally have direct responsibility for the following:

- Undertaking a nutritional assessment.
- Advising on the most appropriate route—enteral or parenteral.
- Estimating nutritional requirements.
- Prescribing PN therapy.
- Assisting with enteral or parenteral feeding access.
- Compounding the PN formulation.
- Monitoring the response to nutritional therapy.
- Supporting the ward staff in the safe administration and monitoring of therapy.
- Providing information and support to the patient.

## Indications

The GIT is the best route for nourishing the patient. PN is indicated for a minority of patients who require artificial nutrition support (Table 6.7). The two categories of patients who might require PN are as follows:

- Intestinal failure—if the absorptive function of the intestine is impaired and persisted for >5 days, and it is anticipated that there will not be a significant improvement. Intestinal failure might be acute (short-lived) or chronic (🕮 p. 386).
- Inaccessible GIT—if the absorption of the intestine is not significantly compromised, but the ingestion of nutrients or the safe placement of enteral feeding tubes is impossible and this has persisted or is likely to persist for 5 days or more.

These categories should be used to guide decision-making not as 'blanket' rules.

---

1 National Collaborating Centre for Acute Care 2006 *Nutrition Support in Adults: Clinical Guideline* 32. National Institute for Health and Clinical Excellence, London. http://www.nice.org.uk/CG32 (accessed 25.06.07).

**Table 6.7** Examples of indications for PN

| Intestinal failure | Example | Considerations |
|---|---|---|
| Acute | Delayed gastric emptying in the post-operative period and gut rest following upper GI surgery | Careful pre-operative assessment and planning for possible enteral access at the time of surgery (e.g. NJ or SJ tube placement) might avoid the need for PN |
| Chronic | Extreme small bowel resection, radiation enteritis, visceral myopathy, scleroderma, high-output fistula | Expert multidisciplinary management is required to minimize symptoms and maximize enteral intake, in addition to preparing the patient for PN therapy at home |
| Inaccessible GIT | Severe mucositis, severe pancreatitis | The use of parenteral nutrition can usually be avoided by the timely placement of enteral feeding tubes |
| | Oesophageal perforation, oesophageal pouch, oesophageal stricture | The use of parenteral nutrition might be indicated if the pathology and clinical condition prohibit a normal oral intake and there are risks associated with enteral tube placement and feeding |

# Parenteral nutrition: central venous catheter access

The NST generally has responsibility for deciding the route for PN delivery and establishing appropriate IV access. Some well-established teams have resources that permit them to place the IV access device, whereas others rely on the services of additional teams (e.g. radiologists or anaesthetists).

The decision regarding the route of parenteral nutrition will mainly depend on the risks associated with potential infection and mechanical complications.[1] The patient's clinical condition, current venous access, nutritional requirements, anticipated duration of therapy, patient comfort, and management of the device should also be considered.

## Central vein catheters

These catheters are designed to provide access to the thoracic vessels, returning blood to the right-hand side of the heart (Fig. 6.8). The catheter tip should lie at the junction of the superior vena cava and the right atrium of the heart. Because the flow and volume of blood are greatest, infused fluids are diluted, enabling large volumes of potentially irritant solutions to be infused.

### Catheter material

There are a variety of different types of catheters, which are chosen for their physical characteristics associated with the type of plastic from which they are manufactured. Important considerations should include:

- Strength (Teflon® and polyurethane).
- Pliability (silicone or polyurethane, which soften within the body).
- Thromboresistant properties (polyurethane–hydromer-coated or silicone elastomer).
- Compatibility with the infusion agent (polyurethane, silicone, and Teflon®).
- Visibility on X-ray.
- Durability (silicone elastomers commonly last for >10 years).

### Number of lumens

National guidelines[1,2] advocate the use of single-lumen catheters for the administration of parenteral nutrition. Multi-lumen catheters are acceptable if a port can be dedicated to the use of parenteral nutrition.[1] Advanced planning for patients anticipated to require multiple therapies (chemotherapy or long-term antibiotic therapy) warrants the placement of long-term multi-lumen central venous catheters (Hickman type).

### Tunnelled catheters

Can be sutured to secure the catheter for short-term use. Catheters intended for use for >3 weeks are recommended to have a Dacron cuff that is positioned on the catheter within the subcutaneous tunnel. Fibrosis

---

1 National Collaborating Centre for Acute Care (2006). *Nutrition Support in Adults: Clinical Guideline 32*. National Institute for Health and Clinical Excellence, London. http://www.nice.org.uk/CG32 (accessed 25.06.07).

2 Pratt RJ, Pellowe CM, Wilson JA, *et al.* (2007). EPIC 2 National evidence-based guidelines for the prevention of healthcare-associated infection in NHS hospitals in England. *Journal of Hospital Infection* **265**, S1–64.

of the cuff anchors the catheter to the subcutaneous tissue within 21 days. This type of catheter has the advantage of ↓ the risk of colonization, avoiding the need of external fixation and ∴ is more comfortable for the patient.

### Non-tunnelled catheters

Catheters should preferentially (if not contraindicated) be placed in the subclavian vessel; then consider the jugular vessel and finally femoral sites.[1]

### Peripherally inserted central catheters (PICCs)

Access the central venous system through the basilic, median cubital, or cephalic veins. Complications associated with the conventional placement of central venous catheters are avoided, but they are not indicated for patients requiring long-term parenteral nutrition who will be responsible for catheter care.

### Totally implanted devices

Also know as 'implantable ports' (Port-a-Cath®). Rather than having an external component, catheter has a titanium reservoir (single or double chamber) that is placed surgically in the subcutaneous pocket of the chest wall, abdomen, or forearm (peripheral vein access). Although promoted to ↓ the issue of altered body image, the placement and removal procedures are surgical procedures that carry the risk of greater scarring compared with conventional central catheter placement.

### Surgical implant

A transthoracic approach to placement of central catheters (superior vena cava or right atrium) might be considered if the central vessels cannot be safely accessed. This requires referral to a vascular surgeon.

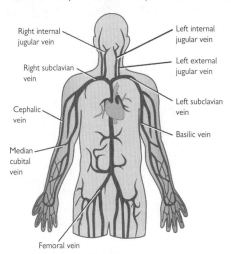

**Fig. 6.8** Venous access sites. Reproduced with kind permission © Burdett Institute 2008.

# Parenteral nutrition: peripheral vein catheter access

Peripheral access is indicated in those patients who are anticipated to need parenteral nutrition for <14 days. PN administration through the peripheral veins is limited by high infusion rates and the need for high levels of electrolytes and hypertonic solutions. The use of glyceryl trinitrate patches over the vein distal to the site of insertion was not investigated by the National Institute for Health and Clinical Excellence.[1]

## Standard peripheral cannula

Peripheral cannulae (18 Fr) are commonly placed in the peripheral veins of the hand. They require vigilance and regular replacement (24–48 h) to prevent thombophlebitis. This site should usually be avoided for the administration of PN in favour of larger vessels.

## Midline catheters

Fine (18–23 Fr) polyurethane–hydromer-coated radio-opaque catheters 15–20 cm long. They are described as midline or medium-vein catheters because they are intended to be placed in the medium veins of the antecubital fossa. These catheters are promoted for peripheral use because they are less thrombogenic and tend to have a lifespan of 5–28 days. They should be removed promptly at the first signs of phlebitis.

## Further reading

Hamilton H (ed.). (2000). *Total Parenteral Nutrition: A Practical Guide for Nurses*. Churchill Livingstone, Edinburgh.

---

1 National Collaborating Centre for Acute Care (2006). *Nutrition Support in Adults: Clinical Guideline 32*. National Institute for Health and Clinical Excellence, London. http://www.nice.org.uk/CG32 (accessed 25.06.07).

# Parenteral nutrition: catheter insertion

Nurses could have responsibility for:
- Preparing the patient for catheter insertion.
- Assisting with catheter insertion.
- Placement of the catheter (including placement of central venous catheters).
- Post-insertion care.
- Patient education and support.
- Ongoing management of the catheter.

Whatever their role, nurses must ensure that they have appropriate knowledge and skills to function autonomously. There are several evidence-based guidelines that must be used to support practice.[1-3] The need for nutrition, although of high importance, should never be considered as an emergency. Care should be taken in the planning and placement of catheters to minimize complications.

## Insertion methods

Catheters are commonly placed percutaneously but can be placed as a surgical procedure (which is described as a 'cut-down procedure'). For non-tunnelled catheters, accessing the subclavian vein is the first choice for placement, followed by the jugular vessel, and then the femoral vessel. Techniques for cannulating the vessel include insertion of a catheter through the needle, over the needle, through a cannula, and over a guidewire.[4] The technique used will be dictated by the make of catheter and operator preference. Short-term catheters are often placed in a clean area of the ward. Long-term catheters are placed under ultrasound guidance[5] or fluoroscopy (to ensure successful placement and ↓ potential life-threatening complications) in vascular suites of the radiology department. Observe the following for placement of central venous catheters:
- Maximal sterile precautions—sterile gown, gloves, and large drapes must be used.
- Skin preparation—chlorhexidine gluconate (2–5%) in 70% isopropyl alcohol.

---

1 National Collaborating Centre for Acute Care (2006). *Nutrition Support in Adults: Clinical Guideline 32*. National Institute for Health and Clinical Excellence, London. http://www.nice.org.uk/CG32 (accessed 25.06.07).

2 Pratt RJ, Pellowe CM, Wilson JA, *et al.* (2007). RPIC 2 National evidence-based guidelines for the prevention of healthcare-associated infection in NHS hospitals in England. *Journal of Hospital Infection* **265**, S1–64.

3 National Collaborating Centre for Nursing and Supportive Care (2003). *Prevention of Health-care Associated Infection in Primary and Community Care*. National Institute for Clinical Excellence, London.

4 Hamilton H (ed.) (2000). *Total Parenteral Nutrition: A Practical Guide for Nurses*. Churchill Livingstone, Edinburgh.

5 National Institute for Clinical Excellence (2002). *Ultrasound Locating Devices. Technical Appraisal 40*. NICE, London.

- Patients are usually sedated and ∴ require oxygen therapy.
- The patient will be placed in the Trendelenburg position (to ↓ the risk of air embolism) unless contraindicated.

## Complications

It is generally accepted that fewer complications occur if the operator is experienced complications related to central catheter insertion include:

- Malpositioned catheters (↑ the risk of thrombosis and arrhythmias).
- Haemorrhage.
- Pneumothorax.
- Air embolism.
- Nerve damage.
- Infection.

Good practice will limit the risks of ongoing complications (Table 6.8).

## Preparation

Once the need for PN has been established, an assessment will be carried out by the practitioner placing the device. This will highlight the individual risks to the patient and ensure patient understanding and comfort. The assessment generally includes a clinical examination (focusing on the cardiovascular, respiratory, and neurological systems; patients who have had multiple catheters might need radiological investigations to establish patency of veins, blood analysis (biochemistry, haematology, and clotting), infection screen, and discussion about specific concerns. Information should be given regarding the catheter, placement procedure, and risks, in addition to what to anticipate following the procedure. Patients having long-term catheters inserted should be consulted about the preferred exit site.

# Parenteral nutrition: catheter care

## Post-procedure care

Monitoring the patient's vital signs and knowing what symptoms indicate procedure-related complications will ensure that any abnormality is identified early. Make observations every 30 min and then less frequently, according to the patient's clinical condition (refer to your local policy). Complications associated with central venous catheters are listed in Table 6.8.

## Dressings

Highly permeable transparent dressings are recommended.[1-3] Replace dressings every 7 days or more frequently if indicated. Catheter sites should be cleaned with alcoholic chlorhexidine gluconate (2.5%) solution.[2]

## Flushing

Catheters should be flushed with 0.9% sodium chloride solution (Table 6.8) using a push–pause technique and positive-pressure clamping.[4]

## Accessing the catheter

Needle-free devices should be used with caution.[2,3] Alcoholic chlorhexidine gluconate (2.5%) solution should be used to decontaminate the hub. Catheters should not be used routinely for blood sampling.

1 National Collaborating Centre for Acute Care (2006). *Nutrition Support in Adults: Clinical Guideline 32*. National Institute for Health and Clinical Excellence, London. http://www.nice.org.uk/CG32 (accessed 25.06.07).

2 Pratt RJ, Pellowe CM, Wilson JA, *et al.* (2007). EPIC 2 National evidence-based guidelines for the prevention of healthcare-associated infection in NHS hospitals in England. *Journal of Hospital Infection* **265**, S1–S64.

3 National Collaborating Centre for Nursing and Supportive Care (2003). *Prevention of Healthcare Associated Infection in Primary and Community Care*. National Institute for Clinical Excellence, London.

4 Goodwin M and Carlson I (1993). The peripherally inserted catheter: a retrospective look at 3 years of insertions. *Journal of Intravenous Nursing* **12**, 92–103.

**Table 6.8** Central catheter complications

| Later complications | Comments |
| --- | --- |
| Catheter-related infection<br>Exit-site infection<br>Tunnel infection<br>Catheter-related bloodstream infection | Care protocols to ↓ the risk of infection are essential. Careful monitoring of the patient's condition will detect potential problems at an early stage, making treatment interventions more likely to succeed. Exit-site infection can be successfully treated using antibiotic therapy and frequent dressing changes. Infection of the subcutaneous tunnel warrants the removal of the catheter. Salvaging catheters should only be attempted for long-term central catheters following consultation with the microbiologist, according to evidence-based protocols |
| Central vein thrombosis | Caused by catheter-tip position (proximal location in the superior vena cava) and the composition of the infusion. Symptoms include neck and face swelling (more noticeable in the morning following infusion), which should prompt upper limb venography. Treat using infusion of thrombolytic therapy |
| Catheter occlusion | Causes include luminal deposits of fibrin, lipid amorphous debris, or kinking. Catheter-care protocols that limit blood sampling, routine withdrawal of blood, and meticulous flushing technique.[4] Ethanol (70%) solution lock can be used to treat lipid occlusions and fibrinolytics can be used to treat blood-related occlusions (identified by recent history of flashback or withdrawal occlusion) |
| Catheter damage | This puts the patient at risk of air embolism, in addition to infection. Damage might be caused by flushing using excessive pressure, incompatible connections, friction between the clavicle and first rib (subclavian catheters), and wear and tear of long-term catheters. Accidental fracture is rare. Patients should br trained to use atraumatic clamps for immediate first-aid management. Long-term catheters can be repaired |

# Parenteral nutrition: formulation

PN solutions are highly complex chemical mixtures that might contain >50 different ingredients. Strict compounding procedures must be followed to ensure that the ingredients are compatible and remain stable in the infusion bag. PN provides energy (in the form of glucose or combined with lipid), nitrogen (as amino acids), water, electrolytes, and micronutrients.

Many hospitals rely on commercially produced solutions and emulsions (containing lipid) that have a long shelf-life. However, these standard bags will require the addition of vitamins, minerals, and electrolytes in an aseptic unit. There is a range of feeds that generally aim to meet these requirements—bags containing 9 g, 11 g, 14 g, or 18 g of nitrogen in a 2–3 L feed. Standard or 'off-the-shelf bags' are used for convenience and can be suitable for patients who do not have unusual electrolyte or fluid requirements.

PN solutions might be compounded on an individual-patient basis if the hospital has a licensed aseptic unit. PN is a fertile medium for microorganisms and meticulous attention is given to aseptic production, which is carried out in laminar flow units under clean room conditions. These aseptic units must meet specific standards.

## Prescribing

Nutrition support teams provide expertise and ∴ have responsibility for estimating requirements (📖 p. 108) and prescribing PN solutions. There is an ↑ number of non-medical supplementary prescribers within NSTs.

### Energy

Once the patient's nutritional requirements have been calculated, this is translated into a formulation usually with a ratio of fat to glucose of 2:3. Care should be taken not to exceed the glucose oxidation rate (4 mg/kg body weight/min). The patient might also be receiving calories from therapeutic agents, e.g. propofol. Feeding in excess will lead to hepatic steatosis (fatty liver). Lipid is commonly provided as soya bean oil emulsified with egg yolk phospholipids. Lipid provides not only energy, but also essential fatty acids, and it is an essential component of infusions intended for peripheral parenteral nutrition because it ↓ the osmolality of the solution. Lipid can be omitted from the infusion or given occasionally if there is concern about the patient's liver function. Lipid emulsions might be unstable in patients requiring large fluid volumes or high electrolyte concentrations. Lipid it can also be administered separately.

### Nitrogen

Provided as a mixture of crystalline amino acids. Several amino acids are unavailable in PN solutions because they are unstable (e.g. glutamine and cysteine). Glutamine is available as a dipeptide solution.

*Electrolytes*

Electrolytes might need to be added following blood biochemistry and urinary sodium analyses. Standard bags will not meet the needs of patients with high-output stomas or fistulas.

*Vitamins and trace elements*

Given intravenously to bypass the selective absorption mechanism of the gut; ∴ ↑ the potential risk of toxicity. Vitamin and mineral requirements are ↑ in stressed and depleted patients. Because specific vitamins are required for the metabolism of energy, additional vitamins are required for patients known to be malnourished at the start of infusion therapy (📖 p. 114).

*Immunonutrition*

Specific nutrients have been investigated for their properties in accelerating recovery and altering the metabolic response to illness.[1] Glutamine is a conditionally essential amino acid (non-essential in health, but essential for immune cells and enterocytes in the metabolically stressed patient). There is some evidence for its use in cancer patients and critical illness, but additional research is needed. Other nutrients with pharmacological effects include arginine and omega-3 fatty acids.

## Storage

PN infusion bags should be kept at low temperature (4–8°C) and used before the stated expiry date.

1 McCowen KC and Bistrain BR (2003). Immunonutrition. *American Journal of Clinical Nutrition* **77**, 764–70.

# Parenteral nutrition: administration

PN should always be administered according to your hospital trust's IV administration policy. PN formulations intended for administration through a peripheral vein can be safely administered through central venous catheters. PN formulations prepared for administration through a central vein must never be infused into peripheral veins.

## Additions to infusion bag

Additions should never be made outside the aseptic unit. This is to avoid compatibility problems and introducing infection.

## Chemical degradation of vitamins

Infusion bags should be covered to limit the loss of ultraviolet-light-sensitive vitamins (A and E).

## Infusion pump

A volumetric pump with alarms for ↑ pressure and air must always used.[1] Accumulation of air in the giving set can be ↓ by allowing the feed to reach room temperature before administration (it must never be artificially warmed).

## Giving sets

Change the giving set every 24 h.[2]

## Continuous infusions

Continuous infusion over a 24-h period is required on commencement of PN therapy. Infusions should not hang for >24 h (the time starts on removal of the bag from the refrigerator).

## Cyclical infusions

Cyclical infusion is advocated to ↓ the risk of abnormal liver function and fatty liver. It will also improve the patient's ability to mobilize and participate in usual activities.[2]

The infusion is delivered over a period of 10–20 h. This type of infusion is used if:
- The patient's condition allows.
- The patient has an appropriate intravascular device.
- The patient can tolerate the ↑ hourly fluid and nutrient delivery.

1 National Collaborating Centre for Acute Care (2006). *Nutrition Support in Adults: Clinical Guideline 32.* National Institute for Health and Clinical Excellence, London. http://www.nice.org.uk/CG32 (accessed 25.06.07).

2 Pratt RJ, Pellowe CM, Wilson JA, *et al.* (2007). EPIC 2 National evidence-based guidelines for the prevention of healthcare-associated infection in NHS hospitals in England. *Journal of Hospital Infection* **265**, S1–64.

# Parenteral nutrition: monitoring

Those responsible for the management of patients receiving PN should ensure they have the appropriate knowledge and skills, beyond those required for fluid therapy. Diligent monitoring by the ward nurse is required for the following reasons:

- To assess whether the patient is safely receiving the PN infusion, as prescribed.
- To assess the effectiveness of treatment compared with the intended goals—the prescription might need to be revised following review by the NST.
- To detect and manage the early signs of complications.

A comprehensive guide to clinical, nutritional, and anthropometric monitoring has been published by the National Institute for Health and Clinical Excellence.[1]

## Complications

These might prolong the patient's hospital stay and, at worst, be life-threatening. Complications can be grouped as outlined below.

### Catheter-related

Strict asepsis is required to prevent catheter-related bloodstream infection, which often leads to the removal of catheters, with an associated interruption in treatment. Frequent need for catheter replacement might damage the vascular system and limit future access.

### Nutritional and metabolic

Patients requiring PN are often already stressed or critically ill. The most common problems are fluid and electrolyte abnormalities: high losses might be associated with the underlying gastrointestinal condition. Retention of fluid might be associated with renal, cardiac, or hepatic failure, or over-prescription of fluid and salt. It will further impair gastric and intestinal motility and delay the progression to oral/enteral intake. The risk of refeeding syndrome should be considered before commencing PN (□ p. 114). Hyperglycaemia, resulting from insulin resistance, is common in the stressed patient. PN solutions must always be administered through a volumetric pump. If the patient is hyperglycaemic and not receiving excess macronutrients, they will need an IV insulin infusion. Care is needed to ensure vulnerable patients do not suffer hypoglycaemia when cyclical infusions are discontinued. Patients who are malnourished at the start of therapy, or take little by mouth in the long term, are potentially at risk of micronutrient deficiencies.

1 National Collaborating Centre for Acute Care (2006). *Nutrition Support in Adults: Clinical Guideline 32*. National Institute for Health and Clinical Excellence, London. http://www.nice.org.uk/CG32 (accessed 25.06.07).

*Effects of PN on other systems*

Abnormalities associated with the hepatobiliary system will also be affected by malnutrition, underlying disease (e.g. inflammatory bowel disease, sepsis, or malignancy), drug therapy, and a limited oral intake (predisposing to biliary sludge). The infusion of excess lipid or glucose will cause hepatic steatosis. Temporary omission of lipid from the infusion, cyclical feeding, and a review of the prescription by the NST is needed. Investigations and biochemistry (ultrasound and biopsy) are rarely indicated. Metabolic bone disease is more of a consideration for patients receiving long-term PN, especially if they have a history of malnutrition or corticosteroid therapy. Intestinal permeability (with associated bacterial translocation) and intestinal atrophy are concerns for patients who do not take an oral diet.

# Home parenteral nutrition

PN is undoubtedly a life-saving therapy for patients with intestinal failure (📖 p. 386) or patients for whom attempts to establish enteral feeding access has failed. Although continuing PN therapy in the community is expensive, home parenteral nutrition (HPN) is a considerably cheaper alternative than a prolonged hospital stay. Patients receiving HPN must be managed by a multidisciplinary team with appropriate expertise. HPN is a complex therapy, with several potentially life-threatening complications (📖 p. 155). Additionally, patients with intestinal failure are likely to have a chronic intestinal condition. HPN has the status of a 'specialized service'.[1]

## Epidemiology

In the UK, there are ~735 adult patients (a point prevalence of 12.3 patients/1 million people in the population) receiving PN therapy in the community.[2] The reasons for HPN include short-bowel syndrome, malabsorption, obstruction, and fistula. The indications for HPN are small bowel infarction (21.4%), Crohn's disease (17%), motility disorders (6.3%), scleroderma (6.3%), and radiation enteritis (1.8%). Although most new patients are aged between 41 and 60, a proportion of patients receiving HPN are between 70 and 90.

Patients might need HPN in the short term (weeks; e.g. patients requiring palliative care), medium term (months to years; those with resolving intestinal failure or awaiting reconstructive surgery), or long term (decades; type III chronic intestinal failure; 📖 p. 387).

## Cost

The HPN package will include the following costs:
• Pharmacy costs of preparing the infusion solution.
• Disposable equipment required for the administration of infusions.
• Dedicated refrigerator for the storage of the PN solution.
• Portable infusion device.
• Servicing and delivery cost.

The average cost of an HPN package is ~£45 000/year, which varies according to the complexity of the PN solution (some patients might only require fluids, vitamins, and electrolytes), frequency of administration (not all patients require a nightly infusion), and need for specialist nursing services. The responsibility for funding HPN lies with the PCT. It is becoming more usual for the strategic health authority to collaboratively commission HPN for several PCTs.

1 DH Specialized Services National Definitions Set (2nd edn). *Home Parenteral Nutrition (Adult). Definition No. 12.* http://www.doh.uk (accessed 26.06.07).

2 Jones B, Holden C, Dalzell M, *et al.* (2006). *Artificial Nutrition Support in the UK 2005.* Report by the British Artificial Nutrition Survey. http://www.bapen.org.uk (accessed 26.06.07).

## Discharge planning

Standards and guidance for the NST initiating HPN include those pro-vided by the British Association of Parenteral and Enteral Nutrition[3] and the National Institute for Health and Clinical Excellence.[4] The clinical responsibility for patients receiving HPN remains with the specialist hospital consultant; good communication is required with the patient's GP and community nursing services.

The majority of patients can be taught how to safely care for their central venous catheter and IV infusion. The time needed to learn the aseptic techniques is ~4–6 weeks. If this aspect of the patient's care is delegated to community nursing teams or specialist nurses employed by an inde-pendent home-care company, the discharging team has a duty of care to ensure they are appropriately trained and competent. In addition to aseptic skills and knowledge of central venous access, the nurse must have a good understanding of intestinal failure and the psychosocial consequences for the patient and family living with a chronic condition.

Patients cannot be discharged home if they require frequent monitoring or changes to their PN infusion. HPN services are usually purchased as a package from home-care companies, which can organize a standard package at 10–14 days' notice. All patients on HPN will need 24-h tele-phone access to their clinical team, monitoring in a nutrition clinic, infor-mation about the national patient support group (PINNT), and an aware-ness of the availability of social and psychological support.

**3** Wood S (1995). *Home Parenteral Nutrition: Quality Criteria for Clinical Services and the Supply of Nutrient Fluids and Equipment.* BAPEN, Maidenhead.
**4** National Collaborating Centre for Acute Care (2006). *Nutrition Support in Adults: Clinical Guideline 32.* National Institute for Health and Clinical Excellence, London. http://www.nice.org.uk/CG32 (accessed 25.06.07).

# Nutrition and the surgical patient

All patients should be screened on admission (📖 p. 104) to identify their risk of malnutrition. Patients who are malnourished and have a functioning GIT should receive pre-operative nutrition support (either oral supplements or enteral tube feeding). Any prolonged or frequent periods of nil by mouth (NBM) required for investigations will compromise the patient's nutritional status and ability to recover post-operatively.

## Peri-operative management

### Fasting recommendations

To ↓ the risk of regurgitation and aspiration, do not expose the patient to dehydration. In healthy individuals, the consumption of clear fluids 2 h before planned surgery and solids (including milk) 6 h before surgery is permitted.[1]

### Gastric decompression

Not routinely advocated in the post-operative period. The presence of a large-bore NG tube is uncomfortable for the patient, and might ↑ the incidence of nausea and vomiting and delay progression to oral diet and fluid.[2]

### Enhanced recovery after surgery

An approach involving holistic peri-operative management of the surgical patient.[3] The aim is to optimize organ function and recovery in the post-operative period. Management includes the following:

- Avoiding the use of bowel prep to clear the bowel.
- Oral fluid and carbohydrate loading pre-operatively.
- Epidural analgesia.
- Minimally invasive surgical techniques.
- Avoiding the routine use of NG tubes for decompression.
- Avoiding IV fluid and sodium overload.
- Offering oral fluid and diet early in the post-operative period.
- Early mobilization.

1 Royal College of Nursing (2005). *Clinical Practice Guideline: Peri-operative Fasting of Adults and Children.* RCN, London.

2 Nelson R, Tse B, and Edwards S (2005). Systematic review of prophylactic nasogastric decompression after abdominal surgery. *British Journal of Surgery* **92**, 673–80.

3 Fearon KC, Linqvist O, von Meyenfeldt M, *et al.* (2005). Enhanced recovery after surgery: a consensus review of clinical care for patients undergoing colonic resection. *Clinical Nutrition* **24**, 466–77.

# Nutritional management of gastrointestinal disease

Diseases of the GIT have a high probability of affecting an individual's dietary intake and nutritional health. Nurses have an important role in providing dietary advice and reinforcing information provided by the dietitian. Dietary modification is used in a variety of GI-related conditions (Table 6.9) to ↓ unpleasant symptoms and maximize the nutritional benefit of food consumed. The nurse's role in health promotion should ensure the following:

• Up-to-date information is prepared in collaboration with the dietetic team.
• Written information is in a form the patient can read and understand.
• Dietary modification is specific to the individual's needs and acceptable in terms of religious, cultural, and economic aspects. It should be realistic and practical to follow.
• The patient understands the scientific rationale and evidence for dietary management.
• Patients are advised that 'nutritionists' are not professionally regulated and have not undergone the professional training required of registered dietitians.

**Table 6.9** Gastrointestinal-related conditions and dietary management

| Condition | Cause | Dietary management/advice |
|---|---|---|
| *Upper GIT* | | |
| Dysphagia | Pharyngeal pouch, achalasia | NBM and enteral feeding for those at risk of aspiration Modified-consistency diet for those with impaired swallow function and oesophageal stent (🕮 p. 204) |
| Gastro-oesophageal reflux (🕮 on p. 334) | Hiatus hernia, weak cardiac sphincter, ↑ intragastric pressure | Meal pattern and size, weight ↓, avoid excess tea, coffee, and alcohol |
| Small stomach syndrome | Following gastric resection, patients might experience early satiety and discomfort | Frequent small meals, avoid liquids with food |
| Dumping syndrome (🕮 p. 368) | Following gastric resection, patients might experience dizziness, faintness, hypotension, sweating, hypoglycaemia | Small meals, avoid liquid with food, limit simple carbohydrates |
| *Pancreas and liver* | | |
| Acute pancreatitis (🕮 p. 430) | Release of activated pancreatic enzymes, causing pain, vomiting, and a diffuse inflammatory process | Most cases are mild/moderate and of short duration (5–7 days) Managed by periods of NBM if symptoms persist In severe cases, nutrition support will be needed |
| Chronic pancreatitis (🕮 p. 432) | Associated with repeated acute episodes and alcohol intake | Enzyme supplementation to assist in pain control and ↓ malabsorption Healthy eating guidance should be followed regarding fat intake and vitamin and mineral supplementation if steatorrhoea persists. Avoid alcohol |

**Table 6.9** (Contd.)

| Condition | Cause | Dietary management/advice |
|---|---|---|
| Liver disease (📖 Chapter 11) | Dietary therapy is used for the management of complications of liver disease | Malnutrition is a common feature of liver disease; nutrition support is the main focus of management. Access to specialist dietitians is essential |
| | Ascites | Sodium restriction |
| | Hepatic encephalopathy | No evidence for routine protein restriction High-fibre diet to speed transit time. Frequent small meals |
| | Steatorrhoea | Cholestasis is rarely severe enough to cause steator-rhoea. If fat restriction is indicated, careful dietetic management is needed to ensure energy require-ments are met. Fat-soluble vitamin and calcium supplementation might also be needed |
| | Gallstones | There is no evidence for the use of low-fat diets. Healthy eating advice should be promoted |
| *Small and large bowel* | | |
| Malabsorption | Coeliac disease (📖 p. 375) | Lifelong exclusion of gluten (wheat, rye, and barley) from the diet. Gluten-free products are available on prescription but not exempt from prescription charges |
| | Extensive intestinal resection and jejunostomy | Short-bowel syndrome (📖 p. 380) |

**Table 6.9** (Contd.)

| Condition | Cause | Dietary management/advice |
|---|---|---|
| | Ileostomy and pouch formation (🕮 pp. 242, 252) | Involvement of the terminal ileum will need intramuscular vitamin $B_{12}$. Following surgery, the range of foods can gradually be ↑. Some foods might cause flatulence and stool odour. Patients should not be given advice that restricts their diet but encouraged to discover their individual tolerance. General advice includes a regular meal pattern, healthy eating, chewing foods well, and drinking at least 2 L/day |
| Inflammatory bowel disease (🕮 p. XXX) | | Patients with Crohn's disease are particularly at risk of nutritional deficiencies. |
| | Crohn's disease | Nutrition support (oral/enteral route) to restore and maintain nutritional status. Liquid diets, with the exclusion of normal food, can induce remission.<br><br>Low-fibre diets are required for those with strictures. |
| | Ulcerative colitis | Remission cannot be induced by liquid feeds. Peri-operative nutrition support for those who are malnourished or have prolonged periods (>5 days) of NBM. Folate may be required for those on sulfasalazine or $B_{12}$ injections, who have terminal ileum involvement. Calcium and vitamin D supplements are required in long-term steroid use |

**Table 6.9** (*Contd.*)

| Condition | Cause | Dietary management/advice |
|---|---|---|
| Irritable bowel syndrome (📖 p. 502) | A combination of chronic or recurring symptoms | Balanced diet/healthy eating. Avoid restricting the diet unnecessarily. Patients who report following exclusion diets should be referred to the dietitian. High-fibre diets might ↑ flatus and bloating |
| Diverticular disease | 📖 p. 476 | Patients on a high-fibre (bran) diet will also need information about ↑ fluid intake. |

## Further reading

British Liver Trust. http://www.britishlivertrust.org.uk (accessed 05.07.07).
British Society of Gastroenterology (2000). *Guidelines for Osteoporosis in Coeliac and Inflammatory Bowel Disease*. BSG, London.
British Society of Gastroenterology (2004). *Guidelines for the Management of Inflammatory Bowel Disease*. BSG, London.
Coeliac Society. http://www.coeliac.co.uk (accessed 05.07.07).
Ileostomy and internal Pouch Support Group. http://www.ileostomypouch.demon.co.uk (accessed 05.07.07).

# Endoscopy

Nursing care/procedures for all common
  endoscopic procedures 174
Sedation and anaesthesia in endoscopy 176
Non-medical endoscopy: practical and legal risks 178
Non-medical endoscopy: consent and sedation 180
Non-medical endoscopy: training and support 182
Oesophageal gastroduodenoscopy: preparations,
  alternatives, and indications 184
Oesophageal gastroduodenoscopy: procedure
  and recovery 186
Endoscopic oesophageal dilatation 188
Wire guidance for oesophageal dilatation 190
Variceal balloon tamponade 192
Oesophageal varices: banding or injecting 194
Foreign-body removal from the upper GIT 196
Percutaneous endoscopic gastrostomy: assessment 198
Percutaneous endoscopic gastrostomy: procedure
  and techniques 200
Jejunal extension using percutaneous endoscopic
  gastrostomy 202
Percutaneous endoscopic gastrostomy and percutaneous
  endoscopic jejunostomy: post-procedure risks 203
Oesophageal self-expanding metal stent 204
Diagnostic endoscopic retrograde
  cholangiopancreatography 206
Therapeutic endoscopic retrograde
  cholangiopancreatography: biliary stent placement 208
Therapeutic endoscopic retrograde
  cholangiopancreatography: stone extraction 210
Therapeutic endoscopic retrograde
  cholangiopancreatography: sphincterotomy 212
Therapeutic endoscopic retrograde
  cholangiopancreatography: biliary duct dilatation 213
Flexible sigmoidoscopy 214
Colonoscopy 216
Colonic stents 218
Polypectomy 220
Capsule endoscopy 222
Cleaning and disinfection of endoscopes: transmission
  of infections 224
Cleaning and disinfection of endoscopes: decontamination 226
Cleaning and disinfection of endoscopes: management 228
Biopsies, aspiration, and handling specimens 230
Other endoscopic procedures 234

# Nursing care/procedures for all common endoscopic procedures

Endoscopy is defined as 'looking inside'. Endoscopic procedures, therefore, are minimally invasive means of examining the internal areas of the body through the use of flexible video endoscopes. The majority of endoscopic procedures focus on varying aspects of the GIT. They can be performed ± sedation or, rarely, under general anaesthetic. Throat spray is used for most upper GI procedures. This is usually determined following agreement between practitioner and patient, and in relation to patient preference and, the difficulty and specifics of the procedure. Endoscopic procedures are associated with small risks of bleeding and perforation, and this risk ↑ if a therapeutic procedure is performed.

## Pre-assessment/admission
- A full, relevant history is taken:
  - Ensure that the preparation and fasting instructions are followed.
  - If the patient has diabetes, check their blood sugar level at admission.
  - History of cardiac problems, especially endocarditis or heart valve replacement.
  - Medication usage—particularly oral anticoagulants, iron supplements, and any drugs that could affect/interact with the sedation used during the endoscopic procedure.
  - Informed consent—obtained by the admitting nurse as per strict procedural guidelines.
- Insertion of a flexible IV cannula for access and administration of sedatives, pain relief, and antispasmodic agents.
- Check whether the patient has loose or broken teeth or dentures before upper GI procedures.
- The patient should be wearing the correct identification bracelet.

## Procedure
- A minimum of two endoscopy assistants (one of whom must be a registered nurse) must be present during all endoscopic procedures:
  - One assistant to monitor the patient's condition.
  - One assistant to aid the endoscopist with practical aspects.
- Correctly position the patient on the trolley (on their left-hand side) for insertion of the endoscope.

The following recommendations are for sedated or high-risk unsedated patients:
- Administration of oxygen through nasal cannulae throughout the procedure.
- Monitoring oxygen saturation and the pulse rate throughout the procedure.
- Additional blood pressure and electrocardiogram measurements might be required.

## Common endoscopic procedures

- Oesophageal gastroduodenoscopy (OGD)—to investigate the oesophagus, stomach, and duodenum.
- Bronchoscopy—examines the upper respiratory system (trachea and bronchi).
- Endoscopic retrograde cholangiopancreatography (ERCP)—examines the biliary and pancreatic ducts and gall bladder.
- Push enteroscopy (PE)—examines the upper GIT similar to OGD, but PE extends further into the proximal jejunum.
- Double-balloon enteroscopy (DBE)— can examine the entire small intestine (through an oral and then a rectal route).
- Flexible sigmoidoscopy—investigates the distal colon (rectum to splenic flexure only).
- Colonoscopy—investigates the entire colon or large bowel.

## Recovery/post-procedure care

- Continuous monitoring of patient observations until fully alert.
- Record and manage any adverse events or complications.
- Provide the patient with specific discharge instructions and emergency contact details in case of complications.
- Check follow-up appointment or management has been arranged.
- Ensure a responsible adult is available to accompany the patient home, if they have undergone sedation.

## Further reading

British Society of Gastroenterology (2003). *Safety and Sedation during Endoscopic Procedures—BSG Guidelines.* http://www.bsg.org.uk (accessed 11.05.07).

# Sedation and anaesthesia in endoscopy

Sedation and anaesthesia are often required during endoscopy 'to help patients accept uncomfortable and distressing diagnostic and therapeutic procedures whilst easing technical difficulties for the operator'.[1] In the endoscopy setting, sedation and anaesthesia are useful for two main reasons:

- To ↓ patient anxiety, thereby enabling their cooperation.
- To produce a more relaxed and amnesic effect.

Sedation and anaesthesia are not always required and their use should be discussed with the patient before obtaining informed consent for the procedure.

## Indications

- Gastroscopy—for which patients may prefer sedation to local anaesthetic throat spray.
- Colonoscopy.
- ERCP.
- Flexible sigmoidoscopy—occasionally.

## General anaesthetic

This option is rarely used in endoscopy, because it ↑ risk of both medical and mechanical complications. For example, because the patient will be unable to move on request throughout the procedure, staff will have to move the patient, which ↑ the risk to both staff and patient. However, young children often have a general anaesthetic for endoscopy to lessen anxiety, especially if colonoscopic screening will become a regular occurrence in their life, e.g. screening in patients with inflammatory bowel disease and other chronic or genetic conditions.

## Local anaesthetic

Lidocaine is an effective local anaesthetic agent which can be used in the following three ways:

- A subcutaneous injection before surgical incision and insertion of a PEG tube into the stomach.
- It is most commonly used in endoscopy, as an anaesthetic throat spray before gastroscopy: 10 mg/spray, maximum dose 20 sprays. The patients is given three to eight sprays at the back of the throat and then asked to swallow. This helps block the gag reflex and ease the passage of the scope. The risks are minimal, but the patient must be advised to refrain from taking hot drinks until the spray has worn off (about 30 min). The administration of local anaesthsia will depend on local policy.
- A topical agent (lidocaine gel) in painful perianal disease, e.g. an anal fissure can cause severe pain and anal sphincter spasm, which could prevent the insertion of the colonoscope.

**1** Fretwell I (2003). The use of intravenous sedation midazolam in the endoscopy unit setting. *Gastrointestinal Nursing* **1**, 31.

## Conscious sedation

The most common form of sedation for endoscopic procedures. Although the patient is conscious, the dose is titrated according to a recognized sedation scale and the state of relaxation of the patient, thereby preventing over-sedation. A state of calm and relaxation is reached, in addition to maintaining the patient's cooperation and participation if a change in their position is required.

For this 'conscious sedation', a benzodiazepine is titrated to the patient's response level. The drug of choice is midazolam because of its rapid onset and short duration of action. It also has amnesic qualities, which aids a speedy recovery. To aid the procedure by inducing a sense of calm and ↑ the patient's tolerance, a 2–3 mg dose of midazolam is often all that is required. However, sedation carries risks and these must be discussed with the patient before gaining their full consent. Flumazenil, a benzodiazepine antagonist, must always be on hand to reverse the sedation if necessary.

Often in colonoscopy, because of looping and stretching the bowel, an analgesic is also intravenously administered concomitantly with sedation. A small dose of an opioid (e.g. pethidine or fentanyl) is administered before sedation.

## Contraindications

- Known benzodiazepine sensitivity.
- Previous history of complications with sedation.
- Patients with respiratory insufficiency or other multiple comorbidity.

## Monitoring the sedated patient

Once the patient is sedated, the endoscopist will be busy with the procedure and ∴ an assistant is required to monitor the patient. The BSG guidelines state that all patients requiring sedation must have an IV access cannula in place throughout the procedure. This enables rapid administration of further sedation or, indeed, reversal drugs. The patient should also have continual administration of oxygen and pulse oximetry monitoring. Because both benodiazepines and opiates can cause respiratory depression, careful monitoring of the patient's respiration rate and oxygen saturation are required.

# Non-medical endoscopy: practical and legal risks

Non-medical endoscopists (such as nurses) have become widely accepted as independent practitioners. They contribute significantly to both upper and lower gastrointestinal endoscopic investigations. Their practice is underpinned by the Nursing and Midwifery Council (NMC) Code of Professional Conduct or the Health Professional Council for Radiographers which provides guidance on the following:

• Development.
• Responsibility.
• Accountability.
• Understanding medico-legal issues.

At present, the status of unaffiliated practitioners, who are not aligned with a professional regulatory body, is under review by the Department of Health.

Professional autonomous practitioners have shown their practice to be:

• Safe.
• Competent.
• Effective.
• Thorough.

The role of the non-medical endoscopist has developed into that of a valuable member of the gastroenterology multidisciplinary team, but it should not be considered as a replacement for another member of the team or as cost-saving.

## Practical and legal risks

Before commencing training, a profile and an approved training protocol, with a named mentor, for the role must be submitted to the senior medical and nursing management for approval, to protect all concerned.

The legal implications of endoscopy practice require full medico-legal cover, with competent knowledge of this by the practitioner before training commences. The local employing trust must also recognize and approve any new role prior to commencing training.

The following must be addressed before training commences:

• The vicarious liability of the trust should be established.
• The common Law of Negligence and Reasonable Care in Practice should be understood (Bolam vs Friern Hospital Management Committee, 1957).
• Review of General Medical Council 'Professional Conduct and Discipline; Fitness to Practice'. Delegation of medical duties.

## Further reading

British Society of Gastroenterology (2001). *Provision of Endoscopy-related Services in District General Hospitals.* BSG Working Party Report. http://www.bsg.org.uk (accessed 11.05.07).

# Non-medical endoscopy: consent and sedation

## Consent and sedation

### Informed consent

The practitioner requires a sound knowledge of the legalities of informed consent and must display sound professional judgement in clinical practice. This is an integral part of the practitioner's role.

Comprehensive understanding of the Department of Health (DOH) guidelines on informed consent is paramount, for example:

- Identify the local trust policy.
- Use the appropriate DOH guidelines[1] in practice to enhance your professional regulatory guidance/past experience.
- Explicit patient information literature identifying the practitioner's role.
- Appropriate knowledge of delegation of duty if informed consent is delegated to others.
- The patient must be aware of a trainee's status.
- Training, with supervision and an audit trail, should follow the training/ practice protocol.
- Support/train and confirm the competence of other professionals delegated to undertake informed consent on your behalf.

The DOH advice states: 'The clinician providing treatment or investigation is responsible for ensuring that the patient has given valid consent before treatment begins'.[1]

### Sedation

Clear guidance and robust protocols with in-depth knowledge must be established before training. The sedation protocol must include the elements in Box 7.1.

Patient-group directives can be established for a specific patient cohort. The practitioner should obtain direction from their local trust pharmacy.

Autonomous practice protocols must be established, with local trust management, before practice commences.

At present, nurses cannot prescribe class A drugs (e.g. opiates), even with a prescribing qualification.

## Further reading

Nursing and Midwifery Council (2008). *Advice on Consent.* http://www.nmc-org.uk (accessed 18.05.08).

---

1 Department of Health (2005). *Good practice in Consent Implementation Guide: Consent for Examination or Treatment.* http://www.doh.gov.uk (accessed 11.05.07).

### Box 7.1 Elements of a sedation protocol

- Type of patient—relevant comorbidities.
- Type of procedure.
- Contraindications/exclusion.
- Dosage—maximum total dose.
- Pharmaceutical formulation and strength.
- Route of administration.
- Monitoring the patient during the procedure.
- Anaphylaxis/reversal treatment available—stating dose/route and aftercare.
- Reporting system for adverse events.
- Documentation/communication of drugs given, with any adverse events recorded on a care protocol in the patient's notes.
- Recovery monitoring before discharge.
- Discharge information/advice for the patient and carers is available.
- Alternative therapies should also be available and documented within the protocol.
- Mentoring continuing professional development, advanced life-support qualification, IV drug/cannulation training, and audit process.

# Non-medical endoscopy: training and support

## Training

Training and educational development must be at the same level as that for a doctor in endoscopic gastroenterology, with a common core standard of anatomy, physiology, and pathology, thereby providing in-depth support in both clinical and managerial care of the patient.

The Joint Advisory Group on Gastrointestinal Endoscopy (JAG) states that all training must be undertaken within these guidelines, whatever the discipline. The JAG course of training is mandatory and provides guidance on the following.
• Curriculum.
• Training structure.
• Experience required for practice.
• Assessments.
• Appraisal.
• Practice documentation.

To underpin this training and achieve a common core standard of practice, a formal university-linked module is recommended. Local trusts will be responsible for supervising the following.
• Personal development plans.
• Further education.
• Audit of practice.
• Annual appraisal.

Practitioners should be encouraged to obtain affiliation to recognized professional societies and attend relevant conferences or courses for continuing professional development (CPD) (Fig. 7.1).

## Practice support

Nurse endoscopists must practice with the same standards of support as any other discipline undertaking endoscopic procedures:
• In designated endoscopy units or safe environments, e.g. the theatre or X-ray department.
• Knowledge of relevant DOH/BSG guidance and health service standards.
• Two endoscopy assistants should be present during the list.
• At least two endoscopy lists per week, but no more than five lists (if in sole clinical practice), to maintain competency. It is suggested that other roles should be developed within the duties to enhance job satisfaction, with sessions allocated appropriately to accommodate quality and safe practice.
• Access to senior colleagues and relevant multidisciplinary team meetings.
• Appropriate IT access.
• An appropriate environment for audit/research and managerial responsibilities.

## Further reading

JAG (2004). *JAG Guidelines for Training, Appraisal, and Assessment of Trainees in Gastrointestinal Endoscopy.* http://www.thejag.org.uk (accessed 11.05.07).

British Society of Gastroenterology (2005). *Non-Medical Endoscopist.* A Report of The Working Party of the British Society of Gastroenterology. http://www.bsg.org.uk (accessed 11.05.07).

Nursing and Midwifery Council (2008). *The Code: Standards of Conduct, Performance, and Ethics for Nurses and Midwives.* NMC, London.

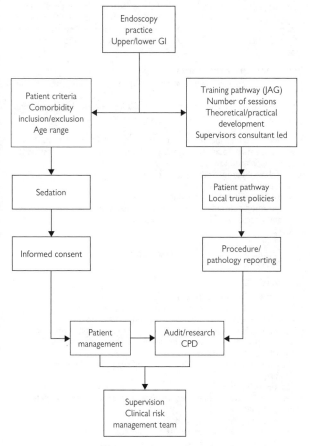

**Fig. 7.1** Practice protocol. Reproduced with kind permission © Burdett Institute 2008.

# Oesophageal gastroduodenoscopy: preparation, alternatives, and indications

Oesophageal gastroduodenoscopy (OGD) investigates the upper GIT from the mouth to the third part of the duodenum. It can be diagnostic or therapeutic and enables examination of the mucosal lining of the oesophagus, stomach, and duodenum. The procedure is undertaken using either local anaesthetic spray on the oropharynx or sedation through IV access.

## Pre-procedure preparation

- Adequate empathetic explanation of the procedure using either of the following methods:
  - Written information or verbal consultation outside the department.
  - Written information with pre-procedure instructions sent to the patient to consolidate informed consent.
- Confirm patient's identity and attach name band. Establish a rapport with patient and planned procedure. The complete health assessment protocol is as follows:
  - Relevant comorbidity.
  - Medication review.
  - Explanation of the procedure.
  - Informed consent—the risks of the procedure should be discussed and alternatives highlighted if the procedure fails.
- Risks:
  - Bleeding.
  - Perforation (1:2000 for diagnostic procedure; 1:260 for dilatation).[1]
  - Aspiration.

## Alternatives

- Barium swallow/follow-through.
- Ultrasound—depending on the presenting symptoms.
- Breath test—depending on the presenting symptoms.
- Oesophageal monitoring—depending on the presenting symptoms.
- Sedation/throat spray should be discussed—consider comorbidities, escort home, and allergies.
- Vital signs should be recorded and blood sugar should be monitored, if appropriate.
- Fasting regimen established.
- Dentures/spectacles identified, removed if necessary, stored safely, and documented.
- IV access obtained, if required.
- Physical and psychological issues documented.
- Hospital gown or appropriate lose clothing to be worn.
- Appropriate storage of personal belongings.

---

1 Quine MA, Bell GD, McCloy RF, *et al.* (1995). Prospective audit of perforation rates following upper gastrointestinal endoscopy in two regions of England. *British Journal of Surgery* **82**, 530–3.

## Indications for OGD

### Diagnostic indications

- Dyspepsia—reflux or *Helicobacter pylori*.
- Haematemesis.
- Dysphagia.
- Coeliac disease.
- Upper GI malignancy.
- Post-gastrectomy.
- Ingested foreign body.
- Peptic ulcer disease.
- Pyloric stenosis.
- Familial polyposis—requires long-term surveillance endoscopy.
- Barrett's oesophagus—requires long-term surveillance endoscopy.
- Vomiting.

### Therapeutic indications

- Dilatation of stricture.
- Haemostasis of bleeding point—injection, argon plasma coagulation, metal clips, and loop diathermy.
- Sclerotherapy for varices.
- Stent placement for obstructing growth—oesophagus, duodenum, or pylorus.
- Laser treatment of malignant area or angiodysplasia.
- Gastrostomy—placement of the feeding tube.

## Contraindications

- Known or suspected GIT perforation.
- Lack of informed consent for a non-urgent procedure.
- Withdrawal of consent after a full explanation.
- An unstable cardiac patient, e.g. recent myocardial infarction (within past 6 weeks), unstable angina, cardiac dysrhythmia, or complete heart block.
- Uncorrected coagulopathy.
- Airway protection—massive GI bleed if semiconscious and not intubated.
- The patient has eaten food within 4 h of scoping or has known achalasia and has not fasted for 24 h.
- Lack of trained personnel to perform and support the procedure.
- High oesophageal obstruction that is not undertaken using fluoroscopy.

# Oesophageal gastroduodenoscopy: procedure and recovery

## Procedure

- Sedation—trained and appropriately authorized personnel (nurse practitioners who work within patient group directives) should titrate the dose according to local policy (e.g. age, comorbidity, conscious level, and contraindicated medication). Trained personnel should spray the patient's throat with local anaesthetic, if required.
- Pulse oximetry monitoring for patients having sedation or who have a history of cardiac disease, anaemia, respiratory disease, or GI bleed—cardiac monitoring might be required.
- Position the patient comfortably on their left-hand side and place a mouth guard between their teeth, having first identified any crowns or loose teeth and removed dentures. Document findings on the nursing sheet, if noted later.
- Place an appropriate pad under the patient's head and left shoulder to prevent saliva leakage.
- Two nurse assistants are required, as follows:
  - One nurse to ensure monitoring and documentation of the patient's airway/vital signs and safety.
  - One nurse for technical support—equipment/specimen handling.
- Technical nurses should have the appropriate equipment ready for the procedure.
- The endoscopist will pass the endoscope through the patient's mouth into the oesophagus, stomach, and down into the second and third sections of the duodenum.
- Careful handling and labelling of any specimens.
- On completion of the procedure, remove the patient's mouth guard and document their vital signs, therapeutic procedures (if any are required), and any drugs used.
- Equipment should be removed to the wash room and relevant articles cleaned or disposed of, according to local policy.

## Recovery

- Check that vital signs are stable, review consciousness level, and check for pain/haematemesis.
- Check toleration of oral fluids. Administer a throat spray, ask the patient to gargle with water, and then ask the patient to sip the water to establish if a reflex is present.
  - The sedated patient should be cardiovascular stable (pulse and blood pressure) and be able to sit up before fluids are offered.
- Offer warm fluids to all patients before discharge, which can help disperse trapped air.
- Remove the IV cannula and check for swelling or erythema—apply an appropriate dressing to the site.
- The patient should have the ability to walk without support.
- Discharge the patient into the care of a relative or friend, if sedation has been given; discharge unsedated patients once stable.

- Provide the patient with relevant information regarding the procedure and instruct sedated patients not to drive or take any responsible action on that day.
- Consultations with sedated patients should take place in the presence of a relative because of possible amnesia from sedation.
- Appropriate follow-up should be arranged before discharge.

## Emergencies

Training in basic life-support procedures and early recognition and prevention must be standard for all endoscopy staff.

# Endoscopic oesophageal dilatation

Oesophageal dilatation has evolved considerably over the years, in addition to development of a large range of purpose-built dilators.

There is a low, but clearly defined, morbidity and mortality attached to this procedure and it should only be undertaken as a planned procedure,[1] assisted by experienced practitioners who can apply expert clinical practice and knowledge.

The first aim of oesophageal dilatation is to alleviate symptoms and improve nutritional intake, in addition to preventing complications (e.g. aspirate pneumonia).

Indications and contraindications for oesophageal dilatation are shown in Table 7.1.

## Patient preparation

- Fasting for 6 h before the procedure; patients who have known achalasia could require a longer period of fasting.
- Informed consent—identify patients at high risk of perforation ± surgical intervention. Risk of perforation during dilatation 1:260. Risk of death 1%.[2]
- Review oral anticoagulation and antiplatelet agents—document the prothrombin time in the medical/nursing notes.
- Administer antibiotic prophylaxis, according to BSG guidelines,[3] to all at-risk patients.
- Use IV sedation, according to local guidance and the BSG guidelines. It is usual to use opiates + benzodiazapines for dilatation. All patients should be classified according to the American Society of Anesthesiologists (ASA) grade I–V scale of physical status.
- Ensure IV access at all times.
- A qualified nurse should administer supplementary oxygen and monitor pulse oximetry.
- Ensure that relevant X-rays are available with patient.

## Dilatation procedure

- The procedure is performed by an endoscopist, with two trained endoscopy assistants.
  - One assistant monitors the patient's comfort and safety.
  - Second assistant manages technical equipment and endoscopic and dilation equipment (Table 7.2).
- A radiologist should be available:
  - X-ray facilities should be available.
- Surgical support: need access to on-call experienced surgeon in case of emergencies.

---

1 Riley SA and Attwood SEA (2004). Guidelines on the use of oesophageal dilatation in clinical practice. *Gut* **53** (suppl 1), 1–16.

2 Quine MA, Bell GD, McCloy RF, *et al.* (1995). Prospective audit of perforation rates following upper gastrointestinal endoscopy in two regions of England. *British Journal of Surgery* **82**, 530–3.

3 British Society of Gastroenterology (2001). *Antibiotic Prophylaxis Guidelines.* BSG, London.

**Table 7.1** Indications and contraindications for oesophageal dilatation

**Indications**

Treatment of symptomatic obstruction—functional or anatomical oesophageal disorders

Acid reflux induced stricture

Malignancy (to aid stent placement, if indicated)

Achalasia

Anastomotic stricture

Corrosive-induced stricture

Sclerotherapy

Radiation

Rings or web (identified by barium X-ray)

**Contraindications**

Active perforation

Recent perforation or upper GIT surgery

Pharyngeal or cervical deformity (↑ risk)

Thoracic aneurysm (large)

Severe cardiac disease (consideration risk vs benefit)

Severe coagulopathy (correction before procedure)

**Table 7.2** Oesophageal dilators

**Push dilators (bougie)**

Weighted mercury or tungsten-filled rubber bougies

Range of sizes (7–20 mm diameter)

**Wire-guided**

Polyvinyl dilators—Savary Gillard range of 5–20 mm diameter each, with a 20 cm tapered tip and a radio-opaque band at the widest point

Eder–Puestow—a series of graduated metal olives of 6.6–19.3 mm diameter mounted on a flexible shaft

Celestin—long tapered radio-opaque bougies. Two dilators ↑ size to 18 mm

Use of push and wire-guided dilators is limited because of decontamination and single-use issues

**Balloon dilators (single use)**

TTS or wire-guided

6–40 mm sizes—the largest size is used for treatment of achalasia

Advantage—single use and various sizes come with guidewire tip insertion built in

# Wire guidance for oesophageal dilatation

Before the procedure, check the following:
- Correct wire—single use.
- Appropriately sized dilators—single use or appropriately decontaminated before use.

❶ If the procedure is controlled using X-rays, radiation-protective equipment should be worn by all staff.

### Rigid dilator

Once the stricture is identified, a flexible wire is guided down the biopsy channel of the endoscope. The assistant has the following responsibilities:
- Support the wire and stop it from migrating up or down the channel once an appropriate length mark is established (markings on wire). The endoscopist will withdraw the scope over the wire.
- A second nurse assisting the airway will hold the wire in place at the mouth as the scope is removed from the external remaining wire. The mouth guard should be removed at this point.
- ▶ Airway maintenance and the availability of suction prevent aspiration.
- An appropriate dilator should be lubricated and placed over the wire by the endoscopist. The assistant maintains the correct positioning of the wire *in situ*.
- This could be repeated three times (the rule of three) using appropriately sized dilators.
- Decontaminate equipment, according to the guidelines, if it is reusable; dispose of single-use dilators.

### Balloon through the scope (TTS) dilator

- Select the appropriate size and check inflation of balloon; lubricate the biopsy channel with silicone. If the dilator is wire-guided follow steps above.
- Check the pressure inflation levels of the balloon and communicate the levels to the endoscopist.
- Inflate the balloon using an appropriate inflation device and communicate the pressure level achieved to commence timing of dilatation.
- Dispose of single-use items—TTS balloons are disposable.

### Complications of dilatation

Perforation:
- Monitor the patient's vital signs.
- Reverse sedation—flumazenil should be available.
- The patient should receive nil by mouth (NBM) until an appropriate X-ray is taken and checked by a doctor.
- Commence IV fluids.
- Cross-match the blood taken.
- Provide antibiotic cover.
- Communicate with the patient regarding their condition and treatment.

- Arrange admission to hospital—check your local policy.
- A surgical opinion should be sought.
- Complete the clinical risk documentation.

## Recovery post-dilatation

- Vital signs monitored and stable?
- Pain-free and no surgical emphysema?
- Tolerating fluids after a period of NBM up to 1 h post-dilatation—check your local policy?
- Able to walk without support?
- No nausea, vomiting, or haematemesis?
- IV cannula removed?
- Discharge/follow-up information given?

# Variceal balloon tamponade

This procedure exerts pressure on identified bleeding vessels, either in the oesophagus or gastric fundal region, after failed endoscopic therapy or drug intervention. Variceal balloon tamponade is rarely used in modern medicine, and should only be inserted by an experienced clinician with the help of an anaethetist to maintain the airway. It requires expert nursing care to ensure patient safety and well-being.[1]

## Balloon tamponade equipment

- Sengstaken (or Minnesota) tube—kept cold; aids placement (Fig. 7.2).
- Lubrication.
- 30 ml syringe.
- Gauze swabs.
- Four artery forceps.
- Drainage bag.
- Adhesive tape/bandage.
- Sphygmomanometer.

## Procedure

The nurse assistant must ensure the following:

- Check balloons for leaks and deflate completely.
- Label lumens.
- Record the level of gastric balloon inflation using a sphygmomanometer before placement.
- Put the patient in a left lateral position—one nurse must be dedicated to this task.
- Cardiovascular monitoring, suction, and oxygen available—there is a high risk of aspiration.
- Lubricate the tube.
- The endoscopist advances the tube through the mouth to 50 cm.
- Secure the tube with the tape or bandage.
- The gastric balloon is inflated. The patient will usually be intubated and paralysed. If not, observe the patient for pain. If the patient is in discomfort, stop, deflate the balloon, and reposition. Slight tension should be applied to maintain the position once the balloon is inflated.
- Measure the balloon pressure, which should correlate with the pre-insertion level.
- Check and record the level of the tube at the patient's incisor. Clamp the lumens—using forceps.
- Attach suction to oesophageal aspiration port using low pressure.
- Attach drainage bag to gastric outlet.

## Post-therapy care

*One-to-one nursing*

- Lay the patient flat, with slight tension on the gastric balloon externally to maintain its position.
- Observe for perforation, rebleeding, or subcutaneous emphysema (chest, abdominal, or pleuritic pain, tachycardia, and pyrexia).

---

1 Shephard M and Mason J (1997). *Practical Endoscopy*. Chapman & Hall Medical, London.

- Cardiovascular monitoring (pulse and blood pressure) should be performed every 30 min initially and then every hour.
- Take the patient's temperature every 4 h.
- Check the balloon pressure every 30 min.
- Deflate the oesophageal balloon for 5 min every hour to prevent tissue necrosis.
- Irrigate the gastric lumen, if required, every 1–2 h with 30 ml of saline.
- Rehydrate the patient intravenously—NBM and mouth care.
- Use sedation, if required.

## Complications

- Aspiration.
- Asphyxia—balloon displacement.
- Perforation.
- Tissue necrosis.

## Removal

- Disconnect suction.
- Clamp gastric and oesophageal aspirate lumens.
- Deflate the balloons.
- The patient should exhale on withdrawal of the tube.
- The patient should receive NBM for 6–8 h.

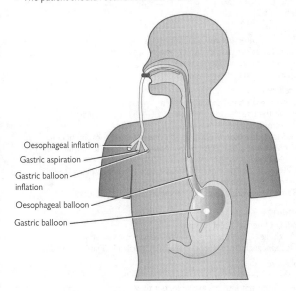

**Fig. 7.2** Oesophageal balloon, with a gastric balloon below. The balloon has three ports: an oesophageal inflation port, a gastric balloon inflation port, and a gastric aspiration port. Sengstaken Blakemore (Minnesota) tube. Reproduced with kind permission © Burdett Institute 2008.

# Oesophageal varices: banding or injecting

## Symptoms
Gastro-oesophageal haematemesis is associated with chronic liver disease, which is caused by morphological changes in the hepatic architecture that lead to venous drain occlusion into the inferior vena cava and portal hypertension. All patients must be resuscitated; in addition, coagulopathy must be corrected before endoscopic therapy. This is a highly skilled procedure requiring:
• Experienced endoscopist and nurse assistant.
• Resuscitation equipment and cardiovascular monitoring.
• Oxygen and suction.
• Documented blood results—cross-match available.
• Expert knowledge and communication skills.

## Sclerotherapy
Injection into varix causing thrombosis.

### Equipment
Similar to OGD (📖 p. 184) (therapeutic scope) and personnel safety equipment.

Additional:
• Two sclerotherapy retractable needles.
• Warmed sclerosant, drawn up into 5 ml syringes.
• Several syringes of sterile water.
• Spare suction liners.

### Procedure
• The patient's head should be slightly raised.
• Prime the needle with the sclerosant—check the needle length (~5 mm; single use).
• Lubricate the biopsy channel—to prevent kinking of the needle.
• Forward and retract needle by answering to 'needle out/in', respectively.
• Communicate the injection volume to endoscopist every 0.5 ml.
• Retract the needle if it is not injecting.
• Remove and dispose of the needle as clinical sharp waste.

## Banding
Banding of oesophageal varices:
• Varical ligation—the occluding of the variceal vessel.
• Oesophageal banding kit—prepacked sterile kit (Plates 1 and 2).

### Procedure
Follow the manufacturer's instructions for loading and firing the band. Several different kits are available, but they have similar components and placement techniques.

- Food bolus—break up or use forceps or suction to grasp the bolus. Take care if bones are involved.
- If present at the same time, the stricture can be dilated to prevent recurrence.
- Soft object—break up with the end of the endoscope, biopsy, or use grasping forceps.
- Use magnetic or rubber forceps for sharp metal objects, e.g. needles or nails.

# Percutaneous endoscopic gastrostomy: assessment

Enteral feeding through a PEG tube is indicated in patients requiring nutritional support for a long period of time if oral feeding is insufficient or impossible. It involves the insertion of a tube through the abdominal wall into the stomach using an endoscopic rather than an open surgical approach. Insertion is straightforward in most patients. PEG has an advantage over nasogastric (NG) feeding as the tube is less likely to become displaced and so the patient will receive the full regimen of feed. Also less trauma to nasopharynx. However, PEG is an invasive procedure, with many complications, and therefore the necessity of the procedure must be carefully considered.

A pre-procedure assessment is crucial to prevent complications, identify ethical appropriateness, and prevent clinical risk. Insertion of a PEG tube is an elective procedure; the indications are shown in Table 7.3.

## Pre-procedure assessment

An appropriately trained nurse should assess the patient using a set protocol obtaining the relevant information:

• Appropriateness of referral.
• Review the multidisciplinary notes.
• Factual information to include:
  • Physical assessment.
  • The patient's condition.
  • Diagnosis.
  • Prognosis.
  • Stability of the patient's condition.
  • Relevant comorbidity.
  • History of any previous surgery.
• Contraindications (Table 7.4).
• The long-term patient management plan—which could influence the choice of feeding device.
• Discharge plan/training requirements.
• Dietitian/speech and language therapy involvement.
• Medications—available in liquid form.
• Does the patient have the ability to give consent? Are the family aware of the procedure?
• If the patient is unable to give consent—a Medical Need Consent Form 4 as provided by the DOH.[1]
• Discuss with family—carer issues, training, understanding of condition.
• Present method of feeding and last feed—implications for the placement date.

---

[1] Deaprtment of Health (2005). *Good Practice in Consent Implementation Guide: Consent for Examination or Treatment.* http://www.doh.gov.uk (accessed 11.05.07).

**Table 7.3** Indications for percutaneous endoscopic gastrostomy

**Swallowing disorder**

Neurological—cerebrovascular accident, multiple sclerosis, motor neuron disease, Parkinson's disease, or cerebral palsy

Mechanical—oropharyngeal or oesophageal cancer/surgery, enteropathy, or planned radiotherapy

Cognitive impairment—head injury

**Other indications**

Severe respiratory distress/long-term ventilation, or intolerance of NG tube

**Table 7.4** Contraindications for percutaneous endoscopic gastrostomy

**Absolute contraindications**

Ascites

Morbid obesity

Peritoneal dialysis

**Relative contraindications**

Proximal gastric obstruction

Ventriculoperitoneal (VP) shunt (potential contraindication if recently sited)

Previous gastric abdominal surgery

Gastrectomy

Ileus

Acute pancreatitis

Untreated clotting disorder

Portal hypertension

Anorexia nervosa

Peritoneal carcinoma

Active sepsis (e.g. respiratory or urinary tract infection)

Active gastric ulceration (within the area of tube siting)

# Percutaneous endoscopic gastrostomy: procedure and techniques

## Pre-procedure clinical requirements

- IV access.
- Prophylactic antibiotic as per BSG guidelines.[1]
- Normal recent clotting documented.
- NBM/feeding tube for 6 h before the procedure.
- Regular mouth care to prevent seeding of a micro-organism causing stoma infection because of the pull-through technique.
- Good basic body hygiene—shower/bath.

## Procedure

There are several types of tubes as per local enteral feeding policy.
A normal OGD is performed (📖 p. 186) as follows:

- Place the patient on their left-hand side initially; they can be placed on their back once a normal gastric outlet is established during OGD.
- ▶ Airway protection.
- Nursing assistance similar to that for OGD (📖 p. 186).
  Three assistants are required for this procedure, in addition to the endoscopist. The first assistant for the gastrostomy placement will be an appropriately trained doctor/nurse. Nurse assistants must have completed the appropriate training, be deemed competent, have the approval of the local trust, and have obtained an appropriately signed relevant practice protocol. Two further nurses are required to assist with this procedure as per recognized working practices.

## Requirements for tube placement

Placement is a sterile technique. Ensure that a tube of the appropriate size and the following relevant accessory equipment are on the dressing trolley:

- Dressing pack.
- Gastrostomy kit.
- Needles—various.
- Syringes—5–10 ml.
- Local anaesthetic.
- Cleansing fluid.
- Dressing or appropriate spray.

## Method of insertion

- The endoscope is directed at the anterior wall.
- Transillumination of endoscopic light must be observed by both the endoscopist and the first assistant on the screen, and also on the abdominal wall, with finger indentation indicating no organ obstruction.
- The position should be marked and the area should be cleaned with antiseptic cleanser.

---

1 British Society of Gastroenterology (2006). *Working Party Consensus on Antibiotic Prophylaxis in Endoscopy*. BSG, London. http://www.bsg.org.uk (accessed 25.10.07).

- Local anaesthetic is infiltrated into the skin subcutaneously, the fascia, and the gastric mucosa.
- Draw syringe plunger back to check for air—to indicate no air-containing organ (i.e. bowel) is overlying the stomach.
- Steps above must be observed to prevent perforation of relevant abdominal organs.
- A skin incision is made, using a surgical blade, into the subcutaneous fat.
- Insert a needle trocar into the marked site and push through the anterior wall, while the endoscopist observes the procedure on a screen.
- The endoscopist places a snare wire over the area of insertion internally.
- The assistant inserts a silk-like thread/suture down the catheter, which is grasped by the snare wire in the stomach.
- The endoscope and snare wire are removed, leaving the wire at the mouth and abdominal exit site—a cheese-wire effect.
- A PEG tube is tied to the wire at the mouth and pulled back through the anterior abdominal wall.
- The internal flange should be felt under the fingers on the abdominal wall and exit site.
- The tube is marked with numbers, which should be documented on the endoscopy report, i.e. ~2–5 cm, depending on patient's weight.
- The outer flange must not be over-tightened, as this could cause compression necrosis.
- Apply the appropriate connections.
- Use a sterile dressing or surgical spray dressing according to local policy.
- Document the tube size, exit site (in cm), dressing applied, and after-care required at the stoma site. An appropriate care protocol should be used.

## Push technique

In the event of a failed endoscopic procedure, or known oral pharyngeal or oesophageal obstruction, the feeding tube is passed through the abdominal wall rather than endoscopically. These types of procedures can be placed either radiologically or by direct surgical gastrostomy. Refer to local guidelines.

# Jejunal extension using percutaneous endoscopic gastrostomy

This procedure is recommended for patients with gastro-oesophageal reflux or known motility disorders to ↓ the risk of pulmonary aspiration.

## Procedure requirements
- An appropriate extension kit for the gastrostomy tube should be available.
- A normal gastrostomy tube will be placed by either PEG technique (endoscopically or push technique) (📖 p. 200).
- Additional equipment—long grasping forceps.

This process requires a three-way line of communication between the endoscopist, the nurse assistant, and the first gastrostomy tube assistant, who must work as a team to achieve successful tube placement.
- If the procedure is wire-guided, flush the wire port with saline to ease removal once the tube is placed.
- Flush the gastrostomy tube with water and insert the extension tube.
- The tube should be picked up by the endoscopist using forceps and fed into the jejunum by advancing the endoscope and forceps appropriately.
- The first gastrostomy tube assistant slowly feeds the tube down the gastrostomy port, while keeping eye contact with the procedure on-screen.
- Once the tube is down into the jejunum, the endoscopist draws back the endoscope, while pushing in the forceps to maintain the position of the tube.
- The endoscopist views the tube at the pylorus and assesses the need to withdraw any excess tube from stomach.
- The guidewire is removed from the extension tube and the endoscope is removed.
- Extension tube connectors are then placed, with care taken not to dislodge the internal extension tube. The extension tube must be cut to size; accurate measurement for fitting is essential.
- Accurate documentation of the type of tube inserted must be made in the patient's notes.

# Percutaneous endoscopic gastrostomy and percutaneous endoscopic jejunostomy: post-procedure risks

The first 36 h after the procedures are the most important, although it takes at least 10 days for the stoma tract to form. Risks are as follows:
- Septicaemia.
- Tissue necrosis—over-tight tube.
- Peritonitis.
- Tube displacement.
- Stoma infection.
- Gastrocolic fistula/bowel perforation.
- Aspiration pneumonia—from endoscopy.
- Bleeding.
- Refeeding syndrome (📖 p. 114).

Post-insertion feeding regimen: check local policy.

## Post-procedure recovery

Similar to OGD (📖 p. 186).
- Oral fluids given only if appropriate.
- Appropriate pain control—if required.
- Observe for abdominal distension.
- Check the wound—if bleeding is present, dress accordingly and observe the wound for haemostasis.
- Vital signs.
- Discharge home for patients needing PEG feeding often needs complex planning (📖 p. 144).

Complications and further investigations if suspected:
- Surgical emphysema.
- Obtain a medical review.
- Chest/abdominal X-ray—according to the patient's clinical condition.
- Gastrograffin X-ray to establish the position of tube.
- Discharge the patient to the ward, with appropriate documentation and aftercare instructions.

## Further reading

Cotton P and Williams CB (1996). *Practical Gastrointestinal Endsocopy* (4th edn). Blackwell Science, Oxford.

Cuffaro G (2004). *Home Enteral Tube Feeding Guidelines*. Haringey Teaching Primary Care Trust/Nutrition & Dietetic Service, London.

# Oesophageal self-expanding metal stent

This procedure aims to maintain the oeosophageal patency of strictures caused by intrinsic or extrinsic malignant tumours. It is usually undertaken as a palliative procedure, but it is also (rarely) used in patients with benign disease. This is a complex procedure that carries a high complication rate.

## Considerations

- The equipment used in the procedure is similar to that for OGD (📖 p.186) ± rigid/balloon dilators of various sizes.
- Two experienced nurses, in addition to the endoscopist, are needed.
- Before insertion of the stent, the stricture should be assessed endoscopically and radiologically—if necessary, it should be dilated to 12 mm in diameter.
- Prosthesis—a knitted titanium wire (various manufacturers produce similar products).
- Two types of stent are available:
  - A covered mesh—a layer of translucent polyurethane covers the midsection. It is indicated for use in oesophageal fistulation. Four radio-opaque markers are required for deployment (markers on ends of the stent and covered area).
  - Mesh only—two radio-opaque markers are required. These stents usually have a metric ruler on the shaft for distance marking.

*Additional equipment needed*
- Guidewire—0.035 in, with a floppy tip.
- Silicone lubricant.
- Radio-opaque markers—if placed using X-rays.

## Contraindications

As for endoscopic dilatation (📖 p.189) plus the following:
- An oesophageal fistula of any type, unless it is covered by a stent.
- Long-term use for a benign stricture.
- A stricture that cannot be dilated to pass the endoscope or delivery system.
- Stent placement within 2 cm of the cricopharyngeal muscle.
- Known oesophago-jejunostomy.
- Necrotic bleeding tumour—active.
- Polypoid lesions.

## Patient preparation

Preparation of the patient is similar to that outlined on 📖 p.188. The patient should be offered specific counselling and access to specialist nursing support.

## Procedure

- Patient is positioned in the ERCP semi-prone position.
- Dilate the stricture—if required (📖 p.188).
- Lubricate the biopsy channel using silicone.
- Pass the guidewire down the scope, through the stricture.
- Pass the delivery system over the wire.

- Measure the length of the stricture, using the scope markings, and place radio-opaque marks externally if joint endoscopy/radiology placement.
- Observe the proximal end of the stricture with the endoscope.
- Position the delivery system in the stricture using the side-marking ruler with measurements obtained from the endoscopic examination.
- Non-covered stent 3–4 cm longer than the stricture; covered stent 5–6 cm to bridge the stricture, once deployed.
- Deploy the stent. Monitor the release of the stent, either endoscopically or fluoroscopically, keeping it within the measured margins.
- For fluoroscopic placement, use radio-opaque markers non-endoscopically through wire-guided technique; check the manufacturer's guidance booklet.
- Only remove the guidewire and/or endoscope slowly, once the stent is fully deployed.
- Use the balloon dilatation of the stent to aid expansion. The procedure is similar to that for balloon dilation. Never use a rigid dilator because it could dislodge the stent.

## Post-procedure care

Care as for any endoscopic dilatation ( p.191), with the following additions:

- Post-anterior and lateral chest film.
- Analgesia 24–48 h post-insertion.
- Clear fluids post-insertion; see local policy.
- The patient should receive NBM if the stent is placed for a fistula—healing must be confirmed.
- The patient should eat in an upright position and drink plenty of fluids during the meal.
- Food should be chewed well.
- The patient should eat slowly and have a fizzy drink following the meal.
- Certain foods should be avoided—chunky, stringy, or fibrous foods (e.g. bread, meat, and raw vegetables).
- Distal oesophageal stents could require acid-suppression therapy.
- Before discharge, dietary advice and contact details should be given to the patient and their carers.

# Diagnostic endoscopic retrograde cholangiopancreatography

Diagnostic endoscopic retrograde cholangiopancreatography (ERCP) confirms or diagnoses biliary pathology or stone obstruction. Therapeutic intervention can be continued, as required, using this basic technique. Experience with, and knowledge of, the equipment is important for both diagnostic and therapeutic use.

## Patient preparation

Similar to OGD (📖 p. 184). Three assistants must be available in the procedure room.

### Special considerations for ERCP

• IV access on the right-hand side.
• Consent: ± therapeutic intervention.
• Prophylactic antibiotics—check local policy.
• Haematological investigation results—full blood count, platelets, clotting time, blood group—cross-match and save.
• Position the patient on their left-hand side in a semi-prone position, with their left arm placed along their back to assist movement onto their stomach during the procedure.

## Indications

• Acute recurrent pancreatitis.
• Confirm malignancy following imaging.
• Unexplained abdominal pain—biliary.
• Deranged liver function.
• Jaundiced—suspected biliary obstruction.
• Confirmation of sclerosing cholangitis.
• Common bile duct stones.
• Confirmation of bile duct patency.

## Contraindications

• Deranged clotting if sphincterotomy is a potential treatment option.
• Recent myocardial infarction.
• Severe respiratory distress.
• Pregnancy—avoid ERCP if possible.

## Equipment

• Duodenoscope—with a 2.8–3.2 mm channel.
• Accessory trolley.
• Medication, contrast medium 10 ml syringes. Saline 20 ml, drawn up in syringe.
• Radiation protection equipment—thyroid shield or apron.
• Reversal drugs available.
• Primed cannula (remove air bubbles)—numerous types of cannula are available.
• Cardiovascular monitor.

## Procedure

- Cardiovascular monitoring is required throughout.
- The cannula is passed down the channel to the ampulla.
- An assistant injects medium slowly under direction of the endoscopist and guided by fluoroscopic imaging.
- Limit the amount of medium injected to a maximum of 3–5 ml. Do not overfill the pancreatic duct because it causes pancreatitis.
- The assistant communicates the amount of medium injected to the endoscopist and documents it in the medical notes.
- Flush cannula with saline if wire-guided access is required before inserting into the ampulla.
- Insert the guidewire down the cannula into the duct. Then withdraw the cannula leaving the guidewire in place, if therapeutic intervention is required. This is done by keeping the wire straight and maintaining the position of the wire in the duct through visual imaging. The endoscopist removes the cannula whilst the assistant inserts the guidewire.
- Further details are outlined in the therapeutic intervention section (☐ pp. 208–13).

## Post-procedure

- Observe the patient for the following:
  - Pain (may indicate pancreatitis: risk 3–5% after ERCP).
  - Vomiting.
  - Bleeding (melaena).
  - Sepsis.
  - Perforation.
- Drug reversal—if required.
- Observe the patient every 30 min for 2 h, then every 1 hour for a further 2 h, and then every 4 h for 24 h.
- The patient should receive clear fluids overnight.

# Therapeutic endoscopic retrograde cholangiopancreatography: biliary stent placement

ERCP is a combined endoscopic and radiological procedure which is undertaken to visualize the biliary and pancreatic ducts. Therapeutic ERCP is a complicated procedure, but it is challenging and satisfying for the nurse assistant.
▶ All members of the multidisciplinary team involved must be fully conversant with the procedure and equipment.

### Biliary stenting
ERCP is the most complicated procedure to assist. Biliary stricture prevents the normal flow of bile. Biliary stenting is performed for the following reasons:
• Biliary strictures.
• Stones.
• Perforation of the duct following surgery.

### Preparation
Similar to diagnostic ERCP (🕮 p. 206) using radiological identification of the stricture through cannulation of the duct and injection of radio-opaque contrast. Often the cause can be identified (stones or tumour).

The endoscopist attempts to clear stones through sphincterotomy, ± stone extraction (🕮 p. 210). The stent is placed only to aid duct drainage in the following situations:
• Unsuccessful removal of stones.
• If the guidewire can pass any of the strictures.

### Aim of treatment
• To relieve obstruction of the biliary tree.
• To provide free bile flow.

### Equipment
• A large-channel duodenoscope—4.2 mm for 10/12 Fr stent. (3.2/2.8 mm scope for 7 Fr stent only).
• Guidewire—a hydrophilic-coated wire is suggested, which is 400–480 cm in length, with an atraumatic tip.
• A stent introducer set.
• Various sized stents or a single-action set.
• Prime the guidewire and stent catheter using saline.

### Procedure
• Introduce the wire down the accessory channel, maintaining fluoroscopic visualization to aid advancement of the wire and stent placement.
• The stent introduction set is mounted over the guidewire—the assistant maintains gentle traction.
• The equipment is held straight to aid process.

- Continue traction to prevent looping of the wire in the duodenum as the stent introducer enters the bile duct.
- Fluoroscopic checks are used to monitor the placement of the guidewire.
- The catheter is guided over the obstruction and the stent is positioned.
- Maintain gentle traction.
- The guidewire is removed at this point for injection of contrast medium and observation of bile drainage.
- Metal expanding stents are placed as outlined in the first two steps.
- Follow the individual manufacturer's guidance.

## Change stent: if blocked or life expectancy expired

- Insert a standard catheter into the stent tip, inject the contrast medium, and check the position of the stent.
- Flush the catheter with saline.
- Introduce the guidewire down the catheter.
- Pass a Soehendra stent retriever over the wire.
- Screw the end into the stent—turning clockwise.
- Once secure, the endoscopist pulls the stent back into the duodenum, while the assistant pushes gently on the guidewire to maintain the position.
- The stent is either removed or left to pass through the gut.
- Normal stenting procedure for replacement.

## Removal

- The stent is removed by a snare, Dormier basket, or grasping forceps using with a scope.

## Complications/nursing care

See diagnostic ERCP (📖 p. 207).

## Further reading

Cotton P, Williams CB (1991). *Practical Gastrointestinal Endoscopy* (3rd edn). Blackwell Scientific Publications. London.
Shephard M, Mason J (1997). *Practical Endoscopy*. Chapman & Hall. London.

# Therapeutic endoscopic retrograde cholangiopancreatography: stone extraction

Biliary stones in the common bile duct (CBD) are the most common cause of biliary disease. There are two types of stone:
- Cholesterol—because of a high concentration of cholesterol in the bile, which is produced by the liver.
- Pigment—made up of bilirubin and inorganic calcium salts.

Patient preparation as per ERCP diagnostic procedure (📖 p. 206).

### Additional considerations
- Sphincterotomy (📖 p. 212).
- Extraction—stones <1 cm might pass spontaneously following sphincterotomy.

## Equipment
- Dormier basket comprising the following:
  - A rectangular or spiral wire basket of six or eight wires.
  - A Luer port for injection of contrast medium.
  - Some baskets are wire-guided.
- Balloons comprising the following:
  - Catheter-tipped—5 Fr or 7 Fr in diameter.
  - Various balloon sizes—8.5–18 mm in diameter.
  - Wire-guided balloons are available.

Check the basket or balloon and prime with contrast medium before insertion.

## Procedure
Sphincterotomy is often required before stones can be extracted.

### Balloon procedure
- Fluoroscopic guidance should be used throughout the procedure.
- Advance the deflated balloon into the CBD above the stones.
- Inject the contrast medium to establish the position of the stones—prevent trapping air in the catheter, because this can mimic stones on imaging.
- Inflate the balloon while observing the imaging screen—inflate the balloon accordingly.
- The endoscopist will retract the balloon slowly, drawing the stones down the duct.
- Repeat the procedure until the duct is clear.
- A wire-guided balloon can also be used for impacted stones or extraction of multiple stones.
- Place the wire into the duct first and then advance the balloon over the wire.

### Basket

Advancement of the basket follows the first three steps above and then the following steps:

- Open the basket in the duct with care not to push the stone further up the duct.
- The endoscopist should pull down to engage the stones—a gentle movement forwards and backwards might be useful.
- The basket should be closed on communication from the endoscopist or before removal of the basket from the duct.

### Mechanical lithotripter

Various types of device are available. Extraction of a large stone is performed using the basket method; check the manufacturer's guidelines for the use of particular accessory baskets.

The following procedure with relevant equipment should be followed:

- A large-channel scope.
- Use fluoroscopic imaging throughout the procedure.
- Sphincterotomy.
- The metal sheath of the lithotripter is passed over the plastic catheter of the basket according to the manufacturer's guidance.
- Attach a torque handle.
- Close the basket slowly using a mechanical torque to crush the stone.
- ❶ The basket could break if the stone is hard.
- The procedure should only be undertaken by an experienced team.

## Post-procedure nursing care

Similar to that for diagnostic ERCP (📖 p. 207).

# Therapeutic endoscopic retrograde cholangiopancreatography: sphincterotomy

Sphincterotomy enables better access to the ampulla and use of a therapeutic accessory. Similar to all therapeutic procedures, a skilled and knowledgeable team is required to perform the procedure.

### Equipment
- A selection of sphincter tomes.
- A selection of guidewires.
- Saline flushes—20 ml.
- Diathermy.

### Patient preparation
Similar to OGD and diagnostic ERCP (📖 pp. 184, 206) with the following additional checks.
- Check whether the patient has a pacemaker or internal metal fittings (e.g. hips or pins)—contact the local cardiology department regarding the suitability of using electrical diathermy with a pacemaker.
- Clotting screening.
- Consent—therapeutic intervention.
- Apply the diathermy plate to the patient's thigh.
- Place the patient's hands and arms on the X-ray mattress.

### Procedure
- Prime the sphincter tome with saline. Check the bowing of the wire at the tip of the sphincter tome.
- Check the diathermy connections are correct and in working order.
- Visual fluoroscopy is required throughout the procedure.
- The endoscopist cannulates the ampulla or passes over the wire *in situ*.
- The assistant bows the sphincter tome slowly according to the endoscopist's instructions.
- The endoscopist cuts through the ampulla with the wire intermittently and the assistant releases and tightens the handle to bow the wire accordingly.
- If the wire cannot be cut, check that the accessory wire is far enough away from the scope—check on screen that the wire is visible at the ampulla opening (prevents internal injury to the duct on cutting blind).
- Observe for excessive bleeding during the procedure.

▶ Sphincterotomy is one of the most dangerous surgical procedures and has high rates of mortality and morbidity.[1]

### Post-procedure nursing care
The post-procedure care required is similar to that for diagnostic ERCP (📖 p. 207); however, a special precaution regarding bleeding must be noted.

1 Cotton P and Williams CB (1991). *Practical Gastrointestinal Endoscopy* (3rd edn). Blackwell Scientific, London.

# Therapeutic endoscopic retrograde cholangiopancreatography: biliary duct dilatation

Biliary strictures are commonly seen in sclerosing cholangitis and post-operative fibrosis, but they can also present as malignant strictures.

## Equipment
- Balloon catheters:
  - 4–10 mm in diameter when inflated.
  - 2–5 cm in length.
  - 5 Fr or 7 Fr gauge.
  - Radio-opaque marks.
- Rigid stepped dilators:
  - 5 Fr, 7 Fr, or 9 Fr gauge stepped.
- Standard guidewire.

## Procedure
Similar to diagnostic ERCP and sphincterotomy with the following additional procedures:
- Pass the guidewire into the CBD.
- The balloon is inserted over the guidewire—flush the internal catheter with saline before handing it to the endoscopist.
- Inflate the balloon to the predetermined pressure.
- Monitor under fluoroscopy for 'waist' (dilation of stricture) disappearance .
- The procedure is painful—limit the dilation time to no more than 10–20 s.
- Rigid dilation, as above.
- Gently insert the catheter up to the maximum gauge of the dilator, using imaging as a guide.

## Intra-procedure
Observe the patient for pain and signs of perforation of the duct on imaging.

## Post-procedure nursing care
The post-procedure care required is similar to that for diagnostic ERCP (📖 p. 207).

## Further reading
Cotton P and Williams CB (1991). *Practical Gastrointestinal Endoscopy* (3rd edn). Blackwell Scientific, London.
Shephard M and Mason J (1997). *Practical Endoscopy*. Chapman & Hall, London.

# Flexible sigmoidoscopy

### Definition
Examination of the left side of the colon from the rectum to the splenic flexure. A long flexible endoscope/camera is inserted into the rectum and guided through the sigmoid and descending colon. The lining of the bowel can be visualized directly. An assessment and diagnosis can be made, and treatment can be performed as necessary.

### Indications
- Outlet-type rectal bleeding—bright red and not mixed with the stool.
- Localized lower-left quadrant pain.
- To further examine/clarify the results, a barium enema/CT scan of the left-hand side of the colon can be performed.

### Complications
- Perforation—1:5000 cases for diagnostic procedure; <1:500 for polypectomy.
- Failure to complete the investigation—requiring retesting or further investigations.
- Haemorrhage from therapeutic procedures (📖 p. 220).

### Special considerations
For patients with infection, such as *Clostridium difficile* in the stool and cytomegalovirus, check with the endoscopist regarding the best time to perform the procedure. If the patient is receiving anticoagulation (e.g. warfarin), biopsy and therapeutic endoscopy might not be possible until the patient's clotting has been corrected. If the patient is to be sedated, a full medical history will also be required.

### Preparation
A purgative/cleansing enema is administered at least 1 h before the procedure, to clean the left-hand side of the bowel. The patient should be advised to refrain from eating and drinking for 2 h before the procedure, if they require sedation. A full medical history must be taken and any significant findings communicated to the endoscopist (e.g. anticoagulant use, epilepsy, diabetes, or cardiac or respiratory conditions). Informed consent must be obtained by the endoscopist.

### Patient explanation/information
The risks and benefits of the procedure must be clearly outlined to the patient before gaining their informed consent. Explain to the patient that, for the endoscopist to view the lining of the bowel, air is inserted through the endoscope/camera. This can cause bloating but will soon pass. It is rarely necessary to sedate the patient for a flexible sigmoidoscopy; sedation adds to the risk of the procedure.

## Procedure

The procedure takes 5–20 min and commences with a digital rectal examination.

- The lubricated sigmoidoscope/colonoscope is inserted into the rectum under direct vision and the rectum is insufflated.
- The endoscopist slowly withdraws the scope, if required, so that the lumen of the rectum is in full view.
- The instrument is slowly advanced, under direct visualization, up to the splenic flexure.
- In the sigmoid colon the circular haustral folds will be visible. Careful examination is required to ensure that no polyps or lesions are missed.
- Once through, the triangular haustral folds of the transverse colon are visible and the insertion is complete.

Careful withdrawal of the scope is required, noting any abnormal mucosal polyps, lesions, or vessels such as angiodysplasias.

Biopsies can be taken of any pathology encountered or inflamed mucosa, which aids diagnosis—note the location and size (in mm). Therapeutic procedures can also be undertaken (📖 p. 220). If the patient is not sedated, they can be discharged as soon as they are dressed and relevant documentation completed. The follow-up plans should be explained to the patient before discharge.

# Colonoscopy

### Definition

An examination of the large bowel, from the rectum to the terminal ileum. Similar to a flexible sigmoidoscopy, a long flexible endoscope/camera (colonoscope) is inserted into the rectum and guided through the sigmoid, descending, round the splenic flexure and transverse colon, around the hepatic flexure, down the ascending colon, and into the caecum. If the ileo-caecal valve is clearly visualized, insertion of the scope into the terminal ileum is possible. The mucosa of the bowel can be visualized directly and an assessment and diagnosis can be made.

### Special considerations

Similar to flexible sigmoidoscopy and sedation (📖 p. 176). Perforation rate <1:1000 for diagnostic procedure. <1:500 risk perforation if polypectomy performed.

### Preparation

Preparation of the bowel is the most important factor in the success of a colonoscopic examination. The bowel lumen must be free of faeces and faecal matter to visualize the vascular pattern and mucosal lining. The patient is required to have a low-residue diet for 2 days before the investigation, and a cleansing solution, such as a phosphate enema or oral sodium picosulfate, is taken in drink form 1 day before the investigation. This induces diarrhoea and facilitates cleaning of the bowel. The patient is advised to take only clear liquids during the preparation procedure and to take NBM for 2 h before the procedure if they are to be sedated.

### Patient assessment

Informed consent must be obtained by the endoscopist. A full medical history must be taken to include:
• Anticoagulant use.
• Epilepsy.
• Diabetes.
• Cardiac or respiratory conditions.
• Allergies.

### Patient explanation/information

The procedure is similar to flexible sigmoidoscopy (📖 p. 215), but the endoscopy will involve the entire large bowel rather than just the left-hand side of the colon. Sedation and analgesia may be administered through an IV cannula. Conscious sedation is required because the patient could be required to move during the procedure, to aid insertion of the colonoscope (📖 p. 177).

### Procedure information

The procedure takes ~20–30 min and commences with a digital rectal examination. The lubricated colonoscope is then inserted into the rectum and insufflated. The instrument is slowly advanced, under direct visualization, along the large bowel. If the ileo-caecal valve is visualized when the scope reaches the caecum, it can be entered. The appearance of the ileal mucosa differs from that of the large bowel because of the presence of villi, which ↑ the absorptive surface area of the ileum significantly. The instrument should be withdrawn carefully; note any polyps, lesions, mucosa, and vessels (e.g. angiodysplasia). Therapeutic colonoscopy can be performed if required (📖 p. 220), after which the examination is complete.

## Pathology

- Diverticular disease is visualized as pockets or 'holes' in the mucosa.
- Sessile (flat) or pedunculated (on a stalk) polyps.
- Cancer.
- Inflammatory diseases, e.g. ulcerative colitis and Crohn's disease (may be seen as ulcers, granular mucosa or 'skip' lesions).
- Vascular pattern differences, e.g. angiodysplasia.

The patient must stay in recovery for up to 2 h, to be monitored following sedation and any therapeutic procedure. The follow-up plans will then be explained to the patient and their relative/carer; consideration should be given to the effect of the sedative on the patient.

## Indications

- Rectal bleeding—which is darker and mixed with the stools.
- Change in bowel habits—especially diarrhoea/looser stools.
- Iron-deficiency anaemia.
- Abdominal pain/mass.
- To further examine/clarify the findings, a barium enema/CT scan can be performed.
- Surveillance for inflammatory bowel disease, cancer, or polyps.
- The procedure can be both diagnostic and therapeutic.

## Complications

- Perforation—<1:1000 (1:500 with polypectomy).
- Failure to complete the investigation—requiring retesting or further investigations.
- Haemorrhage from therapeutic procedures.

# Colonic stents

Up to 30% of patients who have colon cancer present with obstruction (complete or partial/tumour or stricture). Emergency surgery (e.g. stoma formation or resection with an end-to-end anastomosis) has a high rate of morbidity and mortality (up to 20%) and some tumours are inoperable. Stents can be used in emergency situations, with elective surgery at a later date, or as definitive palliation if a decision not to operate has been made. The procedure is expensive, but it is less expensive than surgery.

### Types of stent

Various types of stent are available.
- Self-expanding metal stents are most commonly used.
- Plastic—migrate too easily and can occlude the colonic lumen.
- Rigid—more difficult to place through an obstruction than other types of stent.
- Originally, oesophageal stents were used, but now custom-designed colonic stents are available.

Most patients will be unfit for having an anaesthetic; they need careful nursing because of multiple comorbidities and often have a poor nutritional status. Prior imaging of obstruction is required.

Preparation is not usually required. It is also unusual to sedate the patient; most need no analgesia during stent placement. Most stents are placed under fluoroscopic control; they are deployed over a guidewire. The stent expands during the 48 h following the procedure.

### Complications

- The mortality rate is 2%—lower than that of emergency surgery (20%).
- The risk of perforation is 3%—potentially fatal and more common following balloon dilatation of a stricture.
- Failure to deploy stent—varies, but a rate of 0–30% has been reported.
- Migration (up to 4 weeks later)—re-stenting is often required.
- Bleeding—minor bleeding owing to mucosal pressure is common.
- Faecal impaction.
- Occlusion (all types but plastic most likely).
- Re-obstruction—tumour in-growth of 25% over time.
- No evidence of the promotion of tumour growth or spread—local or metastasis.
- It is easier to place stents in a more distal (lower) position in the colon, but these are more likely to be dislodged and/or cause symptoms, e.g. discomfort, tenesmus, bleeding, or faecal incontinence.

### Post-procedure

- Monitor blood pressure, temperature, and pain—possible perforation or bleeding.
- Expect some abdominal discomfort—mild analgesics or antispasmodics.
- The patient could have repeated bowel actions as the colon decompresses—ensure toilet access for frail patients.

- Stool softeners to keep the stent patent—loose or liquid stool might be needed to prevent blockage (but watch for faecal incontinence).
- Patient/carer education to watch for complications.

## Further reading

Godber SL (2004). Palliation of colonic obstruction by expandable metal stents. *Gastrointestinal Nursing*, **2**, 33–9.

# Polypectomy

Therapeutic endoscopy is now a routine part of endoscopic practice. A polyp is a protuberant lesion in the mucosa, which has different appearances:

- Sessile—without a stalk.
- Pedunculated—on a stalk.

Histologically, polyps have different varieties (Table 7.5). Other conditions, such as familial adenomatous polyposis, can present as a 'carpet of polyps' and require surgical treatment.

## Treatment

Safe polypectomy requires the ability to sever a polyp, while achieving haemostasis and maintaining the integrity of the colon wall.

Sessile polyps can be 'hot biopsied', which involves grasping the polyp with biopsy forceps and pulling it away from the colon wall. An electrical current is applied in addition to a short sharp tug on the forceps, which removes the polyp and ensures haemostasis. Hot biopsy is contraindicated in the right colon (use snare).

Pedunculated polyps require 'snaring', which involves putting a loop of wire (or a snare) around the base of the polyp stalk. The loop is tightened and an electrical current is applied, which severs the base of the polyp and seals the vessels.

## Risks

- Haemorrhage from the polypectomy site.
- Perforation of the bowel mucosa at the site can occur days after the procedure (rate <1:500).

These risks must be explained to the patient; if they experience excessive abdominal pain or haemorrhage, they should to return to the Accident and Emergency Department.

## Post-procedure care

Monitoring the patient's vital signs is of paramount importance, both during and after polypectomy. If haemostasis is not achieved, hypovolaemic shock can result. The patient could require IV fluids to replace any blood loss during the procedure and this must be explained to the patient before the procedure, because afterwards they may be recovering from sedation.

## Follow-up

Depending on the findings at colonoscopy and the histology of the polyps, the patient might require repeat colonoscopy to ensure that there are no further polyps and check the previous polypectomy sites. For adenomatous polyps, the patient should enter a regular surveillance programme to ensure that there is no further growth of polyps. Surveillance for >3 adenomas (any size), or 1> 10 mm (5 yearly).

**Table 7.5** Varieties of polyp

---

**Hyperplastic/metaplastic polyps**

These are hemispherical smooth sessile polyps, which have little or no histopathological potential to develop into any other type of polyp and require no treatment or removal, unless doubt exists regarding their nature

---

**Inflammatory polyps**

Associated with inflammatory bowel disease

---

**Hamartomatous polyps**

These include juvenile polyps and Peutz–Jeghers polyps, which may be harmless unless they are associated with juvenile polyposis syndrome or Peutz–Jeghers syndrome

---

**Adenomatous polyps**

These are neoplastic and therefore have malignant potential. There are four main histopathological considerations:

Size—in mm

Configuration, e.g. sessile, pedunculated, or flat

Growth pattern—tubular, tubular villous, and villous

Degree of dysplasia—mild, moderate or severe, which is an indicator of the extent to which the epithelium lining has undergone changes causing a predisposition to malignancy

---

**Malignant polyps**

These polyps harbour an invasive adenocarcinoma which has invaded the submucosal bowel lining. In general, the bigger the polyp, the higher the probability of malignant change

# Capsule endoscopy

Capsule endoscopy is a non-invasive pain-free fully ambulatory diagnostic procedure specifically for investigating the small intestine. Because only ~5% of all GI abnormalities originate in the small bowel, capsule endoscopy should only be performed if gastroscopy and colonoscopy are both unsuccessful. Owing to the inability to manipulate the movement of the capsule, gastroscopy and colonoscopy remain the 'gold standard' procedures for examining the upper and lower GIT, respectively. Once ingested, the capsule moves along the GIT by natural peristalsis and is eventually excreted by normal bowel motion. In the normal individual, there is a 1% risk of capsule retention, usually resulting from stricturing disease or obstruction. Despite the ease of performing and undergoing capsule endoscopy, it is a time-consuming process. The procedure usually takes about 8 h, which correlates with the estimated duration of transit through the entire small bowel. The capsule takes two colour images per second; ∴ a total of ~50 000–100 000 images can be recorded. A moderately experienced practitioner takes 60 min to complete the review of the imaging video and compile a report; it requires focused attention and specialized training.

## First indications
- Obscure gastrointestinal bleeding (OGIB):
  - Overt—melaena or haematochezia.
  - Occult—faecal occult blood or iron-deficiency anaemia.
- Crohn's disease:
  - New diagnosis.
  - Suspected active episode in a patient with known Crohn's disease.

## Second indications
- Hereditary polyposis syndromes.
- Refractory coeliac disease (exclude small bowel lymphoma or jejunitis).
- Chronic abdominal pain ± diarrhoea.
- Suspected NSAID-induced enteropathy.
- Small bowel transplantation.

## Contraindications
Any of the following conditions (whether suspected or known):
- Obstruction or pseudo-obstruction.
- Fistulas, strictures, or fissures.
- Swallowing disorders.
- Exercise caution with cardiac pacemakers, implanted defibrillators, or other electromechanical devices.
- Pregnancy.
- Caution with previous pelvic or abdominal surgery.
- If unsure if lumen is patent, perform barium follow-through to ensure.

## Potential complications
- Capsule retention owing to stricture or obstruction. If this is suspected, an abdominal X-ray is performed to confirm the location of the capsule and then, if necessary, the capsule is retrieved using endoscopic or surgical means. An estimated 1% risk of occurring in the normal individual (not previously detected by small bowel follow-through or patency capsule).

Rare complications include the following:
- Perforation.
- Aspiration or displacement of the capsule.
- Fracture of the capsule (very rare).

## Procedure
- Preparation—the patient should have a clear fluid diet for 1 day, followed by 10 h fasting before the procedure. Bowel-cleansing agents and prokinetic drugs can also be administered.
- Obtain informed consent.
- Attach a sensor array to the patient's abdomen and fit a data recorder with a belt.
- The capsule is activated once it is removed from the sterile blister pack and ingested (can also be delivered endoscopically).
- The patient should receive NBM for the first 2 h.
- Recommence clear fluids, as desired, for the remainder of the procedure.
- A light diet can be allowed after 4 h.
- Record what the patient has to eat and drink during the procedure on an event form.
- Observe and record any obstructive-type or unusual symptoms.
- Remove the capsule endoscopy equipment when the procedure is completed.
- Connect the data recorder to the workstation to download the data.

## Discharge management
- The patient can return to their normal diet and activities.
- Observe bowel motions for excretion of the capsule.
- Ensure follow-up arrangements are made for discussing the results of the procedure.
- An abdominal X-ray must be performed before MRI scanning if excretion of the capsule is not confirmed.

## Further reading
Melmed GY and Lo SK (2005). Capsule endoscopy: practical applications. *Clinical Gastroenterology and Hepatology* **3**, 411–22.
Rey JF, Gay G, Kruse A, *et al.* (2004). European Society of Gastrointestinal Endoscopy (ESGE): guideline for video capsule endoscopy. *Endoscopy* **36**, 656–8.

# Cleaning and disinfection of endoscopes: transmission of infection

Effective decontamination of reusable medical devices is essential in ↓ the risk of transmission of infectious agents. Decontamination of endoscopes is one of the most important procedures undertaken within the endoscopy department. Cleaning and disinfecting are used in combination to make reusable medical devices safe for further use. A guiding principle for decontamination is that of universal precautions. All patients are considered a potential risk of infection. Because of the complexity of these reusable instruments, decontamination must strictly adhere to local and national guidelines. A review of these guidelines in 2005 was promoted by three relevant developments:

- The Health and Safety Executive (HSE) report on alternatives to glutaraldehyde.[1]
- Variant Creutzfeldt–Jakob (vCJD) disease—the pathogen in humans.[2]
- Updated Medical Device Agency (MDA) bulletin on the decontamination of endoscopes.[3]

A separate review of all three documents is recommended, in addition to the brief details outlined below.

## Transmission of infection at endoscopy

- Limited data are available regarding the absolute risk of transmission.
- Onset following discharge.
- ERCP—septicaemia could be due to endogenous infection, rather than endoscopically induced infection.
- Endoscopically induced infection is usually caused by procedural errors in decontamination:
  - Use of old scopes—more likely to have associated channel and surface irregularities.
  - Inadequately designed or poorly maintained automatic endoscope reprocessors.
  - Substandard disinfection.
  - Inadequate drying and storage.

Transmission of viral infection occurs for the following reasons:
- Failure to brush the biopsy channel.
- Failure to sterilize reusable biopsy forceps ultrasonically or with steam.
- Inadequate chemical exposure.

Three types of micro-organisms are associated with endoscopy:
- Mycobacteria.
- Bacterial spores—*Bacillus* and *Clostridium*.
- Pathological prions—including CJD and vCJD (new guidelines 2005).[2]

1 Health and Safety Executive (2003). *Endoscope Disinfection—Alternatives to Glutaraldehyde*. SIM 07/2003/14. http://www.hse.gov.uk (accessed 02/07/07).

2 Department of Health (2005). *Transmissible Spongiform Encephalopathy Agents: Safe Working and the Prevention of Infection: Guidance from the Advisory Committee on Dangerous Pathogens and the Spongiform Encephalopathy Advisory Committee*. http://www.advisorybodies.doh.gov.uk (accessed 02/07/07).

3 Medicines and Healthcare Products Regulatory Agency (formerly Medical Devices Agency) (2002). *Decontamination of Endoscopes*, DB2002 (05) 2002. http://www.mhra.gov.uk (accessed 02.07.07).

# Cleaning and disinfection of endoscopes: decontamination

If the endoscope is correctly decontaminated and it is assumed that all patients are potentially infectious, there is no need to schedule patients with known infections at the end of an endoscopy list. However, a prevailing infection-control policy should be in place and often includes scheduling patients who are known to have methicillin-resistant *Staphylococcus aureus* (MRSA) at the end of the endoscopy session list.

## Decontamination

Decontamination comprises three basic processes:
- Manual cleaning:
  - Brush the endoscope with a single-use wire brush or purpose-built catheter, exposing all external and internal channels/components to a low-foaming enzymatic detergent.
- Automatic disinfection.
- Rinsing and drying of all exposed surfaces—complying with HTM2030.[1]

All the reprocessing stages must be completed after every use of the instrument, to include any channels not used during a procedure. Decontamination begins as soon as the scope has been removed from a patient.
- Suck water or detergent through the working channels.
- Expel sterile water down the air/water channel by depressing the appropriate button.
- Wipe the insertion shaft down externally—check for any surface irregularities.
- Remove the instrument to the reprocessing room—dismantle the detachable parts.
- Discard the rubber biopsy cap if it was breached by the biopsy forceps.
- Manually clean the air/water button and suction valve before ultrasonic cleaning.
- The water bottle and later-generation scope valves are autoclavable. Older-generation valves should be disinfected (check the CJD policy regarding autoclaving and prion proteins).[2]

The scope is manually cleaned as follows:
- Using a low-foaming enzymatic detergent, clean all external and internal surfaces.
- Accessible channels should be brushed with a purpose-built single-use brush-tip wire.
- Special consideration should be given to auxiliary water channels, the exposed elevator wire channel, and balloon inflation channels (endoscopic ultrasound probes).

**1** NHS Estates (1997). *Health Technical Memorandum HTM2030: Washer Disinfectors.* HMSO, London.

**2** Department of Health (2005). *Transmissible Spongiform Encephalopathy Agents: Safe Working and the Prevention of Infection: Guidance from the Advisory Committee on Dangerous Pathogens and the Spongiform Encephalopathy Advisory Committee.* http://www.advisorybodies.doh.gov.uk (accessed 02.07.07).

## Top ten tips for endoscope decontamination
- Wipe down the insertion tube.
- Flush the air/water channels.
- Aspirate water through the biopsy/suction channel.
- Dismantle the detachable parts, e.g. valves.
- Perform a leak test.
- Manually clean the air/water and suction valves before ultrasonic decontamination or autoclave them, according to the manufacturer's guidance.
- Manually clean the scope with enzymatic detergent and rinse.
- Disinfect and rinse the endoscope in the automatic reprocessor.
- Dry the endoscope.
- Store the endoscope appropriately.

## Disinfection
- Endoscopic automatic reprocessors do not replace manual cleaning/ brushing of all the working channels.
- Automatic endoscope reprocessors flush disinfectant through all the working channels—only use manufacturer's recommended connections.
- Conclude the process by flushing with sterile or filtered water—dry by blowing air through all the working channels.

## Further reading
British Society of Gastroenterology (2005). *Guidelines for Decontamination of Equipment for Gastrointestinal Endoscopy*. BSG, London.

Medicines and Healthcare Products Regulatory Agency (formerly Medical Devices Agency) (2002). *Decontamination of Endoscopes*, DB2002 (05) 2002. http://www.mhra.gov.uk (accessed 02.07.07).

Medicines and Healthcare Products Regulatory Agency (formerly Medical Devices Agency) (2004). *Decontamination and Infection Control*. http://www.mhra.gov.uk (accessed 02.07.07).

# Cleaning and disinfection of endoscopes: management

## Management of cleaning and disinfection

The following procedures and protocols should be followed to ensure maximum safety is attained:

- Trained personnel only.
- Appropriate immunization/assessment by the occupational health department.
- Appropriate protective clothing—single-use nitrile gloves, long-sleeved waterproof gowns, and goggles/face visor.
- Dedicated washing area.
- Automated machine—compatible with HTM2030 guidance.
- Extraction facilities.
- Comprehensive documentation to track scope disinfection and validation available—ongoing review of the traceability of scope accessories that are not decontaminated with the scope.
- Disinfection exposure no more than 3 h before use—check the risk assessment guidance of your local trust.
- HSE-approved vapour mask and spillage kit for emergencies—check the guidance of your local trust.
- Compliance with Health and Safety at Work Act 1974[1] and the Control of Substances Hazardous to Health (COSHH) Regulations 1994.[2]
- All the substances used in the decontamination of medical devices must have a risk assessment by COSHH.

## Management of the process

The *MDA Device Bulletin* includes information regarding compatible processes recommended by the device manufacturers and can be used as a source of reference for all departments.[3]

Ensure decontamination of the instrument before service or repair. All equipment should be decontaminated if possible, unless the insertion tube is leaking (socially clean manual cleaning is required before sending an endoscope for repair). A decontamination certificate must accompany the equipment; (e.g. MHRA DB 2003(5)).

Single-use items must clearly display the International Organization for Standardization (ISO) symbol (Fig. 7.3), with a diagonal line drawn through it.

Store the scopes in a room separate from the reprocessing area; hang the instruments vertically in a dry well-ventilated cupboard.

---

1 Health and Safety at Work Act 1974. Available at: http://www.hse.gov.uk/legislation/hswa.htm (accessed 26.10.07).

2 Control of Substances Hazardous to Health Regulations 1994. Available at: http://www.hse.gov.uk/coshh/(accessed 26.10.07).

3 Medicines and Healthcare Products Regulatory Agency (formerly Medical Devices Agency) (2002). *Decontamination of Endoscopes*, DB2002 (05) 2002. http://www.mhra.gov.uk (accessed 2.07.07).

## Special considerations

### Creutzfeldt–Jakob disease

All personnel involved in the endoscopy must ensure that procedures are in place to minimize contamination and potential risk. Because of the complexity of prion diseases, reading the BSG consensus document on vCJD is recommended.[4]

**Fig. 7.3** ISO symbol for single-use items. Reproduced with kind permission © Burdett Institute 2008.

4 *Endoscopy and Individuals at Risk of vCJD for Public Health Purposes.* A consensus statement from the British Society of Gastroenterology. Decontamination Working Group and the ACDP TSE Working Group Endoscopy and vCJD Subgroup. http://www.bsg.org.uk (accessed 02.07.07).

# Biopsies, aspiration, and handling specimens

The collection of mucosal specimens for examination in the pathology laboratory is an important part of differential diagnosis not only in theatre, but also in the endoscopy department. The two main areas in which cooperation between the clinician and the assistant are of major importance are communication and specimen handling. An experienced assistant can correctly use the equipment and handle specimens and should have sole responsibility for the collection and transfer of the specimens from the clinical environment from which they were taken.

## Communication

**Important communication ponts:**
- ► Anatomical location is of major importance for future treatment.
- Establish the equipment requirements, e.g. forceps, a snare, or a sheathed cytology brush. CLOtest® (urease test strip for *H. pylori*).
- An appropriately labelled container with the correct medium for transport.
- Biopsies from different anatomical sites must be submitted in separately labelled containers and placed in a plastic bag with a pathology request form and adequate information regarding the patient's demographic details and presenting symptoms.
- Check that the patient's demographic details are correct on the container and request form before removing them from the clinical environment.
- Document the area from which the specimen was taken, the patient's demographic details, and the clinician's details in an appropriate book within the department. The book should be kept as an audit trail in case of delayed or lost specimens.

## Procedure for taking specimens

Personal/universal protective equipment must be worn at all times.

### Forceps
- Pass the forceps to the endoscopist, who will pass them down the biopsy channel of the endoscope or laparoscope under direct visualization.
- When the forceps are in contact with the mucosa, the assistant will open and close the forceps on the instruction of the clinician.
- The forceps are then removed from the biopsy channel in the closed position, while the assistant holds a gauze swab over the opening to prevent spillage of gastric contents.
- The specimen is extracted and handled as indicated below (📖 p. 231).

### *Polypectomy*
*Snare*
- As for the forceps procedure.
- On visualization, the endoscopist will ask for the snare to be opened, placed over the polypoid area, and closed to the predetermined mark. Polypectomy assistance should be undertaken by an experienced nurse—check your local trust policy.
- The snare can be removed, as described above (as per forceps removal), and the polyp retrieved using suction into a polyp trap attached to the suction port, appropriate retrieval forceps, or a snare (on removal of the scope).
- The specimen should be handled as indicated in the next section.

## Specimen handling
- Biopsies should be extracted gently from the forceps, with a blunt needle, onto a piece of filter paper which is shaped at one end to differentiate the proximal and distal anatomical orientations—check with your local pathology laboratory for their preference.
- Multiple samples from similar anatomical areas can be placed on one sheet of paper, but place them centrally to enable accurate orientation in the histology laboratory—check with your local pathology laboratory for their preference.
- All the patient's specimen samples should be placed in correctly labelled containers before commencing another patient's samples.
- Place the containers in an appropriate plastic bag, with the appropriate documentation, for transportation.

## Cytology

Cytology specimens can be taken if a biopsy is contraindicated (e.g. anticoagulation therapy) or cannot be obtained.

*Procedure*
- Place a sleeved disposable brush down the biopsy channel.
- On direct visualization and instruction by the clinician, open the brush to enable the head to extend out of the plastic sheath.
- The clinician will brush the surface mucosa and then request that the brush be withdrawn back into the sheath.
- The sheath is then withdrawn from the scope.
- The brush is extended and brushed against two or three glass slides, which are fixed immediately with liquid fixer to prevent the cells drying and damage to the specimen.
- Each glass slide should be labelled with the patient's demographic details and placed in an appropriate slide box for transportation with the correct documentation.
- Alternatively, some clinical areas cut the brush off at the sheath using sterile scissors and place it straight into a specimen pot containing formalin solution.
- All the patient's specimen samples should be placed in correctly labelled containers (pots or slides) before commencing work on another patient's samples.
- Place the containers in an appropriate plastic bag, with the appropriate documentation, for transportation.

## Disposal of single-use equipment

All the equipment used for collecting specimens should be single use if possible.
- Used blunt-ended needles and forceps should be treated as sharps and disposed of in the correct bins provided.
- Reusable forceps should be cleaned and sterilized according to the national guidelines—decontamination of all reusable equipment should be tracked. Single-use items also have tracking labels and these should be placed in the patient's notes.

# Other endoscopic procedures

### Laser therapy

The Nd:YAG laser is most commonly used, but the argon laser can also be used for endoscopic therapy. The procedure takes time and patience.

- Photocoagulation (60°C)—used for inactive potential bleeding (ulcer with visible vessel, Mallory–Weiss tear, neoplasm, haemorrhoids, or angiodysplasia); produces white area with surrounding oedema.
- Photovaporization (100°C) destroys tissue, burns area, produces smoke (used for neoplasms, oesophageal webs, polyps, biliary obstruction).

*Cautions*

- Clotting problems.
- Large blood vessels.
- Poor view.
- Agitated uncooperative patient.
- Cooling agent can produce distension, unless gas is removed.
- The laser can damage the endoscope tip.
- Tumours—usually start at the bottom and work up, so that oedema does not obscure your view.

*Procedure*

- Wear protective goggles to protect your eyes and masks to protect against smoke.
- Two assistants are required.
- Risk of haemorrhage—monitor vital signs during the procedure and for 4 h afterwards.
- Distension can cause a vasovagal reaction—NG tube can relieve distension after the procedure.
- NBM for 4 h following the procedure.

### Endoscopic ultrasound

Less commonly used in the UK than in other countries. Enables detailed observation of local structures and tumours.

### Photodynamic therapy

Some light-sensitive IV drugs collect in malignant tissue—a laser light delivered by endoscope can destroy tumour tissue.

# Stoma care

Stoma care nursing: role of the stoma care nurse *236*
Surgical procedures resulting in a colostomy *238*
Surgical procedures resulting in an ileostomy *242*
Colo-anal pouch *246*
Colectomy with ileo-rectal anastomosis *248*
Kock pouch (continent ileostomy) *250*
Restorative proctocolectomy (ileo-anal pouch) *252*
Formation of a stoma *256*
Stoma reversal *258*
Pre-operative care for the ostomist *260*
Stoma siting *262*
Post-operative care following formation of a stoma *266*
Management of a rod/bridge including removal *268*
Product choice: appliances *270*
Product choice: accessories *272*
Storage, care, and disposal *274*
Discharge planning for the ostomist *275*
Prescription issues and obtaining supplies *276*
Lifestyle issues for the ostomist *278*
Dietary advice for the ostomist *280*
Hints and tips: ileostomists *281*
Hints and tips: colostomists *282*
Complications and problems: mucocutaneous separation *283*
Complications and problems: bleeding *284*
Complications and problems: necrosis *286*

Complications and problems: prolapse *288*
Complications and problems: parastomal hernia *290*
Complications and problems: pyoderma gangrenosum *292*
Complications and problems: peristomal granuloma *294*
Complications and problems: recurrence of disease *295*
Complications and problems: stenosis and dilators *296*
Complications and problems: retraction *298*
Complications and problems: phantom rectum *299*
Complications and problems: constipation and diarrhoea advice for the colostomist *300*
Enterocutaneous fistula management *302*
Catastrophic abdomen *304*
Administration of suppositories and enemas into a stoma *306*
Medina catheter *308*
Skin care: excoriation and allergy *310*
Skin care: trauma and infection *312*
Colostomy irrigation *314*
Antegrade continent enema *316*
Percutaneous endoscopic colostomy *318*
Stomal considerations with chemotherapy and radiotherapy *320*
Palliative care for the ostomist 1 *322*
Palliative care for the ostomist 2 *324*

# Stoma care nursing: role of the stoma care nurse

Stoma care is not new: specialist nurses have worked in stoma care for more than 25 years. Stoma care nurses (SCNs) are expected to demonstrate a high level of clinical decision-making and both monitor and improve standards of care through supervision of practice, clinical audit, and the provision of professional leadership. The development of practice takes place through teaching and the support of professional colleagues.

The SCN role involves the following:
- Having an in-depth knowledge of the physical, psychological, and emotional effects of stoma formation.
- Providing individualized holistic patient care.
- Planning patient care by focusing on the achievement of independence.
- Offering and delivering direct patient care.
- Teaching new skills.
- Providing relevant information at the appropriate time for the patient.
- Coordinating patient care within the multidisciplinary team (MDT).
- Providing continuity of care from admission through to discharge, with follow-up at home.

Five common themes emerge for the nurse specialist role:
- Clinical expert—the expert knowledge and skill of the SCN enables functioning at a high level of practice. Continuity of care commences as soon as the decision is made to form a stoma.
- Researcher—influencing practice and the delivery of care. Research could include new products for patients, audit of the service, or exploring clinical skills to ensure the care provided is evidence based.
- Consultant—working within a multiprofessional setting, the SCN acts as a patient advocate, particularly because s/he tends to hold a deeper understanding of the total patient situation.
- Educator—excellent communication skills are required because the SCN is expected to teach at varying levels and situations. For example:
  - Patients and families.
  - Multidisciplinary care team.
  - General public.
  - Media.
- Clinical lead—using clinical leadership and management skills, the SCN influences the delivery of quality patient care, e.g. facilitation of standard setting and conducting clinical service audits.

## Further reading

Taylor P (ed) (1999). *Stoma Care in the Community—A Clinical Resource for Practitioners*. Nursing Times Books, London.

# Surgical procedures resulting in a colostomy

There are several operations that can result in the formation of a permanent or temporary colostomy.

## Hartmann's procedure

Generally an emergency procedure performed to remove obstructing sigmoid carcinomas, perforated diverticular disease, or sigmoid volvulus. The procedure involves the excision of the sigmoid colon and upper rectum. The rectal stump is either stapled or sutured and placed inside the abdominal cavity or brought out as a mucus fistula on the lower abdominal wall. This procedure results in a temporary stoma; however, because the procedure is performed on an elderly population, a high percentage of patients choose to continue with the stoma (Fig. 8.1).

## Abdominoperineal excision of the rectum (APER)

Performed for carcinoma of the rectum and/or anus/anal canal or anal margin. This is a major procedure, resulting in both a laparotomy and a perineal wound. The lower sigmoid colon, rectum, anal canal, and sphincter muscles are removed, necessitating the formation of a permanent colostomy. The perineum can be closed by different techniques, depending on surgeon's preference (Fig. 8.2).

## Divided colostomy (Devine operation)

This operation was first introduced in 1937. In cases of obstructing carcinoma or colic perforation, a Devine procedure might be carried out. The bowel is divided and both ends are brought out onto the abdominal wall. The proximal end is the opening for faecal output and the distal end is a mucus fistula, which is often placed at the end, middle, or top of the suture line (Fig. 8.3).

## Trephine procedure

If the formation of a stoma is confirmed before surgery, it is possible to form the stoma before opening the abdomen. This is known as the 'trephine colostomy'. The advantage of creating a stoma this way is that the layers of the anterior abdominal wall retain their anatomical relationship without sliding onto one another, ∴ providing a more satisfactory stoma. Currently, this procedure is not in common practice.

## Soave

This is a pull-through procedure performed for the surgical management of Hirschsprung's disease, a congenital defect of the large bowel (Fig. 8.4).

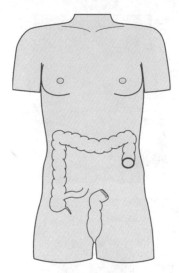

**Fig. 8.1** Hartmann's procedure. Reproduced with kind permission © Burdett
Institute 2008.

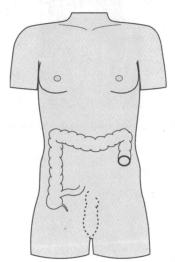

**Fig. 8.2** Abdominoperineal excision of the rectum. Reproduced with kind
permission © Burdett Institute 2008.

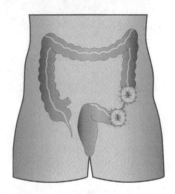

**Fig. 8.3** Divided colostomy (Devine operation). Reproduced with kind permission © Burdett Institute 2008.

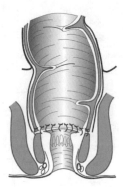

**Fig. 8.4** Soave. Reproduced with kind permission © Burdett Institute 2008.

# Surgical procedures resulting in an ileostomy

There are a number of operations that can result in the formation of a permanent or temporary ileostomy.

## Anterior resection

An anterior resection is often performed to remove a rectal cancer and can result in a temporary ileostomy. An anterior resection is a sphincter-saving operation, where the rectum and some of the sigmoid colon are removed. The amount of rectum removed differs, because of the variation in the type of operation:

• Anterior resection.
• Low anterior resection.
• Ultra-low anterior resection.

For the lower resections, a defunctioning loop ileostomy is common. This enables the colonic anastomosis to heal without faeces passing through the anastomosis (Fig. 8.5).

## Panproctocolectomy

The anus, rectum, and colon are removed. This surgery results in a permanent end ileostomy. This operation can be performed on those with a diseased colon and poor anal sphincters (Fig. 8.6).

## Subtotal colectomy

A subtotal colectomy is performed when the rectum is retained, but the colon is removed (ascending, transverse, descending, and sigmoid) and a temporary end ileostomy is formed. A subtotal colectomy is commonly performed for diseases, such as ulcerative colitis, in which the colon is diseased. Usually, this operation is performed in the emergency setting and as the first part of a series of operations, such as the following:

• Ileo-anal pouch formation.
• Anastomosis of the ileum to the rectum (ileo-rectal anastomosis).
• Removal of the rectum and a permanent ileostomy formation.

The formation of the temporary ileostomy enables the diseased bowel to be removed and the patient to regain their health. This then allows the surgeon to plan the next phase of surgery, which reduces the risks, such as anastomatic leaks (Fig. 8.7).

## Restorative proctocolectomy

📖 p. 252.

## Further reading

Blackley P (1998). *Practical Stoma, Wound and Continence Management*. Research Publications Vermont, Australia.

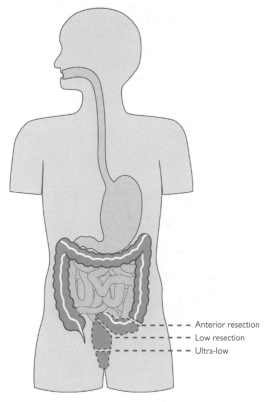

**Fig. 8.5** Anterior resection. Reproduced with kind permission © Burdett Institute 2008.

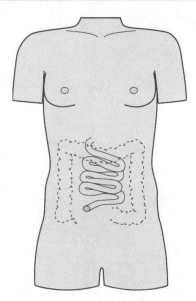

**Fig. 8.6** Panproctocolectomy. Reproduced with kind permission © Burdett Institute 2008.

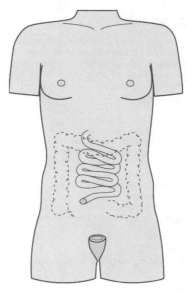

**Fig. 8.7** Subtotal colectomy. Reproduced with kind permission © Burdett Institute 2008.

# Colo-anal pouch

A colo-anal pouch is a surgical procedure that restores faecal storage capacity when the rectum is surgically removed. However, this procedure might not be suitable or appropriate for all patients having a proctectomy. The colo-anal pouch is formed from the large bowel. Usually, when it is first formed, a temporary ileostomy is required to protect the anastomosis in the colo-anal pouch (Fig. 8.8).

## Advantages

The aim of forming a colo-anal pouch is to ↓ the urgency and faecal leakage possible after a straight anastomosis when the rectum is removed, e.g. when low anterior resection is performed.

## Disadvantages

There are a number of potential complications associated with colo-anal pouch formation, including:
- Incomplete bowel evacuation.
- Difficulty in passing faeces from the colo-anal pouch.
- Constipation.

## Bowel function

There might be problems when the colo-anal pouch is initially used, including:
- Diarrhoea.
- Urgency.
- Evacuation problems.
- Faecal leakage.

These problems often resolve during the first few months. The following can assist in improvement of bowel function:
- Recommending or manipulating the diet.
- Anal leakage can be helped by performing anal sphincter exercises to strengthen the muscles.
- A small pad can be worn if leakage occurs.
- Bulking agents can assist in 'normalizing' bowel patterns.

## Long-term function

The long-term function of a colo-anal pouch is usually good. The bowels are generally opened once or twice daily on average, and not usually at night. Faeces are usually formed and most people are continent. However, if long-term function is poor, a colostomy is an alternative option. Most people can return to work ~6 weeks after stoma closure. In the long term, after healing and recuperation, resumption of all activities is possible, including swimming and bathing.

## Further reading

Williams J (ed) (2002). *The Essentials of Pouch Care Nursing*. Whurr, London.

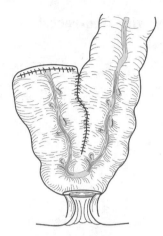

**Fig. 8.8** Colo-anal pouch. Reproduced with kind permission © Burdett Institute 2008.

# Colectomy with ileo-rectal anastomosis

Performed less often with the advent of restorative proctocolectomy, this procedure is a compromise to avoid a stoma in patients with ulcerative colitis (UC) or familial adenomatous polyposis (FAP). The colon is removed and the ileum is anastomosed to the rectum, hence the term ileo-rectal anastomosis (IRA) (Fig. 8.9). In both situations, disease is present, and because of the proximity to the anal verge, regular surveillance is obligatory. Surveillance is of paramount importance in long-term preventative disease management. Destruction of adenomas might be necessary for patients with FAP, whereas early detection of dysplasia is necessary for patients with UC.

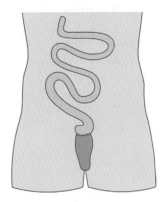

**Fig. 8.9** Colectomy with ileo-rectal anastomosis. Reproduced with kind permission © Burdett Institute 2008.

# Kock pouch (continent ileostomy)

Originally created in the late 1960s, this procedure is not now considered the first surgical choice for patients with UC or FAP (Fig. 8.10). The procedure is ∴ performed less often, but there are still patients living with Kock pouches in the community. The reservoir is created from small bowel that resides in the abdominal cavity. A channel is created from small bowel, which runs from the pouch to the abdominal surface. Within the channel, a nipple valve is formed to maintain continence and a flush stoma is visible on the abdominal surface.

A medina catheter is used to intubate and empty the pouch. Until it is established, the patient can wear a stoma cap for protection and collection of any mucus secretions. During intubation, the length of time taken to drain faecal matter varies, depending on the consistency of the stools. It can be assisted through irrigation. Problems and suggested action are highlighted in Table 8.1.

## Equipment required for intubation
- Medina catheter.
- Lubricating gel.
- Soft wipes.
- Stoma cap or cover.
- Bladder syringe and water (if irrigation is required).

## Further reading
Williams J (2002). *The Essentials of Pouch Care Nursing*. Whurr, London.

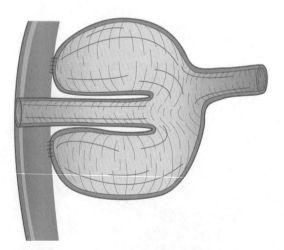

**Fig. 8.10** Kock pouch. Reproduced with kind permission © Burdett Institute 2008.

**Table 8.1** Complications of the Kock pouch

| Problem | Action |
| --- | --- |
| Nipple valve necrosis | Regular observation of stoma ensuring good perfusion |
| | Necrosis will de-slough eventually |
| Nipple valve ischaemia | Regular observation of stoma ensuring good perfusion |
| | Surgical revision |
| Pouch/enterocutaneous fistula | Treat conservatively by inserting Medina catheter in the long term |
| | Maintain skin integrity |
| | Drainable appliance to collect effluent |
| | Surgical revision |
| Stenosis of nipple valve | Dilatation |
| | Surgical revision |
| Difficult intubation | Surgical revision |
| Sliding nipple valve | Surgical revision |
| Pouch leakage | Stoma plug can be useful |
| Prolapsed pouch | Surgical revision |
| Pouchitis | Antibiotics |
| | Topical steroids |
| | Temporary loop jejunostomy |
| Recurrent Crohn's disease | Topical steroids |
| | Immunosuppressants |
| | Removal of pouch |
| Obstruction | Abdominal X-ray to confirm |
| | NBM |
| | Reintroduce fluids |
| | Reintroduce diet |

# Restorative proctocolectomy (ileo-anal pouch)

Acting as a reservoir, the pouch is constructed from loops of small bowel and anastomosed to the anal canal (Fig. 8.11). The anal canal is stripped of its mucosa to prevent recurrent disease. The newly formed pouch is protected by a loop ileostomy, which is closed from 12 weeks following pouch formation. Defecation occurs 3–7 times/day, with a porridge-like stool consistency.

### Indications for surgery
- UC/indeterminate colitis.
- FAP.

### Patient criteria
- Good understanding.
- Motivated.
- Psychologically prepared.
- Age (6–80 years).
- Good anal sphincter control.
- Not obese.

### Surgical stages
Stage 1: Total/subtotal colectomy with ileostomy ± mucus fistula.
Stage 2: Completion proctectomy, formation of ileo-anal pouch, and loop ileostomy.
Stage 3: Closure of loop ileostomy.

Stages 1 and 2 can be undertaken at the same time.

### Complications
- Pouchitis—inflammation within the pouch causing symptoms similar to inflammatory bowel disease (IBD). The aetiology is unknown, but pouchitis is more likely to affect those with UC. It affects 10–20% of all pouches, and the incidence
  ↑ over long-term follow-up. The complication is not associated with any particular configuration, and treatment is fairly straightforward with antibiotic therapy.
- Cuffitis—inflammation of the columnar cuff, which is situated above the anal transition zone.
- Outflow problems—difficulty in evacuating: either incomplete emptying or inability to evacuate because of stenosis.
- Incontinence—usually passive (often nocturnal).
- Pouch vaginal fistula—associated with stapled surgical procedures.
- Pelvic abscess—because of delayed healing or long-term steroids before surgery.
- Retained rectal mucosa—poor surgical procedure, resulting in pouchitis-like symptoms.
- Perianal skin soreness—caused by a combination of frequency, leakage, and poor skin care.

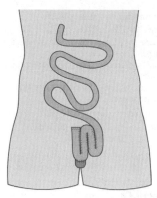

**Fig. 8.11** Restorative proctocolectomy. Reproduced with kind permission © Burdett Institute 2008.

## Lifestyle issues and an ileo-anal pouch
### Sex and pregnancy
Sexual difficulties are linked to anxiety, fear of failure, or concern about the partner's feelings.
- ♂—difficulties include erection and ejaculation problems.
- ♀—vaginal dryness.

Fertility is known to decrease by 50%; therefore patients should be referred for specialist advice.

### Contraception
Oral contraceptives are fully effective (in addition to the morning-after pill); uterine devices are contraindicated.

### Pregnancy
Can expect to go to full term with minimal problems, except ↑ in defecation. Caesarean section is recommended.

## Some hints and tips
Some pouch patients will encounter the problems in Table 8.2.

**Table 8.2** Problems related to the ileo-anal pouch

| Problems | Solution |
|---|---|
| Evacuation of pouch ↓ or stops | Consider what has been eaten |
| | If no abdominal pain present, drink fluids only for 24 h and then reintroduce diet |
| | If vomiting, seek medical attention |
| ↑ defecation | Consider what has been eaten |
| | Administer anti-diarrhoeals |
| Incomplete emptying of pouch content | Consider stenosis |
| | May need urea and electrolytes, examination under anaesthetic (EUA) |
| | Dilatation |
| | Biofeedback therapy |
| | Medina catheter |
| Perianal soreness | Basic personal hygiene |
| | Use moist toilet paper |
| | Keep anal area dry |
| | Use of barrier cream/film |
| | Avoid perfumed talcum powder |
| | Avoid excessive use of creams |
| Rectal burning/itch | Warm bath |
| | Instil haemorrhoid preparations into pouch |
| | Instil aloe vera gel into pouch |
| Fatigue | Long-term intestinal absorption could altered—annual full blood count (FBC) from 5 years post-pouch is a necessity |
| | Lack of mineral salts—check urea & electrolytes; 1 L of rehydration solution daily |
| Incontinence | Wear small pad/liner |
| | Administer anti-diarrhoeals |
| | Anal plug |
| | Medina catheter |
| | Dietary restrictions |
| | Biofeedback therapy |
| Wind | Avoid high-fibre diet, i.e. bran, beans, and pulses, and excessive fruit and vegetables |
| Bleeding | Not common; might occur if straining |

# Formation of a stoma

There is no rule regarding the length or shape of a stoma. An ileostomy positioned on the right side of the abdomen should ideally be no longer than 3 cm in length, with the apex pointing slightly downwards. This is achieved by the creation of the '554' ileostomy (Fig. 8.12). Two sutures are placed at the upper edge of the divided ileum, on either side of the mesentery. A serosal bite 5 cm proximal is followed by a subcuticular bite. When these two stitches are tied, it results in a superior margin on the stoma of 2.5 cm and, if a single inferior suture takes its serosal bite at 4 cm rather than 5 cm, the stoma has an inferior margin of 2 cm and an apical opening that points slightly downwards.

When a loop ileostomy is formed, it is essential that the afferent loop (active) forms a spout as a means of preventing sore skin.

Colostomy construction is more difficult than an ileostomy. This is usually because patients are older and fatter, creating a more bulky colon. Consequently, the bulky colon is difficult to bring through a small opening in the abdominal wall. To ensure adequate length, mobilization of the splenic flexure and the entire left colon might be necessary. A slight rim is recommended and, to do this, the basic steps are to take bites of the divided colon edge, followed by serosal bites ~1 cm proximal, and then subcuticular bites of the skin. This results in a 0.5 cm rim.

Transverse loop colostomy is easy to both create and close, and it does not have to be placed in the right upper quadrant where it might interfere with the waistline or rib margin.

Stoma formation is usually the last part of a sometimes long surgical procedure. It is vital that it is well constructed so the patient does not have management problems that can lead to reduced quality of life.

## Mucus fistula

A mucus fistula is the exteriorized rectal stump that is retained in some surgical procedures, e.g. subtotal colectomy. The rectal stump produces ~5 ml of mucus, which appears as a thick, white, or yellowish discharge.

There is still debate as to whether a mucus fistula should be brought out onto the surface of the abdomen or over-sewn and secured to the anterior abdominal wall. Unlike a stoma, a mucus fistula is not sited before surgery. Because of its shortened length, it is located in the suture line or at a distance proximal from the stoma and lies flush to the skin. Patients are not usually prepared for a mucus fistula and ∴ do not cope well with having what they see as two stomas.

The decision to create a mucus fistula occurs at the time of operation and depends on the following factors:
• The general condition of the patient.
• The state of the diseased bowel.
• The surgeon's preference.

Sizes vary from 10 to 30 mm in diameter. All the post-operative complications that can affect a stoma can affect a mucus fistula. Therefore it is important to monitor and treat the mucus fistula with as much attention as the stoma. If necrosis of the stoma occurs, it is unlikely that the mucus fistula will be affected, and vice versa. In the case of the patient with severe

UC, it is in the patient's interest to form a mucus fistula. This prevents the risk of pelvic infection and enables steroid treatment, both distally and rectally, until a decision is made to remove the rectum.

## Further reading

Williams J and Nicholls R (2001). Controversies relating to ileal anal pouch surgery. In: Williams J (ed) *The Essentials of Pouch Care Nursing*. Whurr, London.

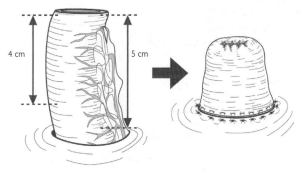

**Fig. 8.12** '544' ileostomy. Reproduced with kind permission © Burdett Institute 2008.

# Stoma reversal

### Reasons for stoma formation
- Protect anastomosis—loop ileostomy/colostomy.
- In the event of a perforated bowel and risk of contamination, no anastomosis is formed and an end stoma is brought out, e.g. Hartmann's procedure.
- Disease.
- Functional problems.

### Criteria for reversal
- An intact anastomosis is demonstrated radiologically.
- Patient fitness.
- Patient choice.

On average, the bowel anastomosis heals after ~4–6 weeks from the original operation.

### Pre-operative preparation
- Pre-operative assessment.
- Loop ileostomies require no bowel preparation, just clear fluids for 24 h pre-operatively.
- Loop colostomies require bowel preparation, e.g. oral sodium picosulfate.

No major abdominal incision is required for the reversal of loop stomas because the surgery is performed at the site of the stoma. It results in a small transverse wound at the stoma site.

At the time of the operation, an EUA is performed before stoma reversal to confirm that the anastomosis has healed.

### Post-operative management
- Post-operative assessment.
- IV fluids until oral fluids are tolerated.
- Oral fluids can be commenced once the patient is awake.
- Food can be taken once fluids are tolerated.
- Discharge home when bowels are opened.
- Average length of hospital stay is 3–5 days.

### Pre-operative preparation for reversal of Hartmann's procedure and end stomas
- Pre-operative assessment.
- Bowel preparation.
- Patients must be counselled and sited for a temporary loop stoma because an anastomosis is formed during this operation.

### Post-operative management
- This operation requires a laparotomy and ∴ is, managed as major abdominal surgery.

## Specific potential risks/complications following stoma reversal

- Ileus.
- Anastomotic leak.
- Wound infection/fistulae.

Because the peristomal skin has long-term exposure to gut flora, there is a high risk of wound dehiscence/infection.

## Bowel function following closure

### Loop stomas

The majority of patients who have a loop stoma reversed have had their rectum removed and ∴ the implications for bowel function are long term. Frequency, unpredictability, and incontinence are often reported as the common problems. The term 'anterior resection syndrome' is used to summarize these problems.

### End stomas

For those patients whose rectum is still intact, bowel function might differ from pre-surgery function. However, the long-term implications are minimal. Bowel function might be looser and more frequent than before, and antidiarrhoeal medication might be required.

Stoma reversal is not without its potential complications and risks. Patients must be fully informed about the risks, in addition to the potential outcome of bowel function, before considering reversal. The majority of patients prefer to live without a stoma. However, some opt to keep it if their quality of life has not been affected.

# Pre-operative care for the ostomist

Whether the stoma is temporary or permanent, the patient must be prepared both physically and psychologically. Preparation for stoma formation begins once the decision has been made to create the stoma. Good communication is very important to establish a comfortable rapport with the patient and their family, and to facilitate the adaptation period following formation of the stoma.

The SCN undertakes much of the pre-operative care, including giving the information regarding the stoma and its siting. A thorough assessment of the patient identifies any potential post-operative concerns that might occur when they are discharged home. The aim of the pre-operative assessment is to ensure the patient is fully informed with regard to the stoma surgery, while ensuring a seamless transition from the hospital to home. It might be appropriate to offer the patient a visit from an ostomist who is in a similar situation, to discuss the practicalities of living with a stoma.

The patient might not have even heard of a stoma. Therefore it is, important to explain the many issues related to the stoma, including the following:
• What the stoma will look like?
• How big the stoma will be?
• Will the stoma be visible by others?
• Where the stoma will be placed in the abdomen?
• Will the stoma smell?

Before abdominal surgery, it is usual to prepare the bowel; this varies according to the surgeon's preference. The patient might be required to take a bowel-cleansing solution, to ensure the bowel is clear. Generally, the patient has NBM for at least 4 h to prevent aspiration of stomach contents during surgery.

▶ Discuss the expectations of how life with a stoma will be. The patient is expected to become independent in the care of the stoma before discharge.

Preparation before surgery generally ensures that the patient copes better with the new stoma. To do this, pre-operative information must be accurate and appropriate. Information (verbal, written, or video) required pre-operatively can include the following topics:
• The stoma itself.
• Demonstration and discussion of stoma appliances.
• Post-operative expectations.
• Past medical history.
• Current medication/allegeries.
• Coping mechanisms.
• Clothing.
• Occupation.
• Religion and culture.
• Fertility and sexual issues.
• Diet.
• Exercise and sport.

## Further reading

Davenport R (2003). Pre-operative stoma care. In: Elcoat C (ed) *Stoma Care Nursing*. Hollister, Reading.

# Stoma siting

▶ The choice of position for a stoma is crucial if the patient is to live a full and active life. It is generally accepted that the responsibility for siting a stoma lies with the SCN.

### Criteria for choosing a stoma site

To ensure the ostomist has a secure and leak-proof appliance, the stoma should be situated on a relatively smooth abdominal surface and positioned to avoid discomfort or hindrance of any activity.

### Basic guidelines for stoma siting

Explain each stage in the procedure to the patient and gain their cooperation. The patient should appreciate and understand why the site has been chosen and the importance of its accurate placement. A detailed patient history should be obtained before carrying out the procedure. Check the patient has signed a consent form, identifying the type of stoma to be formed (Figs 8.13 and 8.14).

Gather the following equipment together:
- Tape.
- Indelible pen.
- Stoma appliance.
- Transparent adhesive dressing.

Introduce yourself to the patient and explain the procedure. Position the patient comfortably on the bed, ensuring privacy at all times. Using the flat of the hand, identify the rectus sheath muscle by getting the patient to lie flat and put chin onto chest, thereby tighting up the rectus sheath muscle and making it easier to identify. An incision will be made through this muscle for the stoma to be bought through. Identify an imaginary line between the umbilicus and the iliac crest on the appropriate side of the abdomen where the stoma is to be created. Make a provisional mark using tape. Check this provisional mark while the patient stands, sits, lies flat, and bends.

Move the provisional mark appropriately until a suitable position is determined. Once an appropriate site is identified, mark it with a permanent marker. It might also be necessary to mark an additional site choice or, indeed, highlight problem areas. Record the site marked within the patient's notes.

Refer any difficulties to the consultant.

### Anatomical features to avoid

Secure fitting of a collecting appliance is complicated in some areas (Table 8.3). Also remember that the patient could gain or lose weight, or, in the case of a child, grow.

### Additional points

Further consideration of a patient's cultural and religious beliefs is required. Patients with disabilities, such as someone who is wheelchair-bound, should be sited whilst seated in their wheelchair so as to achieve optimum independence.

## Further information

Phillips R, Myers C, Kelly L (1997). *The Principles of Stoma Siting* (video). Dansac Ltd, Cambridgeshire.

---

**Table 8.3** Sites to avoid

- Bony prominences—iliac crests, symphysis pubis, and rib cage
- Natural waistline
- Skin creases and folds
- Umbilicus
- Large pendulous breasts
- Previous scarring
- Any other irregularities in the contours of the abdominal wall, i.e. fat folds and bulges
- Groin areas
- Current fistula
- Primary incision site
- Areas of problematic skin disorders, such as eczema and psoriasis

**When not to site**

- Following any pre-operative medication
- Presence of a distended abdomen
- A child <7 years should only be sited at the request of the surgeon; otherwise no site should be marked

---

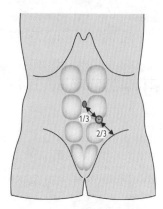

**Fig. 8.13** Siting for left iliac fossa stoma. Reproduced with kind permission
© Burdett Institute 2008.

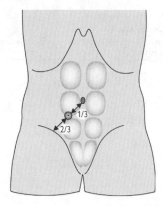

**Fig. 8.14** Siting for right iliac fossa stoma. Reproduced with kind permission
© Burdett Institute 2008.

# Post-operative care following formation of a stoma

## Aim

A safe discharge home. The ostomist should be able to care for the stoma, eat, drink, mobilize, and ensure their stoma is functioning.

## Observation of stoma

▶ Assess the newly formed stoma regularly for any signs of complications. The stoma must be checked for the following:

• Colour—red or pink.
• Warm—body temperature.
• Output.
• Shape and size.

Fluids and diet are usually allowed soon after surgery, depending on the patient's condition, but might be delayed for several days after surgery. The first output from a stoma could take several days. The usual sequence of events for faecal stoma output is flatus and then stool (initially loose), which could take several days. The first stool passed is usually offensive in odour.

## Post-operative stoma care teaching

Ideally, the patient will be independent with their stoma care before discharge. A practical guide to teaching will facilitate this and enable the healthcare professional to ensure the following occurs:

• Collecting all the necessary equipment.
• Removing the appliance.
• Clean the skin—gently but thoroughly.
• Measuring the stoma size.
• Cutting the appliance 2–3 mm larger than the size measured.
• Securing the appliance to the abdomen.

Other issues that should be discussed in the post-operative period:

• Selecting an appliance.
• Practical advice on appliance changing.
• Dietary advice.
• Problem prevention and solving.
• Who to contact in case of difficulty.
• Obtaining further supplies.
• Resuming activities after surgery.

The stitches around the stoma are usually soluble, taking 2–6 weeks to disappear. The rod or bridge, if used, is usually removed from under the stoma 3–10 days following surgery.

## Appliances

In the immediate post-operative period, the appliance used over the newly formed stoma should be clear to enable visualization of the stoma. In the long term, a comfortable leak-proof appliance should be found to contain the effluent. For a colostomy, the appliance should be closed at the bottom to contain the soft or formed faeces.

An ileostomy appliance is ideally suited to a looser faecal output that requires drainage several times daily. The newer fastenings are clipless, making it simpler for those with dexterity issues.

Stoma appliances are available in one or two pieces to suit the various needs of the individual patients. The choice is ultimately that of the patient, with guidance from the SCN.

## Further reading

Metcalf C (1999). Stoma care: empowering patients through teaching practical skills. *British Journal of Nursing* **8**, 593–600.

# Management of a rod/bridge including removal

A rod or bridge is used to support a loop stoma in the immediate post-operative period (Fig. 8.15). The rod is placed under the loop of bowel on top of the skin and prevents the bowel from retracting into the abdominal cavity. The rod is usually in place for 3–7 days to enable the tissues surrounding the stoma to heal, anchoring the stoma in place.

## Management
- Examine the stoma closely post-operatively.
- Both ends of the rod should always be visible.
- Ensure the stoma is in the middle of the rod and the ends of the rod are not rubbing against the stoma, causing damage.

## Removal
- Confirmation that the rod is to be removed should be sought from the surgeon.
- Consent should be obtained from the patient before removing the rod. The patient should be advised that this is a painless procedure.
- One end of the rod swivels to straighten, enabling the rod to be easily pulled through and removed.

## Further reading

Porrett T and McGrath A (2005). *Stoma Care*. Blackwell, Oxford.

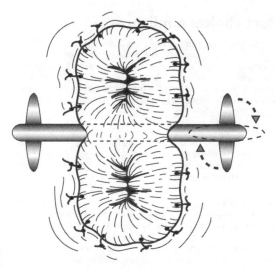

**Fig. 8.15** Rod or bridge supporting a stoma. Reproduced with kind permission © Burdett Institute 2008.

# Product choice: appliances

There are many different types of appliances and accessories available for patients with a stoma. Appliances come in varying sizes and shapes, with different closure methods, clear or opaque covers, and as one-piece or two-piece systems. The product choice is based on the type of stoma, the output from the stoma, how easily the patient can manage the appliance, and patient choice. The stoma care nurse assists the patient in this choice.

## Appliances

### One-piece appliances

One-piece appliances incorporate the bag and flange (base plate) together. Patients remove the whole appliance when it is changed. Advantages of this type of appliance are its flexibility and discreteness underneath clothing. This style of appliance is available in closed or drainable, and clear or opaque forms.

### Two-piece appliances

Two-piece appliances consist of a flange (base plate) and a bag that come separately and can be joined together by a clipping mechanism.

An advantage of this style of appliance is being able to leave the flange in place for several days, while being able to change the bag as required. This style of appliance is available in closed or drainable, and clear or opaque forms.

### Convex appliances

Convex appliances are used to ↑ the profile of the stoma or an end pointing downwards. They are often used if the stoma is retracted, flush with the skin, stenosed, or the stoma output is high. The convex appliance applies pressure to the peristomal skin and pushes the stoma out and into the appliance. This encourages the faeces to fall out into the appliance rather than tracking underneath the appliance onto the skin. A belt can also be attached to apply additional gentle pressure, further ↑ the profile of the stoma and securely holding the appliance in place.

### Biodegradable appliances

Following removal of the outer lining, the inner biodegradable lining can be flushed down the toilet. Waste material passes into an inner liner, which is inside a protective pouch (outer liner). To discard, remove the inner liner and flush it down the toilet; the liner naturally dissolves once in contact with water for prolonged periods in the sewage system. The clean outer lining can then be disposed of in the normal way.

### Fistula/wound appliances

There are now many appliances available for successfully managing an enterocutaneous fistula. When selecting the appliance, the following considerations should be made:
• Size of wound.
• Size of fistula.
• Volume of output from fistula.
• Flexibility.
• Patient comfort.
• Ease of management.

# Product choice: accessories

In most instances, accessories (e.g. paste, barrier protection, or washers) will also be used to ↑ the wear time of the appliance and protect the abdominal skin.

### Skin barriers

Sprays, creams, and wipes are available from a variety of different product companies. They are designed to protect the skin from proteolytic enzymes in faeces, other body fluids, adhesive trauma, and friction. Can be used on healthy or excoriated peristomal skin. Applied at each appliance change, but some can provide protection for up to 72 h.

### Paste

Highly effective filler and sealant. Can be placed in skin creases, folds, and dips to create an even surface. Because some pastes contain alcohol, they should not be used on excoriated skin, wounds, or ulcers. Can be used at each appliance change. It is not necessary to remove all traces of old paste. To spread the paste easily, use a wet finger.

### Seals/washers

Available in large, small, or thin sizes. Can be used to add convexity around a stoma, as a packing agent in skin folds, scars, or creases (similar to paste), or to provide extra skin protection around an enterocutaneous fistula.

### Powder

Designed for use on weepy skin. Forms a protective barrier against proteolytic enzymes in faeces and other body fluids. Applied onto wet areas and any excess is brushed off to enable the appliance to adhere securely.

### Protective wafers

Available in small, medium, and large sheets of hydrocolloid. Can be placed over large areas of peristomal skin that is excoriated or where an allergy has occurred. Provides protection to the skin and enables healing to take place.

### Adhesive removers

Designed to aid the removal of appliances or accessories such as paste from the patient's abdominal skin. Dissolves the adhesive of the appliance. Useful when patients are required to change their appliance frequently. The skin must be washed thoroughly after removal because some products can leave a residue that impairs the adhesion of the next appliance.

### Retention strips

Designed for use as an extension of the flange, providing extra adhesion. This could ↑ the appliance's wear time. Can also protect the edges of the flange from disintegrating when patients swim or during hot weather.

## Deodorant

Masks the odour of faeces. Available in atomizers or powders that can be sprayed or placed inside the appliance. If the appliance is securely in place, without leakage, there will be no associated odour. There should only be odour when the appliance is changed or emptied.

## Absorbing agents

Designed to rapidly absorb fluid from faecal effluent. Recommended for patients with an ileostomy to transform liquid effluent into effluent that is ↑ solid. This can ↓ appliance leakage problems associated with liquid effluent. Sachets are placed into the bag whenever the appliance is emptied.

## Belts/support garments

Various belts and support garments are available as a means of providing support for the stoma, particularly in the case of parastomal hernia, whilst also providing additional security to a stoma appliance. It is necessary for the SCN or a trained individual to fit such a garment.

## Further reading

Porrett T and McGrath A (2005). *Stoma Care*. Blackwell, Oxford.

# Storage, care, and disposal

Stoma appliances can deteriorate over time if not stored correctly. They should be stored in cool dry place, away from heat and direct sunlight. Patients should only order supplies as required. Stockpiling ↓ the effectiveness of appliance.

Disposal of used appliances brings about environmental concerns. Experts have suggested that used appliances (urine and faeces) are not classed as 'clinical waste' and are ∴ low risk, requiring disposal in heavy plastic bags. At home, the patient can safely dispose of appliances in household waste.

## Ileostomy

Drainable appliances should be emptied into the toilet and rinsed through. It is not necessary to clean the appliance thoroughly. The used appliance should then be wrapped securely in a plastic bag and placed in the domestic waste.

## Colostomy

Closed appliances should be cut at the bottom and the contents shaken down the toilet and flushed.

Delivery services supply disposal bags as part of their service. Nappy sacs or old carrier bags can also be used.

## Further reading

Black P (2000). *Holistic Stoma Care*. Baillière Tindall, Edinburgh.

# Discharge planning for the ostomist

Discharge planning is no different than that for any other surgical patient; it should commence on admission. The goals for a safe discharge home include the patient being independent and confident with their stoma care. If a patient cannot perform their own stoma care when discharged, community nurses or the family can assist. Before discharge from hospital, a patient should ideally fulfil certain criteria:

• Be independent in changing their stoma appliance.
• Tolerate food and fluids.
• Stoma active.
• Mobilizing independently.
• Have an understanding of what to do if problems or queries occur.
• Be capable of obtaining further supplies.
• Have an awareness of their limitations immediately after surgery.

On discharge, tiredness is expected. Mobilization is advisable, but exercise should not be undertaken too soon. It is expected that it will take ~3 months to feel really well following stoma-forming surgery.

Many activities should not be recommenced for 6 weeks following surgery. The list below is only a guide; each patient needs an individual assessment.

• Exercise (except walking).
• Driving.
• Working.
• Lifting.
• Sexual intercourse.

Issues to be discussed by the hospital staff before discharge home:

• Reintroducing foods to the diet.
• Practical stoma-care issues.
• Disposal of used appliances.
• Obtaining further supplies, including prescription information.
• Storage of appliances at room temperature.

When an ostomist is discharged home, they are usually given a limited supply of stoma equipment (~2 weeks' supply). Ongoing supplies are required following discharge from hospital; these are available using a standard prescription form. Obtaining further supplies of stock with a prescription is currently possible from a pharmacist, a dispensing GP, or a delivery company. If the ostomist has a permanent stoma, they can apply for a prescription exemption certificate. This is not available to those who have a temporary stoma.

## Further reading

O'Connor G (2003). Discharge planning in rehabilitation following surgery for a stoma. *British Journal of Nursing* **12**, 800–7.

# Prescription issues and obtaining supplies

Prescription prepayment certificates (PPCs) help people who require large quantities of, or regular, prescriptions to ↓ the cost when they are not entitled to free prescriptions on other grounds. PPCs are available for periods of 4 months or 1 year. PPCs save patients money if they regularly need more than one prescription/month.

Applications for PPCs can be obtained from the following locations:
• The Internet—at http://www.ppa.nhs.uk.
• By posting form FP95, which is available from local pharmacies.
• A pharmacy registered to sell PPCs.
• By telephone—on 0845 850 0030 (calls are charged at the local rate).

## Obtaining supplies

There are two options for receiving ongoing stoma supplies in the community. It is the patient's choice which option they use. In either case, a prescription for the stoma products is required.

### Option 1: supplies delivered by a dispensing appliance contractor (DAC)

Patients are given 2 weeks of stoma supplies on discharge from hospital. The SCN rings the DAC to organize a delivery to be sent to the patient's house as soon as possible. The patient must contact their GP within 5 working days of discharge to obtain a prescription and post it to the DAC in a prepaid envelope. Each month, for as long as they have a stoma, the patient must obtain a prescription from their GP and post it in the prepaid envelope to the DAC. Deliveries usually arrive within 2 working days. This service is free of charge. Patients also receive free wipes and rubbish bags with their delivery.

It might be possible for the DAC to write directly to the GP requesting the prescription. The SCN will arrange this. If using this method, the patient rings the DAC when they have ~2 weeks of supplies left. The DAC then writes to the patient's GP, requesting a prescription.

### Option 2: supplies obtained from a pharmacist

Patients are given 2 weeks of stoma supplies to go home with on discharge from hospital. The patient must contact their GP as soon as possible for a prescription. This prescription is then taken by the patient to a pharmacist to receive the supplies. This can take several days. Each month, the patient must contact their GP, obtain a prescription, and take it to the pharmacist. This continues for as long as they have a stoma.

## Payment for stoma supplies in the UK

Stoma appliance prescriptions are free for the following patients:
• Aged >60 years.
• Aged 16–18 years and in full-time education.
• The stoma or fistula is permanent.
• The patient or their partner is receiving Income Support, income-based Job Seeker's allowance, or Pension Credit Guarantee, or has an NHS Tax Credit Exemption Certificate.

Patients are required to pay for prescriptions for the following reasons:
• The stoma is temporary.
• They are <60 years of age.

# Lifestyle issues for the ostomist

## Travel

There is no reason why an ostomist cannot travel; however, they must make preparations.

- Advise the use of a travel certificate explaining the patient's condition—certificates are available in various languages.
- Check with the airline to see if an extra weight allowance is available.
- Take the majority of appliances as hand luggage.
- The change in air pressure within the cabin can create wind, so avoidance of fizzy drinks and eating too quickly should be advised.
- In the case of the colostomist, take drainable appliances in case of diarrhoea.
- To prevent dehydration, drink plenty of bottled water.
- Avoid risky foods that could lead to diarrhoea—raw vegetables, unclean fruit, salads, shellfish, cream, ice cream, ice in drinks, and tap water.
- Replace salt and potassium by adding salt to food, and drink fruit juices and savoury drinks.
- Use anti-diarrhoeals to assist with ↑ output from the stoma.
- Be aware of storage of appliances, especially in hot weather.
- Use of RADAR key whilst in the UK—allows access to disabled toilets.
- Ensure adequate travel insurance is taken out prior to travelling.

## Clothing

A well-sited stoma is not visible under clothing, and most people can wear the same clothes that they wore before their stoma-forming surgery. There are, however, clothing companies that specialize in garments that help to disguise the stoma appliance. Hints and tips might include:

- If a stoma requires siting near the waistline, it might be necessary to adjust clothing by wearing braces instead of belts, looser clothing, and higher-wasted skirts/trousers.
- Pleating in both trousers and skirts will hide any bulges.
- Track suits are baggy and comfortable to wear, which tends to hide bulges or weight gain/loss.
- Boxer-style swimwear for ♂ and patterned swimsuits for ♀ hide bulges. Also, a wrap, tankini, or skirt can be useful.
- Lycra underwear gives extra support for both ♂ and ♀. There are companies that produce underwear with pockets in to secure the bag.

## Exercise and sport

As a result of surgery, the abdominal muscles might be weakened. It is advisable to take short walks to begin with, preferably accompanied, because walking is an excellent exercise. The aim is to take a walk each day, ↑ the distance as the individual feels able. Abdominal exercises should strengthen the muscles, but these should not be attempted for at least 6 weeks after surgery. Swimming is a good way of improving overall fitness.

## Support garments and shields

A support belt or girdle is useful to wear during strenuous work and certain sporting activities, such as golf. For physical and contact sports, it is advisable to wear a shield. A prescription is required.

## Driving

Driving can recommence 6 weeks after surgery, but it is always advisable to check the insurance policy and with the insurer before returning to driving. ► The individual should have the ability to do an emergency stop and be aware that, if this action was to take place, it might cause pain or potential damage to the abdominal muscles that are not yet healed. Seatbelts can be a cause of worry, especially if they cross the stoma when worn. It must be noted that stoma patients are not exempt from wearing a seatbelt. A device can be obtained from most high street motor accessory stores that helps keep the seatbelt away from the stoma.

## Employment

Once physically fit, the individual should be fit enough to resume their normal work, usually ~6 weeks after surgery. Information on rights to pay during illness and general advice about returning to work can be found at http://www.dwp.gov.uk.

## Drugs

Many drugs can affect stoma function and some medications might not be completely absorbed. Patients should be advised to discuss this issue with the SCN, GP, or pharmacist before commencing a new drug.

## Sex and pregnancy

In most cases, a normal sexual relationship can be resumed, although it might take some time to recover fully from the surgery. Stoma patients might prefer to use a smaller appliance and some ♀ might wear a lace 'body' to disguise the stoma bag. Ileostomists can have a normal pregnancy and delivery; they might need appliance alterations because the stoma will change shape because of the growing abdomen.

## Information

- Ileostomy and internal pouch support group (http://www.the-ia.org.uk).
- Red Lion Support Group (http://www.redliongroup.org).
- National Association for Colitis and Crohn's (NACC) (http://www.nacc.org.uk).
- Colostomy Association (http://www.colostomyassociation.org.uk).
- Citizens Advice Bureau (CAB).
- Sexual problems of the disabled (SPOD).

## Further reading

Elcoat C (2004). *Stoma Care Nursing*. Hollister, Reading.

# Dietary advice for the ostomist

## Healthy diets

A healthy diet is important for all ostomists. This includes a balance of all the major food groups (protein, carbohydrates, fats, vitamins and minerals) (📖 p. 58).

Following abdominal surgery, it is important to reintroduce food into the digestive tract cautiously. The timeframe varies for each patient, frequently following a gradual ↑ in intake from the day after surgery.

## Dietary advice for colostomist

The diet for a colostomist is similar for that of a person before stoma-forming surgery. Each person needs individual assessment of his/her dietary requirements, but the general advice should be:
- Eat a varied diet.
- Avoid constipation.
- Drink ~1.5–2 L daily.

## Dietary advice for ileostomist

The dietary advice for an ileostomist in the long term is to eat a varied, balanced diet. Note that some foods might potentially cause problems, such as obstruction. The general advice for an ileostomist should be:
- Chew food well—to ↓ the risk of obstruction.
- High-fibre foods should be taken with caution.
- Drink ~1.5–2 L daily.
- Ensure adequate salt intake (particularly if stools are loose or during hot weather).
- Some foods thicken a loose output, e.g. carbohydrates.

## Further reading

Taylor P (2003). Other considerations in stoma care. In: Elcoat C (ed) *Stoma Care Nursing*. Hollister, Reading.

# Hints and tips: ileostomists

### High output

High volumes (≥2000 ml) of effluent from the stoma can lead to severe dehydration and electrolyte imbalance. Rapid transit of nutrients and secretions in the duodenum and jejunum lead to malabsorption of essential nutrients, electrolytes, and gastrointestinal secretions, producing a high output from the stoma. Consequently, vital nutrients and salts, such as sodium, potassium, and magnesium, are lost and need appropriate replacement.

### Clinical signs of sodium depletion

- Thirst.
- Lethargy.
- Cramps.
- Dark sunken eyes (panda eyes).
- Rapid low, weak pulse.
- Dizziness on standing.

### Treatment of high output

- Oral fluid restriction—500–1000 ml (any fluid, but avoid caffeine).
- Commence oral hydration solution (📖 p. 393).
- Avoid drinking and eating at the same time.
- Anti-diarrhoeals.
- Oral supplement drinks can be useful.
- Sprinkle a little extra salt on meals.
- Chew foods well.
- Avoid fibrous foods.
- Use a high-output appliance.

# Hints and tips: colostomists

## Constipation

Hard pellet-like stool, which may present as overflow diarrhoea. General advice includes:

- ↑ intake of fluids.
- ↑ intake of fruit and vegetables.
- ↑ mobility/gentle exercise.
- Administer prescribed aperients.
- If prolonged, seek medical advice.

## Pancaking

Soft sticky stool that collects around the stoma instead of dropping into the appliance. General advice includes:

- Grease the inside of the appliance with lubricating gel or baby oil.
- Screw up a piece of tissue and place it inside, at the top of the appliance, so as to prop open the aperture.
- ↑ fluid intake.
- Renew the appliance (ineffective filter).

## Wind and odour

Normal bacteria in the bowel digest fibre, producing gas as a by-product. General advice includes:

- Check that the appliance is fitted correctly.
- Use of deodorants.
- Place a soluble aspirin in the appliance.
- Put a few drops of vanilla essence in the appliance.
- Strike a match before emptying the appliance.
- Avoid foods high in fibre that have a tendency to cause more wind (📖 p. 76).

## Skin care

The peristomal skin should look like the skin elsewhere on the abdomen. If not, general advice includes:

- Check the appliance fits properly.
- Observe the patient's technique for changing the appliance.
- Redness/rash could indicate irritated skin.
- Refer to stoma care nurse specialist (📖 p. 236).

## Further reading

Breckman B (2005). *Stoma Care and Rehabilitation*. Churchill Livingstone, Edinburgh.

# Complications and management of problems: mucocutaneous separation

Mucocutaneous separation is the disruption of the suture line between the stoma and the abdominal skin, which usually occurs in the early post-operative period (Plate 3). The causes are linked as follows:

• Infection.
• Delayed healing.
• Tension on the suture line.
• Acute abdominal distension associated with post-operative paralytic ileus.
• Trauma caused by removal of the stoma rod or bridge.
• Difficulty exteriorizing the stoma during surgery.
• Rapid retraction of the stoma after surgery.

If the separation is minimal and does not cause difficulties in appliance adhesion, the flange can be successfully placed over the area of separation. However, if the separation presents as a cavity with a large amount of exudate, management is more complicated. Small clean cavities can be irrigated with normal saline and then confined within a protective paste or powder to promote healing. Sometimes, a small amount of de-sloughing agent or dressing can be used and lightly packed into the cavity. The use of a two-piece appliance might be helpful, to observe the cavity or ↓ the number of times that the flange is removed from the skin. The flange should be cut large enough to ensure that it can adhere to the healthy peristomal skin. Extensive wound infection is remarkably infrequent, even if the effluent is allowed to drain into the cavity.

## Further reading

Breckman B (2005). *Stoma Care and Rehabilitation*. Churchill Livingstone, Edinburgh.

# Complications and management of problems: bleeding

## Normal

The mucosa of a healthy stoma is moist and red in appearance. The colour results from the prolific blood vessels in the bowel. The bowel is not designed to be exteriorized as a stoma and can be easily damaged. There is a risk of the stoma bleeding, some of which is of no consequence, whereas other bleeding can indicate a serious complication.

When a stoma is newly formed, it is common to pass a small amount of fresh or old blood into the appliance. A haemoserous fluid might also be passed, usually in small amounts of <100 ml/day and generally only for a few days after the stoma is formed. This is normal and requires no intervention.

When cleaning a newly formed stoma, small amounts of blood may be seen on the cleaning cloth. This is normal and may be referred to as 'contact bleeding'. However, if bleeding still occurs when the stoma is cleaned several months after it is formed, it could be an indication of the following:

• Excessive cleaning.
• Anticoagulants.

In this situation, the cleansing technique should be reviewed and a more gentle action used. There is no need to actually clean the surface of the bowel and this should be discouraged.

## Abnormal

Bleeding from the bowel lumen could be an indication of a new bowel cancer, varices, or ulceration. If fresh or old blood is observed passing out of the bowel lumen in an established stoma, this requires investigation and the patient must see their GP or surgeon for advice.

Some ostomists are prone to the formation of granulomas on the stoma junction with the skin. This is often because of pressure or friction on the stoma edge and takes some time to occur. Granulomas are usually minor and might not require treatment.

It is possible that there is no bleeding and that the discoloration seen through the stoma is due to excessive consumption of certain foods, e.g. strawberries, red jelly, food colouring, beetroot, and tomato sauces. Certain drugs can discolour the faeces. Ferrous sulphate tablets, for example, can make the stool darker, which could look like old blood to an ostomist. It is advisable to inform the ostomist that certain foods, drinks, and drugs could discolour the faeces. In general, there should be no more than a few spots of blood when cleaning at any stage. Patients should contact their nurse for advice if bleeding occurs.

## Further reading

Porrett T (2005). The immediate post-operative period. In: Porrett T and McGrath A (ed) *Stoma Care*. Blackwell, Oxford.

# Complications and management of problems: necrosis

Necrosis of the stoma is localized death of tissue as a response to injury during surgery (Plate 4). The bowel mucosa quickly displays signs of necrosis if this is to occur, within days of the stoma being formed. Necrosis is fairly uncommon and can be left untreated or might require surgical resection. Signs of necrosis are outlined in Box 8.1.

## Stoma temperature

If the temperature of the stoma, when felt through the appliance, is cooler than the rest of the abdomen, it is an indication that there might be potential problems with the viability of the stoma. In this situation, the SCN or surgeon should be informed and the stoma should be checked every hour.

## Stoma colour

The usual colour for a stoma is red or pink. If the patient is slightly anaemic, the bowel mucosa could be paler in colour. If the bowel is dark red after surgery, it could just be that the bowel was 'bruised' during surgery. If the colour of the stoma is becoming ↑ dark or brownish, there might be problems with the blood supply and the surgeon should be informed. It is sometimes possible, if necrosis is not extensive, that a pink glow can be seen through the necrotic bowel. Surgery is not usually required. The surface of the stoma will simply 'slough off'. In the event of the stoma becoming darker in colour, check that the appliance is not too tight, which might cause the problem.

## Treatment

*Minimal necrosis*

Usually no treatment is required. The dark surface becomes loose, often within a few weeks, and this surface will 'slough off'. During this period, the appearance and shape of the stoma will alter, and the patient should be advised of this. Once this process is complete, the stoma will have a healthy red bowel at the surface.

*Extensive necrosis*

Surgery might be required, in which necrotic bowel is excised and a new stoma is formed. Complications could occur following de-sloughing of a necrotic stoma: the bowel surface might be considerably lower than the skin, the spout of the stoma might be lost, or the stoma might now be retracted, which could lead to leakage of the appliance.

Another potential problem can occur when the skin heals around the stoma: the skin around the stoma might contract, leading to a narrowing, or stenosis, which can cause evacuation problems. A rare condition, in which discoloured colon appears like a necrotic bowel, is called 'melanosis coli'. The bowel is dark brown or black in colour as a result of years of laxative usage. The colostomy remains this colour and no treatment is required.

## Further reading
Breckman B (2005). Problems in stoma management. In: Breckman B (ed) *Stoma Care and Rehabilitation*. Churchill Livingstone, Edinburgh.

---

### Box 8.1 Signs of stoma necrosis

There are a number of signs that a stoma is becoming necrotic. Thus it is important to inspect the stoma regularly in the post-operative period for the following:

- Temperature—stoma should be warm. A cool/cold stoma indicates poor blood supply.
- Colour—Stoma should be reddish/pink. Dark purple/brownish colour indicates poor blood supply.

# Complications and management of problems: prolapse

A prolapsed stoma is caused when a length of bowel telescopes out onto the exterior of the abdomen (Plate 5). This is largely because of inadequate fixing of the stoma to the abdominal wall at the time of surgery and can occur at any time following stoma-forming surgery. It is generally advised that the stoma is sited and created through the rectus muscle as a means of ↓ the risk of a stomal prolapse.

A prolapse is more commonly seen in patients with a loop colostomy, especially those with a transverse loop. If the stoma becomes difficult to manage or presents problems with leakage and odour, the SCN will need to advise. The prolapse can be managed by using a larger appliance to accommodate the extra bowel.

In some cases it might be possible to reduce the prolapse manually:
• The patient lies flat.
• A cold compress can be placed over the stoma as a means of ↓ its size.
• A stoma shield with a belt is applied to support the prolapse.

Caster sugar can also be added to the patient's current appliance as a means of ↓ the size of the prolapse through osmosis. Neither of these management methods is particularly successful.

▶ Ensure that the prolapsed bowel does not become damaged by friction or change colour. Most patients do not require surgery unless the prolapse causes intolerable discomfort or the bowel becomes obstructed or damaged. A small amount of bleeding could occur if the bowel is handled frequently and should not cause alarm. Primarily, all the patient requires is support and reassurance that this is not a serious condition. It is advisable to contact the GP or SCN as soon as possible so that they can be aware of and review the situation.

## Further reading

Collett K (2002). Practical aspects of stoma management. *Nursing Standard*, **17**, 45–52.

# Complications and management of problems: parastomal hernia

Bulging of the intestine through an abnormal opening in the muscle wall (Plate 6). There are three main types of parastomal hernia:
- Interstitial—the hernia sac lies within the abdominal wall.
- Subcutaneous—the hernia passes through the abdominal wall and into subcutaneous tissue.
- Intrastomal—the hernia passes through the abdominal wall, subcutaneous tissue, and stoma.

## Signs and symptoms

Can cause pain and discomfort around the stoma site because of the stretched abdominal wall and peristomal skin. The degree of hernia can vary from a slight bulge on coughing or straining of the abdominal wall to, in severe cases, a large painful bulge where the stoma might become retracted underneath the prominence. There might be a dragging or heavy sensation around the stoma. Some hernias can become strangulated and cause an obstruction of the bowel. Several predisposing factors should be considered (Box 8.2).

## Management

Abdominal supports can be used to disguise and support the weight of the hernia. These might be in the form of a belt or underwear and are available on prescription. The SCN can measure, fit, and order the correct size. The hernia could cause problems with the stoma appliance, e.g. the bulge can cause the appliance to lift off and, possibly, leak.

A new bag, or a bag with a larger flange, can be recommended by the SCN. Sometimes, the skin around the stoma can become sore.

## Surgery

In some cases, the hernia might become unmanageable, cause frequent obstructions, or prevent a patient irrigating the stoma, ∴ creating physical or psychological distress. In these situations, the surgeon might decide to operate, to repair the hernia. The most common method used to repair the hernia is a mesh. The mesh reinforces the weak muscle and gives extra support. Sometimes, the stoma is resited on the other side of the abdomen. According to the literature, surgical results are less than satisfactory and many hernias tend to recur within a couple of years.

## Further reading

Carne PW, Robertson GM and Frizelle FA (2003). Parastomal hernia. *British Journal of Surgery*. **90**, 784–93.

## Box 8.2 Predisposing factors for hernia

- ↑ age.
- Multiple operations.
- Wound infection.
- Heavy lifting.
- Obesity.
- Malnutrition.
- Peristomal infection.
- Steroid therapy.
- Poor abdominal wall support.
- Wide abdominal defect.
- Urinary retention (straining).
- Sited outside rectus muscle.
- ↑ abdominal pressure, e.g. coughing.
- Construction defects.
- ↓ muscle tone.
- Collagen defects/disorder.

# Complications and management of problems: pyoderma gangrenosum

Pyoderma gangrenosum (PG) is a rare debilitating skin disease, which is often associated with IBD (Plate 7). Although several theories exist regarding the aetiology of PG, the cause is still unknown. Pathergy, where lesions develop as a result of minor trauma, might have a role in 30% of cases. If PG develops in the peristomal area, treatment must not interfere with the security of the stoma appliance.

## Diagnosis

No single test diagnoses PG. Diagnosis is made on the clinical presentation and exclusion of other causes. Blood tests might be essentially normal. Skin biopsies exclude other causes, such as malignancy or infection. Colonoscopy determines any active underlying disease. Signs and symptoms of PG are outlined in Box 8.3.

## Treatment options

### Mild or limited disease

- Topical steroids (Haelan® tape, Trimovate®, and betamethasone valerate 0.1%):
  - Consistent, effective treatment.
  - Lengthy treatment period because of slow healing.
  - Area can deteriorate before improvement is seen.
- Oral steroids:
  - Improvement is usually rapid.
  - If prolonged therapy, consider steroid-sparing agents.
- Intra-lesional injections:
  - New lesions might develop at the injection site.

### Severe or widespread disease

- Systemic steroids:
  - Toxicity.
  - Steroid tapering after disease control.
- Immunosuppressants:
  - Used if the patient is intolerant to steroids.
  - Therapeutic action can take several weeks.
  - Risk of bone-marrow suppression.
- Antibacterials:
  - Used as adjunct therapy to steroids, either topically or systemically.
  - Limited success because PG is not bacterial in nature.
- Alternative therapies (hyperbaric oxygen, nicotine patches, and thalidomide):
  - Used if standard therapy fails.
  - Response is variable because therapies are based on anecdotal reports and small case studies.

### Surgery

There is much debate regarding the success of surgical debridement in PG. Although many case reports describe debridement as ineffectual and detrimental, others describe the successful treatment of PG by debridement. Surgery might be advised to refashion a short spouted or retracted stoma to prevent trauma to the skin from faecal leakage.

## Further reading

Lyon CC and Smith AJ (2001). *Abdominal Stomas and their Skin Disorders: An Atlas of Diagnosis and Management.* Martin Dunitz, London.

---

### Box 8.3  Signs and symptoms of PG

- Well-defined, circular, full-thickness wound.
- Punched-out lesions.
- Striking blue borders.
- Skin bridges.
- Irregular border.
- Rapidly spreading ulceration.
- Extreme pain.
- Overhanging edges.
- Necrotic centre.
- Purulent exudates.
- Satellite lesions.
- Surrounding erythema.

# Complications and management of problems: peristomal granuloma

A chronic inflammatory lesion (Plate 8). Peristomal granulomas form around the mucocutaneous junction of the stoma. The formation of granulomas can occur soon after formation of the stoma, but generally occurs after many years. Another term used to describe these masses is 'over-granulation tissue'.

## Appearance

A granuloma appears as a 'cauliflower-like' mass or nodule of granulation tissue. Granulomas are friable and tend to bleed easily if touched, such as when cleaning the stoma.

## Causal factors

Granulomas are often formed as a result of trauma, which could be a consequence of the appliance rubbing the mucocutaneous junction or persistent faecal contact. The growth of the tissue is a response of the body to protect the area.

## Treatment

The treatment for granulomas that are assessed to result from trauma from the appliance flange is resizing of the stoma appliance aperture to ensure no further friction. If the granulomas have occurred as a result of faecal contact, the skin needs protection from faeces. Checking that the appliance is providing a good seal is essential.

Treatment of the actual granulomas can include the following:
• Silver nitrate to cauterize the mass (if bleeding is a problem).
• Protective powder, paste, wipes, or spray (could be useful if pain is an issue).

If the granulomas do not cause any problems, they do not require treatment. Therapy will be of limited long-term benefit if the source of the trauma is not resolved, because recurrence is likely.

Note that care must be taken to exclude cancerous growths or other gastrointestinal disorders.

## Further reading

Lawson A (2003). Complications of stomas. In: Elcoat C (ed) *Stoma Care Nursing*. Hollister, Reading.

# Complications and management of problems: recurrence of disease

### Recurrent disease associated with a stoma

Cutaneous metastases might develop around or on the stoma. This is rare but requires prompt attention if observed. Recurrent disease can present as granulomatous warts or could cause stenosis if the cancer obstructs the lumen of the bowel. Recurrence can occur if there is inadequate clearance during the surgical excision of the cancer (Plate 9). There could also be metastatic spread through the lymphatic system or peritoneal deposits at the time of surgery, which can lead to a cancerous growth near the stoma. The cancer could cause a localized obstruction.

### Treatment

The treatment of any metastatic disease in or around the stoma depends on the patient's condition and prognosis. Surgery, chemotherapy, or radiotherapy might be appropriate treatments of choice. If these modalities of treatment are not deemed suitable, the nursing care of this rare patient group is as follows:
- Psychological support.
- Symptom control.
- Finding a suitable appliance.

Crohn's disease can occur at any position in the GIT. Therefore it is possible to develop Crohn's ulcers on or near the stoma. These will generally need systemic therapy and might be associated with Crohn's disease in other parts of the GIT. Medication, such as steroids, might be useful when applied topically.

# Complications and management of problems: stenosis and dilators

Stenosis occurs when the outlet of the stoma becomes narrowed, ↓ its elasticity (Plate 10). Patients with a stenosed stoma might experience pain and abdominal cramps when faeces are pushed through the bowel. Stool consistency is described as 'ribbon-like'. Stenosis, or narrowing of the stoma, is usually seen in the longer term rather than the early post-operative period. The causes of stenosis include:

• Scar tissue.
• Mucocutaneous separation.
• Pelvic sepsis.
• Infection.
• Poor surgical technique.

If the stenosis is not severe, a patient can be taught to dilate the stoma regularly under the supervision of the SCN. Dilation should be done at every appliance change, or as necessary, to prevent further narrowing. Some patients can use their fingers to dilate their stomas. However, some strictures can be too tight or the patient cannot insert their finger, so a metal dilator might be required (Fig. 8.16). Metal dilators (Hegars dilator, and St Mark's rectal cone: Roberts Surgical Healthcare, Kidderminster, Worcestershire) must be prescribed and can be ordered from most pharmacies. Faeces should be kept soft to aid movement through the bowel, and patients might need to be referred to the dietitian or GP for dietary advice or a laxative prescription. Some patients prefer a two-piece appliance for simple access to the stoma when dilating regularly.

## How to use a dilator

• Wear disposable gloves.
• Lubricate the little finger or dilator with a water-based lubricant.
• Insert into the stoma as far as is comfortable.
• Slowly remove the finger or dilator. It might be more comfortable to rotate the finger or dilator slightly when pulling out.
• Clean around stoma with warm water.
• Apply a protective wipe or spray to shield the peristomal skin.
• Remove gloves and wash hands.

If the stenosis is very tight, the stoma could become obstructed and the patient will require surgical intervention to locally mobilize and resect the narrowed portion. If the stenosis occurs through the abdominal wall, the stoma might have to be relocated to the other side of the abdomen.

## Further reading

Metcalf C (2001). Stoma care complications. *Nursing Times*, **97**, 43–4.

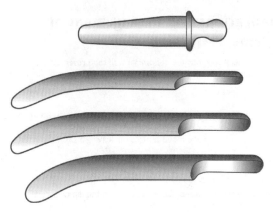

**Fig. 8.16** Dilators. Reproduced with kind permission © Burdett Institute 2008.

# Complications and management of problems: retraction

Retraction of the stoma into the abdominal wall can present as a shallow dip surrounding the stoma or a cavity with the stoma at the base (Plate 11).

## Causes
- Tension on the bowel at time of surgery—as healing occurs, the stoma is pulled into the abdominal wall by contracting tissues.
- Stomal necrosis—necrotic tissue sloughs off, leaving a small retracted stoma.
- Weight gain.

## Presenting problems
- Appliance leakage because of faeces leaking into the dip or recess surrounding the stoma.
- Skin excoriation because of repeated skin contact with faeces.
- Pain from skin excoriation.

## Treatment
- Convex appliance to ↑ the profile of the stoma. There are varying depths of convexity to treat this problem. It is advisable to start with the shallowest convexity.
- Washer or paste to fill in the dips or recess.
- A belt can provide additional traction to hold the appliance in place.
- If successfully managed conservatively, surgical refashioning of the stoma is not required. However, in some instances, because of the depth of the retraction and appliance leakages, this option might be appropriate.

# Complications and management of problems: phantom rectum

Pain or sensations related to a rectum that has been surgically removed. This is a complex and not fully understood sensation, but methods can be employed to help resolve it.

## Proctectomy

If the rectum has been removed (e.g. following a panproctocolectomy), it is common to have pain or discomfort at the site immediately post-operatively. This will improve in time, although analgesia is useful initially.
▶ If new pain occurs in this area, a nursing or medical review is required. This might be a symptom of a recurrence of disease, e.g. cancer, if the initial surgery was for resection of a cancer.

Although the rectum has been removed, it is possible to encounter feelings that there is still a rectum there. This is called a 'phantom pain' and might never completely resolve.

## Phantom rectal pain

Phantom rectal pain is poorly understood. However, there are many ways to try and treat it, so if one therapy is unsuccessful, another might work. One choice is medication, which includes analgesia or medical treatments that are usually taken to control epilepsy or depression. The pain control team might be required if these therapies are unsuccessful. A simple technique is to sit on the toilet and gently bear down. Although nothing will be passed, it can help to relieve symptoms.

## Alternative therapies

There are many potentially effective alternative therapies. This can include acupuncture, relaxation techniques, reflexology, aromatherapy, and homeopathy. Patients should be advised to have a medical review before commencing these therapies, to ensure that nothing sinister is occurring at the site where their rectum was.

# Complications and management of problems: constipation and diarrhoea advice for the colostomist

Bowel dysfunction with a stoma can make stoma management quite difficult.

## Constipation

Constipation can be seen as incomplete or infrequent passage of hard stools or difficulty in passing stools. The cause of constipation can be either mechanical or functional. Mechanical reasons can include intestinal obstruction, diverticulitis, or tumours. Narrowing of the colonic lumen, because of recurrence of carcinoma, adhesions, or stricture, can also cause a slower transit of faeces through the colon. Functional causes include reduced motility such as in immobile people.

Constipation is only encountered with a colostomy; failure of an ileostomy to function is usually because of obstruction and is a much more urgent condition.

Advice can be given on eating a healthy balanced diet. Encouraging a diet that contains fruit, vegetables, and plenty of fluids is required. Anecdotally, ↑ exercise or mobility can help. It can be useful for the nurse to assess the medication taken because some, such as various forms of analgesia, can lead to constipation.

Oral laxatives can be useful to soften or bulk the faeces, but ideally they should not be taken in the long term. Suppositories and enemas can be difficult to administer, because there are no sphincter muscles to retain the medication (📖 p. 306).

## Diarrhoea

Frequent passage of loose watery stools. There might also be associated abdominal cramp and generalized weakness.

▶ It is essential to establish the cause of the diarrhoea and treat it.

Causes include infection, IBD, gastrointestinal tumour, anxiety, and irritable bowel syndrome. Treatment might include:
• Antibiotics for gastrointestinal infection.
• Anxiety can be treated with relaxation therapy.

The symptoms of diarrhoea could lead to dehydration and electrolyte imbalance. If the illness is prolonged, these symptoms might require treatment. If vomiting occurs, IV fluids in hospital might be required.

If the cause of diarrhoea is found to be permanent following an extensive bowel resection, e.g. because of ↓ bowel length, the following might be useful:
• Loperamide taken 30–60 min before meals.
• Codeine phosphate—to thicken the faeces.
• 2–3 L of fluid daily (unless fluid restriction is required).
• Dietary manipulation.
• Salt intake should replace that lost in the stools.

Dietary advice can be given. This advice might be to ↓ foods that cause loose stools, such as spicy or high-fibre foods. Also ↑ consumption of low-residue foods, such as carbohydrates, might be useful.

## Further reading

Lawson A (2003). Complications of stomas. In: Elcoat C (ed) *Stoma Care Nursing*. Hollister, Reading.

# Enterocutaneous fistula management

Enterocutaneous fistula (ECF) is a rare complication and can be described as an abnormal track between the bowel and the skin (Plate 12). ECF most commonly develops after abdominal surgery, but can also develop as a result of inflammation, malignancy, radiotherapy, ischaemic bowel, and trauma. Post-operative ECF usually develops through a dehiscent surgical wound and arises from the small bowel, producing 2–5 L of faecal fluid in 24 h.

▶ See also catastrophic abdomen (📖 p. 304).

### Aims of management
- Fit and maintain an appropriate appliance.
- Protect the surrounding abdominal skin.
- Psychological support.

### Appropriate appliance selection
Consider the following points:
- Size of the wound or fistula.
- Volume—the amount of faecal effluent coming out determines the type of the appliance used.
- Flexibility—the appliance should be moulded to fit the contours of the abdomen in different positions, such as sitting and standing.
- Ease of emptying—the patient must be able to empty the appliance during the day and attach a night-drainage system overnight.

### Skin care
Healthy, intact skin around an ECF is vital to maintain an intact appliance (Box 8.4). Skin that becomes excoriated will cause the appliance to leak, which will cause further trauma to the skin, causing more leaks, and so on. This vicious circle will continue until the skin is protected and allowed to heal.

Appliances can be left in place for several days. The frequency of changes will depend on patient choice, patient comfort, and the condition of the skin surrounding the fistula. If the skin is healthy and shows no signs of excoriation, appliances can be left for as long as possible. However, if the skin shows signs of excoriation, the appliance should be changed more frequently, such as every third or fourth day. Establishing a routine for appliance changes (e.g. every third day) will ↓ the risk of unexpected leakages.

### Further reading
Myers C (1996). *Stoma Care Nursing: A Patient-centred Approach.* Arnold, London.

## Box 8.4  Skin care for ECF

- Thoroughly clean the skin with warm tap water.
- Thoroughly dry the skin. If the skin already has moist excoriation, a hairdryer can be used to dry it. A cool setting should be used and the hairdryer continuously moved for 5–10 min to enable the skin to dry.
- Barrier protection—intact healthy skin does not require any form of barrier protection, because the appliance will protect the skin from the corrosive effluent. However, if the skin is excoriated, barrier protection can be used to provide the skin with another layer of protection.
- Appliance template—the size and shape of the wound surrounding the fistula can change dramatically from week to week. A new template of the wound should be made each week to ensure the appliance correctly fits the wound and protects the skin from faeces.
- Skin creases—fill any creases or dips with paste or seals, or both, to provide a flat surface for the appliance to adhere to. Paste can be accurately applied with the use of a 10 ml syringe. Seals can also be used around the fistula to provide the skin with another layer of protection.
- The patient should lie flat after the appliance change for up to 1 h, with their hands holding the appliance in place. Heat from the abdomen and their hands will mould and secure the appliance in place.
- Appliance leaks—leaking appliances should be changed as soon as possible and should not be patched.

# Catastrophic abdomen

There is no precise definition of the term 'catastrophic abdomen' because it is a colloquial term used when things go wrong. A patient who has had abdominal surgery might develop a fistula through the wound, which is an abnormal connection between two epithelized surfaces, e.g. skin to bowel, otherwise known as an 'enterocutaneous fistula'.

Generally, 5% of fistulae occur spontaneously, e.g. in Crohn's disease/intraperitoneal abscesses, or radiation enteritis (damaged intestinal wall/poor nutritional state/high-dose steroid), and 95% of fistulae occur following operative surgery, e.g. a breakdown of intestinal anastamosis Common places for fistulae to exit are laparotomy wounds and drain sites.

## Nursing challenge

Catastrophic abdomen can present a nursing challenge because the patient might have large amounts of fluid discharging from their abdomen. Generally, the higher the fistula is in the GIT, the more fluid is lost.

## Major considerations

*Nursing assessment*

- Make a full assessment of the fistula—the patient must have an appliance that is clean, dry, and comfortable. The skin around the fistula must be protected. Consider the way the patient moves, contours of the skin, size and shape of wound area. How does the fistula changes in shape when the patient sits up? You might need to apply stoma paste to any creases that form, to prevent seepage.
- Management of the fistula—the losses from the fistula must be recorded on a fluid-balance chart because the patient is at great risk of fluid and electrolyte imbalance.
- Assess nutritional status—there can be a huge loss of protein through effluent. Ensure involvement of the hospital dietitian. Sometimes enteral nutrition is given distal to the stoma.
- Medication can be given to ↓ gastric secretions, e.g. octreotide (unlicensed use), an $H_2$ receptor antagonist, or a proton-pump inhibitor.
- Psychological care—healing of a fistula varies, and treatments can be prolonged. Therefore patient psychological needs should be addressed.[1]

*Practical management*

- For a patient who is discharging faecal fluid around a tube, the nursing emphasis must be to cleanse and dry the skin and to apply a drainable stoma appliance, which has been cut close to the tube size to ensure that there is close fitting of the appliance around the tube.
- For skin that is excoriated, either calamine lotion (to soothe and dry the skin surface) or a stoma powder (e.g. Orahesive®, which helps to provide a better surface for an appliance to adhere to) is useful.
- For skin that is unbroken, it might be appropriate to use a barrier (e.g. Cavilon) after cleansing to protect the skin—a skin protector applied around the edge of the fistula to provide an additional seal (e.g. Salts Cohesive seals/Dansac seal) is advisable.

---

1 Burch J (2003). The nursing care of a patient with enterocutaneous faecal fistulae. *British Journal of Nursing* **12**, 736.

*Further surgery*
Surgical closure might be necessary if the fistula fails to heal after conservative treatment. In laparostomy, however, the abdomen is purposely left 'open'.

# Administration of suppositories and enemas into a stoma

## Suppositories

If suppositories are inserted into a colostomy and just left, they will expel immediately, because of the absence of sphincter control. Before insertion of the suppository, the stoma should be examined digitally to determine the presence of hard stools. The suppository must be held in place, either by a piece of gauze over the colostomy or by the patient holding a hand over the appliance for about 20 min to allow time for it to dissolve.

▶ An ileostomy does not become constipated and ∴ it is inappropriate to insert a suppository or enema into this particular type of stoma. If there is no output, it is more likely to be a blockage, and instilling any substance into the stoma may lead to perforation.

## Enemas

Similarly, if an enema is instilled into a colostomy, it will ooze out immediately. ∴ the following procedure is recommended:

- Initially, examine the stoma digitally to identify the direction of the colon and rule out the presence of a local tumour.
- Clean the stoma and peristomal skin as usual.
- Insert a medium-sized Foley catheter well into the stoma and inflate the balloon to 5 ml so it will aid retention of the enema.
- Apply a drainable bag over the stoma and pass the catheter into the bag so it can be reached through its outlet. Instil the warmed enema gently, then clamp the catheter, tuck it into the bag, and apply its clip.
- After 10 min, deflate the balloon, remove the catheter, and re-clamp the bag.
- Allow faeces to pass freely.

An arachis oil enema can be instilled through the colostomy, preferably in the evening. Turning the patient onto their right side to sleep enables the oil to penetrate across the transverse colon. This might need to be repeated on the next evening. Note that anyone with a nut allergy should not be given an arachis oil enema.

## Further reading

Breckman B (ed) (2005). *Stoma Care and Rehabilitation*. Churchill Livingstone, Edinburgh.

# Medina catheter

A Medina catheter is a flexible plastic tube (FG30), which is 30 cm in length with a bullet tip (Fig. 8.17). At the top end, there are three eyelets: two oval eyelets on either side of the tube, and one small round eyelet on the tip. These eyelets assist the emptying mechanism, whereas the bottom end is funnel-shaped to assist drainage.

The Medina catheter is used to aid the evacuation of faeces from a Kock pouch (continent ileostomy) on a daily basis or from an ileo-anal pouch when there are difficulties with evacuation. Although the catheters are soft, when new they often feel less malleable and stiff. Regular use will soften them, making them more flexible. The life of a Medina catheter can vary from a few weeks to a few months. However, it is recommended that a new catheter be supplied daily while the individual is an in-patient. Most patients keep two or three catheters on the go at any one time, but they are advised to renew them monthly (Table 8.4).

## Guidelines for storing and cleaning

- Wash the catheter with soap and water.
- Rinse the soap and water through the inside of the catheter.
- Rinse well.
- Hang the catheter to drip dry over a clean surface, such as a paper towel.
- When dry, store in a clean zip-lock-type plastic bag.

**Table 8.4** Prescription details

| Name | Astra Tech code no. | Description |
|---|---|---|
| Medina catheter (ileostomy catheter straight) | M8731 | Sterile |
| | | Funnelled end |
| | | Single/packet |
| Medina catheter (ileostomy catheter straight) | M8730 | Non-sterile |
| | | Non-funnelled end |
| | | 5/packet |
| | | Short-extension tubing |

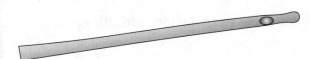

**Fig. 8.17** Medina catheter. Reproduced with kind permission © Burdett Institute 2008.

# Skin care: excoriation and allergy

Intact healthy skin is essential for the stoma appliance to adhere to the patient's abdomen. The most common stoma-related skin problem is excoriation caused by faeces leaking onto the skin; however, it can also be caused by trauma, infection, and pre-existing skin conditions.

## Excoriation

Skin excoriation from faecal leakage and allergy to an appliance have similar characteristics. ∴ a through history of the presenting condition and clinical examination must be undertaken to make a diagnosis. Signs and symptoms of skin excoriation are outlined in Box 8.5 (see Plate 13).

*Treatment of excoriation*
- Review whether the appropriate appliance is being used and change as necessary.
- Review how the patient changes the appliance.
- Assess the patient's abdomen in varying positions, looking for skin creases and dips that could be causing the leakages.
- Use barrier accessories to protect the skin.
- Use accessories that will ↑ the profile of the stoma.

## Allergy

An allergy to an appliance is very rare and only accounts for 0.6% of skin complications (Plate 14). For an allergy to occur, the allergen penetrates the epidermis and combines with the skin's natural proteins. This molecule travels to the regional lymph nodes where it is presented to the T cells, which make antibodies to that molecule. These memory-specific T lymphocytes enter the circulation, and when they encounter the allergen again, they react with it, causing inflammation. Signs and symptoms of skin allergy are outlined in Box 8.6.

*Treatment of allergy*
- Change the appliance to a different brand. Often, this alone enables the allergy to heal and no further treatment will be required.
- Place protective wafers directly onto skin and then place the offending appliance on top.
- Topical steroids.

## Box 8.5  Signs and symptoms of skin excoriation

- Excoriation only occurs in areas where there is faecal contact with the skin.
- Occurs within a few hours of exposure.
- Acute phase:
  - Usually at its worst 24 h after exposure—itch.
  - Well-defined erythema.
  - Clustered papulovesicles.
  - Wet weeping skin.
  - Areas of denuded skin.
- Chronic phase:
  - Dryness.
  - Lichenification.
  - Fissures.

## Box 8.6  Signs and symptoms of skin allergy

- Can occur after years of using the same appliance.
- Can occur on parts of the body that did not come into contact with the allergen.
- Inflammation occurs within 12 h of exposure.
- Inflammation is at its worst 3–4 days after exposure.
- Itch.
- Pain.
- Erythema.
- Margins are indistinct and blurred.
- Papules and vesicles are often seen.
- Small wheals.
- Might have blister formation.
- Lesions can become painfully eroded and crusted.

# Skin care: trauma and infection

## Trauma

Skin excoriation can be caused by trauma to the skin (Box 8.7 and Plate 15), as a result of too frequent appliance changes or a poor changing technique. Repeated appliance changes strip the skin of the outer cells that provide protection.

### Treatment
- Ensure the appropriate appliance is being used.
- Reassess the patient's changing technique. Closely observe the patient's technique for removing the appliance. Patients should gently remove the appliance with one hand, while supporting the skin with the other hand. Excessive rubbing of the skin by overly vigorous cleaning will damage the skin.
- Question why the appliance is being changed frequently. Provide support, advice, and education to patients who report only feeling clean when the appliance is changed or are finding it difficult to come to terms with their stoma.

## Infection

For signs and symptoms, see Box 8.8.

### Treatment
- Advise patients to shave once a week with a new razor in the direction of hair growth.
- Topical or oral antibiotics.

## Pre-existing skin conditions, e.g. eczema and psorasis

### Signs and symptoms
- Present on other parts of body.
- Plaques.
- Scaly dry thickened skin.

### Treatment options
- Treat dermatological condition.
- Topical steroids.
- Review appliance.

## Further reading

Lyon CC Smith A (2001). *Abdominal Stomas and their Skin Disorders: An Atlas of Diagnosis and Management*. Martin Dunitz, London.

## Box 8.7  Trauma: signs and symptoms

- Similar appearance to excoriation.
- Weeping areas.
- Bleeding.
- Areas of skin might be denuded or ulcerated.

## Box 8.8  Infection: signs and symptoms

- Pustules at the base of hair follicles.
- Multiple lesions.
- Itch.
- Individual lesions are painful.

# Colostomy irrigation

Instilling a measured amount of water into the colon through the colostomy. The goal is not to wash out the entire colon, but to induce a reflex peristaltic wave and evacuate faeces from the distal colon. This can offer a safe way of controlling how and when the colostomy works; it is not suitable for everyone. Irrigation is appropriate for end colostomy with a formed stool.

## Considerations during patient assessment

- Is there any active disease, such as Crohn's disease, diverticular disease, or radiation colitis?
- Evidence of cardiac or renal disease.
- Evidence of parastomal hernia, stenosis, or prolapse.
- Presence of loose stools.
- Good manual dexterity and eyesight.
- Motivation.

Irrigation is time-consuming and can take up to 1 h to complete. It should be done daily for at least a fortnight, until regulation is achieved; thereafter, it can then be performed every 48–72 h. The suggested total amount of liquid is 500–1200 ml.

An irrigation set includes a cone, tubing, an irrigation bag or a water reservoir, and irrigation sleeves. The hook for hanging the irrigation bag should be secured to the wall at shoulder height (as measured when sitting on the toilet). Lubricating gel is used to help insert the cone into the stoma more easily. A colostomy bag or cap should be worn following irrigation. Only tepid tap water should be used for irrigation. Problems can occur and Table 8.5 offers suggested management.

## Advantages

- Full control of bowel function.
- Confidence in personal appearance ↑.
- No need to wear an appliance.
- Freedom to relax more in social activities.
- ↓ in wind, irregular bowel motion, and odour.
- ↑ confidence regarding ↓/no appliance leakage.
- No need to dispose of used appliances—but a stoma cap is still needed.
- ↓ equipment to carry around.
- An irrigation kit comes in a small bag.
- Available on prescription.

## Disadvantages

- Time-consuming—can take up to 1 h/day or alternate days.
- Irrigate at about the same time each day.
- Inadequate toilet facilities (only one bathroom in a shared/family home) could make this procedure difficult for the colostomist and their family members.
- Irrigation can be difficult if away from the home environment.
- The procedure cannot be stopped and started, it must be continuous.

## Further reading
Williams J (2004). A stoma for incontinence? In: Norton C, Chelvanayagam S (ed) *Bowel Continence Nursing*. Beaconsfield Publishers, Beaconsfield.

**Table 8.5** Problem-solving in irrigation

| Problem | Suggested action |
| --- | --- |
| Unable to administer fluid | Move cone around while irrigating |
| Patient feeling very tense | Deep-breathing exercises |
| | Stop the procedure and try again later |
| Abdominal pain | Check height of reservoir |
| | Slow down the rate of fluid through the flow regulator |
| Bleeding from the stoma | Gently massage stoma with a lubricated gloved finger to dilate the aperture |
| | Be gentle throughout procedure |
| Scorched bowel | Ensure tepid water is instilled (recommended temperature 37°C) |
| Difficult evacuation | Water too cold or patient constipated |
| Dehydration/fluid retention | ↓ alcohol intake |
| Breakthrough of stool | ↓ amount of water administered |
| Seepage of water | ↓ amount of water used for irrigating |

# Antegrade continent enema

Antegrade continent enema (ACE) assists bowel emptying using irrigation (Fig. 8.18). Indications:
• To resolve constipation.
• To resolve faecal leakage from the anus.

### Surgical procedure

Surgically formed by creating a small passage between the bowel and the skin using the appendix or a small tube of bowel as a conduit. The opening is called an 'ACE stoma'.

### Post-operative care

A Foley catheter is inserted into the ACE stoma to prevent its closure. This catheter is usually left *in situ* for 4–6 weeks. Irrigation can commence 4 days post-operatively. Once Foley catheter removed, use a straight Nelaton catheter.

### Equipment required

• Regular-sized catheter (often size 8-12 FG).
• Administration set, with integral tubing and regulating clamp.
• 50 ml bladder syringe, with catheter tip.
• Solution of choice.
• Spigot.

### Common irrigating solutions

• Tap water.
• Phosphate enema.
• Saline.
• Arachis oil (not to be used in patients with a nut allergy).

### Complications

• Stenosis.
• Leakage/seepage of faeces.

If completely unsuitable, the use of the ACE stoma can simply be stopped or it can be reversed by another operation.

### Irrigation procedure

• Sit the patient comfortably on the toilet.
• Insert a small amount of phosphate enema (50 ml) into the catheter using a syringe.
• After a few minutes, insert the saline over of a period of 30–45 min).
• Faeces might be passed from the anus within ~10 min.
• Advise the patient to wear a pad in case of anal leakage.

Each day, gradually ↑ the enema and saline volumes until a good faecal output is achieved. For the best results, irrigate at the same time each day. Irrigating 30 min after a meal can be useful, so evenings can be a good time to irrigate. Most people use 200–500 ml of irrigation solution. Common problems and possible solutions are given in Table 8.6.

**Table 8.6** Problem-solving in ACE irrigation

| Problem | Action |
| --- | --- |
| Difficulty in inserting catheter | Initially insert smaller catheter, then proceed to standard size. If persistent, leave catheter in and spigot end |
| Abdominal pain | Should be temporary and resolve spontaneously |
| No result/soiling between irrigations | Ensure good irrigation routine. Do not repeat irrigation. Review irrigation regimen |
| Stenosis of stoma | Might require examination under anaesthetic (EUA)—dilatation |
| Gastroenteritis | Irrigation should be stopped until recovered |

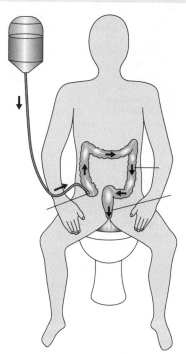

**Fig. 8.18** Irrigating ACE. Reproduced with kind permission © Burdett Institute 2008.

# Percutaneous endoscopic colostomy

A percutaneous endoscopic colostomy (PEC) is a relatively new procedure. It is designed to assist bowel emptying by irrigation and is suitable for people with the following:
- Constipation.
- Incontinence.
- Megacolon (for bowel decompression to release gas).
- Recurrent sigmoid volvulus (for fixation, not bowel emptying).

## Procedure
The PEC tube is inserted endoscopically. The tube is pulled through the skin into the distal colon and fixed.

## Irrigation
Irrigation usually commences 24 h after insertion of the tube and is carried out daily or on alternate days. This is not required for those with megacolon or volvulus. The procedure is as follows:
- Collect irrigation equipment.
- Fill the reservoir with 500 ml of warm tap water.
- Sit the patient on the toilet.
- Run the water into the PEC (this takes 5–10 min)—some people use a phosphate enema with less water.

Evacuation usually occurs within a few minutes and is completed in ~20 min. The major aim of a PEC is continence for 1–2 days or resolution of constipation.

## Disadvantages
There are a number of disadvantages of a PEC. There is a risk of infection. Minor infection and slight discharge do not require treatment, whereas severe infection is rare but would require antibiotic therapy and, possibly, hospital admission.

The tube might become dislodged. In the long term, this is of no consequence if the opening is reintubated within a few hours—a urinary catheter (14 Fr Foley) is ideal in the short term. The tube must be replaced every 6 months. Thus repeated out-patient appointments are necessary for the duration of PEC use.

If the PEC does not work, the hole generally heals over after removal of the tube. Removal of the PEC tube should not be done for at least 1 month after initial insertion.

# Stomal considerations with chemotherapy and radiotherapy

## Chemotherapy

Patients with a stoma who are undergoing chemotherapy often complain of diarrhoea. Patients using a closed appliance who experience diarrhoea during their treatment might need to temporarily use a drainable appliance or a two-piece appliance, whereby the flange can be left in place for several days but the bag changed as needed. If patients complain of constipation, a high-fibre diet and fluid intake should be encouraged. Stool softeners and aperients can also be prescribed.

In some cases, the stoma can become oedematous and inflamed. Because the stoma has no nerves, this will not cause the patient any pain but can lead to leakage of the appliance because the swollen stoma can push the appliance off. Patients should be advised to ↑ the aperture of their appliance while the stoma is oedematous.

Some patients might complain of pruritus, with an overwhelming urge to scratch. Avoiding perfumed products, wearing cotton clothing to avoid friction, and ↑ fluid intake to hydrate skin could alleviate this urge. Local anaesthetic creams or antihistamines can also help.

## Radiotherapy

Skin reactions after radiotherapy depend on the total dose of radiation, size of the area treated, and condition of the skin before commencing radiotherapy. Box 8.9 outlines the classification of skin damage following radiotherapy.

### Prevention and treatment

Patients undergoing radiotherapy should seek advice in relation to skin care from the centre providing their treatment, because there are varying recommendations.

### Preventive measures

- Wash the skin within the treatment area with a mild soap.
- Perfumed products should not be used on the treatment area.
- Moisturizing creams should be used to hydrate the skin, but avoid creams with alcohol, petroleum, or lanolin, and metallic-based creams, such as zinc creams.
- Loose clothing, preferably made from natural fibres, should be worn to prevent friction over the treatment area.
- Patients who shave their abdomen to ensure the appliance adheres to their skin should use an electric razor rather than a wet razor to avoid friction while receiving radiotherapy.

### Treatment

- Soothe erythema by placing the moisturizer in the fridge before use.
- Exudate should be blotted dry with sterile gauze.

- Moist desquamation should not be routinely cleaned unless there is evidence of infection.
- Repeated appliance changes will further traumatize already damaged skin; ∴ the patient should either change appliances less frequently or use two-piece appliances, where the base plate can be left in place for several days and the bag changed regularly.

### Further reading

Lyon CC, and Smith A (2001). *Abdominal Stomas and their Skin Disorders: An Atlas of Diagnosis and Management.* Martin Dunitz, London.

---

#### Box 8.9 Classification of skin damage following radiotherapy

- Erythema—red, dry, hot, and itchy skin (appears similar to sunburn); the skin might have a rash-like appearance or spots. Occurs 2–3 weeks after commencing radiotherapy and resolves 2–3 weeks after therapy ceases.
- Dry desquamation—red, dry, flaky, peeling, and itchy skin. It is often the precursor of moist desquamation. Occurs 2–3 weeks after commencing therapy.
- Moist desquamation—painful peeling skin that sloughs off, exposing the dermis. Bleeding could occur. Exudate could be serous, white, yellow, or green.

# Palliative care for the ostomist 1

Palliative care is 'the active, holistic care of patients with advanced, progressive illness. Management of pain and other symptoms and provision of psychological, social, and spiritual support is paramount. The goal of palliative care is the achievement of the best quality of life for patients and their families.[1]

## Common symptoms related to the ostomist

- Pain.
- Constipation.
- Diarrhoea.
- Intestinal obstruction.
- Malabsorption.

## Management of pain (📖 Chapter 21)

The patient's pain should be assessed using a recognized pain assessment tool (e.g. the McGill Pain Questionnaire or Brief Pain Inventory) to determine cause, intensity, and severity. This should be an ongoing activity, to monitor the effectiveness of interventions.

The analgesic ladder (📖 p. 694) is the mainstay of treating pain:

- Start with a non-opioid drug and titrate the dose against the patient's response.
- Move up the ladder if the patient's pain persists despite the maximum dose of analgesia.
- Do not 'side-step' if analgesia is ineffective—move up the ladder.
- Use the oral route unless the patient's condition requires an alternative.
- Give analgesia regularly.
- Use adjuvant drugs to supplement the non-opioid/opioid analgesic regimen, to treat each pain.

## Tenesmus

Tenesmus is the painful sensation of rectal fullness. The patient might experience spasms of the smooth muscle or neuropathic pain, which causes stabbing or continuous pain. Treatment (note some of these are unlicensed uses)

- Treat underlying constipation.
- Non-steroidal anti-inflammatory drugs (NSAIDs).
- Opioids.
- Steroids.
- Neuropathic agents, e.g. gabapentin.
- Radiotherapy for symptom management (may debulk tumour).
- Benzodiazapines.
- Calcium-channel blocking agents (which ↓ smooth muscle spasms), e.g. nifedipine.

---

1 World Health Organization (1990). *Cancer Pain Relief and Palliative Care.* Geneva: WHO Technical Support Senes 804. WHO, Geneva.

# Palliative care for the ostomist 2

## Constipation
Finding a balance between 'soft' and 'liquid' stool can be difficult to achieve. General advice includes:
- Use softeners or osmotic agents, e.g. docusate sodium.
- Be cautious with stimulant laxatives, e.g. bisacodyl or senna.
- Avoid danthron-containing products, which are only licensed for use in terminal illness and can cause 'burns' if in contact with the peristomal skin.
- Maintain adequate intake of fluids.
- Dietary modification.
- For faecal impaction, suppositories can be given.

## Diarrhoea
A full assessment, coupled with the patient history, should help to establish the cause; treat accordingly. General advice includes:
- Rehydrate—either orally or parenterally.
- Check for infection (in stool specimen) and treat accordingly.
- Consider the drug regimen.
- Check feeding regimen.
- Abdominal X-ray to exclude 'overflow'.
- Loperamide.
- Codeine phosphate (30–60 mg four times daily).

## Malignant obstruction
This can be partial or complete and could be caused by occlusion (e.g. tumour or impacted faeces) or a lack of normal peristalsis, or both. General advice includes:
- Establish the cause.
- Surgical opinion.
- NBM/intravenous infusion.
- Consider the patient's nutritional status.
- Treat symptoms—pain, spasm, nausea, and vomiting. The oral route should be avoided (the level of absorption could be difficult to determine). Use of a syringe driver/pump is recommended. Avoid metoclopramide and domperidone because they can worsen colic.
- Frequent/large vomits might require the insertion of a nasogastric tube.
- The administration of a somatostatin analogue might be necessary, to ↓ intestinal secretions (e.g. octreotide (unlicensed use), 300–1200 mcg/day).

## Psychological care
The impact of symptoms might be significant for the patient and their family. ▶ Seek expert advice (palliative care nurse specialist or specialist registrar/consultant) if symptoms are not controlled by simple measures. Assessment of the patient's psychological state, with appropriate intervention, should be an integral part of their care.

## Further reading

Doyle D, Hanks G, Cherny N and Calman K (2005). *Oxford Textbook of Palliative Medicine* (3rd edn). Oxford University Press.

# Oesophagus and stomach

Structure and function  328
Dysphagia (difficulty in swallowing)  330
Dyspepsia (indigestion)  332
Gastro-oesophageal reflux disease  334
Oesophagitis  336
Key drug treatment for dyspepsia, gastro-oesophageal
    reflux disease, and related pathology  337
Barium swallow/meal  338
Oesophageal manometry  339
24-h ambulatory pH monitoring  340
Oesophageal cancer  341
Barrett's oesophagus  342
Bolus obstruction (food/foreign bodies)  344
Oesophageal rings and webs  345
Oesophageal and gastric varices  346
Oesophageal diverticula  347
Oesophageal spasm  348
Mallory–Weiss tears  349
Achalasia  350
Nausea and vomiting  352
Hiatus hernia  354
Haematemesis  356
Gastroenteritis  358
Gastritis  361
Gastric ulceration  362
Helicobacter pylori  364
Pyloric stenosis  366
Gastric cancer  367
Gastric dumping syndrome  368
Gastric polyps  369

# Structure and function

## Oesophagus

The oesophagus is a muscular tube that begins at the pharynx and ends at the stomach. It lies behind the trachea and close to the greater vessels and the left atrium of heart. The oesophagus wall comprises six layers (Fig. 9.1). The upper third is striated muscle and the lower two-thirds are smooth muscle. The lower muscle is involved in tonic contraction, as part of the lower oesophageal sphincter (the cardiac sphincter). The vagus nerve penetrates the oesophageal muscle directly and through intrinsic nerves in the myenteric nerve plexus located between the longitudinal and the circular muscle layers and the submucosal plexus (Fig. 9.1). The oesophagus is lined with tough stratified squamous epithelium, changing abruptly at the squamo-columnar junction (the 'z line') to columnar epithelium. This junction is above the gastro-oesophageal junction and usually easily identifiable endoscopically. The gastro-oesophageal junction is seen where the gastric folds begin: 'nip' of the diaphragm often visible. Submucosa contains lobulated glands that secrete lubricating material.

The oesophagus propels food, fluid, and saliva to the stomach by a coordinated wave of contraction behind the food bolus, with relaxation ahead of it (peristalsis); it is an involuntary action.

## Stomach

The stomach is a J-shaped organ which lies in the abdomen and is adapted for mechanical churning, storage, and digestion of food. It comprises five distinct regions (Fig. 9.2). The stomach wall comprises seven layers; an additional oblique muscle layer supports mechanical churning function and enables expansion. There is an arterial blood supply through the coeliac artery, with venous drainage into the hepatic portal vein. The stomach is innervated by parasympathetic nerves through the vagus nerve and sympathetic fibres from splanchnic nerves. It is lined with a non-stratified epithelium. Mucosa covers coarse folds (rugae) with smoother antral mucosa. Tubular structures (gastric glands) have specialized cells for production of hydrochloric acid (HCl, in the parietal cells), pepsin (chief cells), and mucus (goblet cells). The stomach mixes food thoroughly by a churning action against a closed pyloric sphincter. The pylorus opens only to let semiliquid (chyme) through. Rhythmic electrical activity produces peristaltic waves three times per minute. Gastric secretion is stimulated by the anticipation or presence of food.

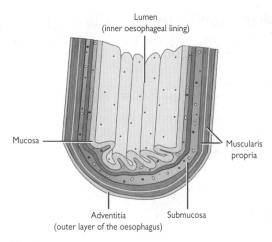

**Fig. 9.1** Oesophagus layers. Reproduced with kind permission © Burdett Institute 2008.

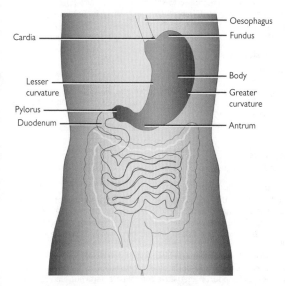

**Fig. 9.2** Five regions of the stomach. Reproduced with kind permission © Burdett Institute 2008.

# Dysphagia (difficulty in swallowing)

Acute or progressive; needs urgent investigation to exclude malignancy (oral, pharyngeal, or oesophageal).

## Causes

Numerous, including the following:
- Malignant stricture—oesophageal (📖 p. 341), gastric (📖 p. 367), or pharyngeal cancer.
- Benign stricture—oesophageal web (📖 p. 345), shatzki ring (📖 p. 345), or oesophagitis (📖 p. 336).
- Pharyngeal pouch.
- Oesophagitis or oesophageal candidiasis.
- Extrinsic pressure (lung cancer or aortic aneurysm).
- Achalasia (📖 p. 350).
- Oesophageal spasm (📖 p. 348).
- Globus hystericus.
- Corkscrew.
- Nutcracker oesophagus.

## Clinical features

Key questions will facilitate prompt diagnosis.
- What was the speed of onset of symptoms?
- Were symptoms in response to solids, semisolids, or fluids?
- Are symptoms constant, intermittent, worsening, or painful—odynophagia (📖 p. 334)?
- Are other 'alarm' symptoms present (i.e. weight loss or anaemia)?

## Investigations

- Upper GI endoscopy ± biopsy.
- Blood tests (anaemia).
- Barium swallow (useful in motility disorders).
- ENT opinion—if a pharyngeal cause is suspected (confirmed on barium swallow).
- Oesophageal manometry—if barium swallow is normal (📖 p. 339).

## Treatment

Treat underlying cause.

## Nursing management

Dependent on underlying diagnosis. Risk of regurgitation of food and consequent aspiration, particularly in elderly or patient nursed prone with reflux. Dysphagia will interfere with the delivery of food to the stomach and ∴ there is a risk of malnutrition, which should be managed as follows:
- Assessment of the extent of malnutrition.
- Dietetic opinion and appropriate nutritional support.
- Education and support if alternative enteral/parenteral nutrition is required in long-term dysphagia or during treatment (oesophageal cancer).
- Reassurance and empathy (for pain and anxiety).

# Dyspepsia (indigestion)

Non-specific group of symptoms relating to the upper GIT. ▶ Detect and distinguish organic disease from non-ulcer dyspepsia, which is a functional disorder without evident pathology but causes significant and persistent symptoms.

## Common symptoms

Epigastric, upper abdominal, or retrosternal discomfort related to meals, specific foods, hunger, or the time of day. Bloating and fullness can be associated with heartburn, flatulence, or early satiety.

## Investigations

Not all patients need investigation—follow NICE (2004) guidance[1] for indications (Fig. 9.3). However, investigations can be useful for the following reasons.

- Blood tests could indicate an organic cause, e.g. anaemia or abnormal liver function.
- Endoscopy will show pathology.
- Ultrasound of gall bladder and/or pancreas is performed if endoscopy is normal.
- A history can identify risk factors—including NSAID use.

## Organic pathology

Lesions identified on routine investigation include the following:

- Peptic (gastric or duodenal) ulceration (📖 p. 362).
- Gastric cancer (📖 p. 367).
- Oesophagitis (📖 p. 336).
- Gastritis (📖 p. 361).
- Duodenitis (📖 p. 382).
- Cholelithiasis (📖 p. 442).

## Treatment

Treat pathology as indicated. Persistent symptoms, despite treatment, indicate a functional component, e.g. a motility disorder. Explanation and reassurance is imperative, especially where the cause is functional.

## Nursing management

Provide education and reassurance on the following:

- The nature of dyspepsia.
- The treatment of dyspepsia.
- The rationale behind lifestyle changes to manage symptoms (📖 p. 335).

Provide support in making changes, including referral to appropriate agencies (e.g. smoking cessation or weight-loss programmes).

---

1 National Institute for Health and Clinical Excellence (2004). *Dyspepsia: Managing Adults with Dyspepsia in Primary Care*. http://guidance.nice.org.uk/CG17/ (accessed 14.05.07).

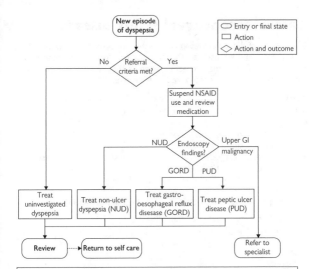

1. Immediate referral is indicated for significant acute gastrointestinal bleeding.
   Consider the possibility of cardiac or biliary disease as part of the differential diagnosis. Urgent specialist referral* for endoscopic investigation is indicated for patients of any age with dyspepsia when presenting with any of the following: chronic gastrointestinal bleeding, progressive unintentional weight loss, progressive difficulty swallowing, persistent vomiting, iron deficiency anaemia, epigastric mass, or suspicious barium meal.

   **Routine endoscopic investigation of patients of any age, presenting with dyspepsia and without alarm signs, is not necessary. However, in patients aged 55 years and older with unexplained** and persistent** recent-onset dyspepsia alone, an urgent referral for endoscopy should be made.**

   Consider managing previously investigated patients without new alarm signs according to previous endoscopic findings.

2. Review medications for possible causes of dyspepsia, for example, calcium antagonists, nitrates, theophyllines, bisphosphonates, steroids, and NSAIDs. Patients undergoing endoscopy should be free from medication with either a proton pump inhibitor (PPI) or an H$_2$ receptor (H$_2$RA) for a minimum of 2 weeks.

   * The Guideline Development Group considered that 'urgent' meant being seen within 2 weeks.

   ** In the referral guidelines for suspected cancer (NICE Clinical Guideline no. 27), 'unexplained' is defined as 'a symptom(s) and/or sign(s) that has not led to a diagnosis being made by the primary care professional after initial assessment of the history, examination and primary care investigations (if any)'. In the context of this recommendation, the primary care professional should confirm that the dyspepsia is new rather than a recurrent episode and exclude common precipitants of dyspepsia such as ingestion of NSAIDs. 'Persistent' as used in the recommendations in the referral guidelines refers to the continuation of specified symptoms and/or signs beyond a period that would normally be associated with self-limiting problems. The precise period will vary depending on the severity of symptoms and associated features, as assessed by the healthcare professional. In many cases, the upper limit the professional will permit symptoms and/or signs to persist before initiating referral will be 4–6 weeks.

**Fig. 9.3** NICE indications for investigations for dyspepsia.

# Gastro-oesophageal reflux disease

Dysfunction of the lower oesophageal sphincter predisposes to the reflux of acid from the stomach to the oesophagus. Because the oesophagus does not have the same protective lining as the stomach, complications can be caused if reflux is prolonged or excessive.

## Symptoms

- Burning retrosternal discomfort (heartburn).
- Belching.
- Regurgitation of acid, bile, or food.
- Excessive salivation (water brash).
- Painful swallowing (odynophagia) or food sticking (dysphagia) resulting from oesophagitis or stricture.
- Asthma (commonly nocturnal), whereby the volume of reflux leads to minimal inhalation of gastric contents.
- Chest pain, which can be difficult to distinguish from angina.

Symptoms are exacerbated by the following:
- Hiatus hernia (📖 p. 354).
- Obesity.
- Smoking.
- Alcohol.
- Bending and lifting.
- Tight clothing.
- Large meals—especially late at night.
- Pregnancy.
- Drugs, e.g. tricyclic antidepressants, nitrates, anticholinergics, and bisphosphonates.
- *Helicobacter pylori* (📖 p. 364)—the role of *H. pylori* in GORD is controversial.

## Complications

- Oesophagitis (📖 p. 336).
- Oesophageal ulceration (📖 p. 336).
- Iron-deficiency anaemia.
- Benign strictures.
- Barrett's oesophagus (📖 p. 342).
- Oesophageal adenocarcinoma (📖 p. 341).

## Investigations

- Upper GI endoscopy should be preformed as indicated by the NICE guidelines (📖 p. 333).
- Barium swallow will show hiatus hernia.
- 24 h pH monitoring (📖 p. 340) ± manometry (📖 p. 339) will distinguish GORD from other causes.

## Treatment

Drug treatment should be guided by the severity of the symptoms and adjusted according to the response (📖 p. 337). In very severe cases that do not respond to other management, surgery (fundoplication) is occasionally considered.

## Management and nursing intervention

Advise patients to avoid known precipitants they associate with their dyspepsia, where possible. These include smoking, alcohol, coffee, chocolate, fatty foods, and being overweight. Raising the head of the bed and having a main meal well before going to bed may help some people (NICE 2004). However, the evidence for these interventions is lacking. The mainstay of treatments remains drug therapy (📖 p. 337). Nurses can teach patients to take medication as required rather than continuously, and may help patients to wean from drugs once symptoms are controlled.

## Further reading

National Institute for Health and Clinical Excellence (2004). *Dyspepsia: Managing Adults with Dyspepsia in Primary Care.* http://guidance.nice.org.uk/CG17/ (accessed 14.05.07).

# Oesophagitis

Inflammation resulting from the prolonged exposure of oesophageal mucosa to refluxed gastric contents (as in GORD).

## Symptoms

The severity of inflammation does not always correlate with symptoms. Patients might be asymptomatic, but the condition can include symptoms of GORD (📖 p. 334). Severe oesophagitis could cause dysphagia from strictures (rare).

## Investigations

Isolated symptoms of GORD do not need investigation. Upper-GI endoscopy should be performed as indicated by the NICE guidelines (📖 p. 333). Inflammation is graded endoscopically according to severity using the Los Angeles classification.[1]

### Grade A

One or more mucosal breaks no longer than 5 mm, none of which extends between the tops of the mucosal folds.

### Grade B

One or more mucosal breaks >5 mm long, none of which extends between the tops of two mucosal folds.

### Grade C

Mucosal breaks that extend between the tops of two or more mucosal folds, but which involve <75% of the oesophageal circumference.

### Grade D

Mucosal breaks that involve at least 75% of the oesophageal circumference.

## Treatment and nursing management

As for GORD (📖 p. 335).

## Further reading

National Institute for Health and Clinical Excellence (2004). *Dyspepsia: Managing Adults with Dyspepsia in Primary Care.* http://guidance.nice.org.uk/CG17/ (accessed 14.05.07).

1 Lundell L, Dent J and Bennett J (1999). Endoscopic assessment of esophagitis: clinical and functional correlates and further validation of Los Angeles classification. *Gut* **45**, 172–80.

# Key drug treatment for dyspepsia, gastro-oesophageal reflux disease, and related pathology

## Compound alginates

Examples include Gaviscon® Advance and Rennie® Duo. These agents form a 'raft' that floats on the surface of the stomach contents, ↓ reflux and protecting the oesophageal mucosa. Used in managing mild symptoms.

## Type 2 histamine (H₂) receptor antagonists

Ranitidine is in this class of drugs, which ↓ gastric acid output as a result of H₂ receptor blockade. By suppressing acid secretion, they might relieve symptoms of GORD and permit ↓ in antacid consumption. They are used to heal gastric and duodenal ulceration (including NSAID-induced ulceration) but are not beneficial in bleeding peptic ulcers.

## Proton-pump inhibitors (PPIs)

Omeprazole is in this class of drugs, which inhibit gastric acid by blocking the proton pump in the gastric parietal cell. These agents are used in treating refractory/severe symptoms of GORD or in those with a proven pathology (e.g. oesophagitis), in addition to short-term treatment of gastric and duodenal ulceration. PPIs are licensed for ulcer healing and are the only acid suppressant that has been shown to significantly reduce re-bleeding rate in peptic ulcer disease. When symptoms abate, treatment is titrated down to a level that maintains remission (e.g. by dose reduction, intermittent usage, or substitution for a H₂ receptor antagonist). These agents are used in long-term treatment of NSAID-associated ulceration in which NSAIDs must be continued and in Barrett's oesophagus (📖 p. 342).

## Motility stimulants

Metoclopramide is in this class of drugs. Dopamine antagonists can improve gastro-oesophageal sphincter function and accelerate gastric emptying. They are used in some patients with non-ulcer dyspepsia (📖 p. 332) or as an accessory treatment for GORD (📖 p. 334).

## *Helicobacter pylori* eradication therapy

Acid inhibition using a PPI, in addition to antibacterial treatment comprising two antibacterial agents. The treatment choice is dependent on allergy to any component (e.g. penicillin) and previous treatment. Eradication is successful in >90% of cases.

# Barium swallow/meal

X-ray examination that can be used to determine the cause of odynophagia (painful swallowing), high dysphagia (difficulty swallowing), abdominal pain, vomiting, and weight loss, assessing suspected dysmotility disorders or suspected complicated hernia (strangulation or paraoesophageal), or if upper GI endoscopy is unsuccessful. Any significant suspected pathology should be followed up with upper GI endoscopy, where possible, to obtain histological evidence.

## Procedure

The patient drinks a preparation containing a radio-opaque metallic compound, barium sulphate, which shows up on X-ray. X-ray tracks the path of the liquid through the oesophagus and stomach into the duodenum; the focus of examination depends on its indication.

## Risks

Generally considered a risk-free procedure. However, there can be an occasional allergic reaction to barium, leading to anaphylaxis and aspiration of barium (where swallow is compromised).

## Nursing management

Ensure that patients have sufficient information to make a valid consent to undertake procedure. Advise patients to drink plenty of fluids post-procedure (to avoid constipation); warn patients that stools will have an altered colour (white/light coloured) for 1–3 days post-procedure.

# Oesophageal manometry

A pressure transducer placed into the oesophagus measures the function (competence) of the oesophageal body muscle at the lower oesophageal (cardiac) sphincter. The procedure is straightforward but should be performed in specialist centres where there is expertise to interpret the results.

## Indications

- Patients with persistent or disabling symptoms, principally.
- Dysphagia (with normal upper GI endoscopy).
- Diffuse oesophageal spasm.
- Achalasia (📖 p. 350).
- Chest pain of uncertain cause.
- Before anti-reflux surgery (predicts obstructive complications, which are more likely if sphincter function is impaired).
- To facilitate accurate placement of pH electrodes for 24-h ambulatory pH monitoring (📖 p. 340).
- NB: little use in reflux disease (it will predict those more likely to have severe disease).

## Method

The catheter is swallowed, sips of fluid are given, and the pressure during swallowing action is observed, recorded, and analysed.

## Nursing management

Ensure that the patient has adequate information to give informed consent (information might not be available locally). The procedure is uncomfortable; gagging and sore throat post-procedure can occur.

# 24-h ambulatory pH monitoring

A highly sensitive and specific test in the diagnosis and quantification of oesophageal acid exposure. Episodes of low pH in the distal oesophagus are correlated with symptoms (e.g. heartburn, chronic cough, and chest pain). The patient records meals and time spent in recumbent position, to see whether reflux symptoms are actually caused by acid reflux.

## Indications

- Definitive diagnosis of gastro-oesophageal reflux in patients with severe symptoms and normal upper GI endoscopy.
- Diagnosis of GORD as a cause of atypical symptoms (e.g. angina-like chest pain or respiratory or laryngeal symptoms).
- If surgical treatment is contemplated.
- Assessment of complex oesophageal disorders.
- Assessment of the effects of medical or surgical treatment if the patient remains symptomatic.

## Method

The pH probe is placed transnasally and sited 5 cm above the lower oesophageal (cardiac) sphincter—optimally identified manometrically ( p. 339). The probe is attached to a small recording device, which is worn around the waist; the procedure is completed on an out-patient basis, with the patient undertaking normal activities and returning after 24 h for removal of the probe. The patient also completes an events diary, including meals, symptoms, and periods spent in a recumbent position. The recording is analysed by downloading information into a computer program to give the frequency, duration, and pattern of reflux, which is correlated with the patient information.

## Nursing management

Ensure that the patient has adequate information to give informed consent (information might not be available locally). It is an uncomfortable procedure of long duration; ensure the patient has contact numbers for support (out of hours).

# Oesophageal cancer

Classified as 'adenocarcinoma' or 'squamous cell carcinoma'. Squamous cell carcinoma arises in the normal oesophageal mucosa; adenocarcinoma is caused by spread from the stomach or a malignant change in Barrett's oesphagus (📖 p. 342). Adenocarcinoma of the oesophagus now has the most rapidly ↑ incidence of any solid tumour in the Western world. Risk factors for oesophageal cancer include smoking (especially a risk for squamous carcinoma), GORD (adenocarcinoma; 📖 p. 334), alcohol, obesity, and achalasia (rare; 📖 p. 350).

## Clinical features

Progressive dysphagia and weight loss are typical, in addition to odynophagia (pain on swallowing). Hoarseness of voice, hiccups, and oesophago-bronchial fistula (because of local spread) can also occur.

## Diagnosis

- Upper GI endoscopy and biopsy (confirms diagnosis).
- Barium swallow.
- Endoscopic ultrasound (for staging).
- CT scan and endoscopic ultrasound ± laparoscopy (to assess resectability).

## Treatment

Early disease can be cured (oesophago-gastrectomy), but the majority of cases are non-resectable. Palliative treatment includes endoscopic dilatation, mesh-stent placement across the tumour, laser treatment (de-bulk tumour), chemotherapy or radiotherapy. There is no single best treatment.

## Nursing management

Must be coordinated through specialist multidisciplinary teams and a key worker (normally a specialist nurse). Dietetic input is essential, because dysphagia prevents adequate nutrition and post-operatively altered anatomy affects nutritional intake. Because of the high morbidity and mortality, early support (psychosocial and symptomatic) is needed from relevant agencies (e.g. Macmillan nurses). Post-operative recovery is prolonged and problematic, requiring reassurance, support, and early identification of complications (e.g. anastomotic leak—potentially life-threatening emergency).

# Barrett's oesophagus

Describes the replacement of the stratified squamous epithelium normally lining the upper oesophagus with an abnormal columnar epithelium (abnormality of intestinal metaplasia in this columnar epithelium; diagnosed on histology of biopsy sample). Identified as a pre-malignant condition for oesophageal adenocarcinoma (□ p. 341). Linked to chronic GORD (□ p. 334), which is easily identified on endoscopy, although most people will not know that they have it. Malignant degeneration follows a stepwise progression in individuals with specialized intestinal-type epithelium from metaplasia (normal tissue in an abnormal place) to dysplasia (abnormal tissue in an abnormal place) to invasive adenocarcinoma. Progression in not inevitable and the time taken for progression to cancer is unknown, but is probably about 1% per year.

## Investigation

Barrett's oesophagus is identified on endoscopy and confirmed histologically. The recommended method for clinical detection of early cancer is serial biopsy of Barrett's epithelium. Endoscopic surveillance programmes for this group of patients have been developed and refined over time (Fig. 9.4); however, their benefits remain unproven.

## Treatment

Management of symptoms is important, requiring ongoing review and early identification of any changes, especially 'alarm' symptoms.

Long-term treatment with PPIs is recommended, although there is no evidence for this.

## Nursing management

Surveillance is an intervention that can alter patients' life experiences and outcomes, potentially creating a group of 'worried well'. Nursing management centres on reassurance and education regarding the nature and progression of Barrett's oesophagus. Assessment of risk factors and appropriate lifestyle advice are equally important.

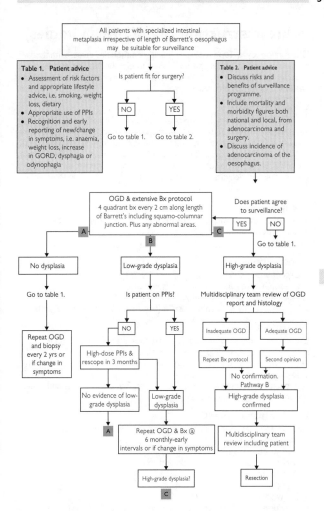

**Fig. 9.4** Algorithm for assessment and management of Barrett's oesophagus (Bx, biopsy). National Institute for Health and Clinical Excellence (2004). Dyspepsia: Managing Adults with Dyspepsia in Primary Care. http://guidance.nice.org.uk/CG17/ (accessed 14.05.07).

# Bolus obstruction (food/foreign bodies)

Obstruction by a food bolus is most common in those with known strictures, but fish bones and swallowed foreign bodies can also become impacted in the oesophagus. Young children, the mentally ill, and prisoners swallow a variety of objects.

## Clinical features

Often sudden and complete dysphagia for solids, liquids ± saliva, either at the cricopharyngeus or the gastro-oesophageal junction. Check the duration of symptoms, predisposing disease (e.g. carcinoma, stricture, or Schatzki ring (□ p. 345), type of food consumed (e.g. toast, meat, or fibrous foods), presence of other object (e.g. money, pen-top, batteries, or dentures), weight loss, and dehydration (if presentation is delayed, e.g. in the mentally ill).

## Complications

- Risk of aspiration with bolus obstruction at the cricopharyngeus.
- Risk of perforation with bolus obstruction at the gastro-oesophageal junction.

## Investigations

- Urgent upper GI endoscopy.
- Chest X-ray (e.g. obstruction or aspiration).
- Bloods (e.g. anaemia or dehydration).
- Barium swallow is often not useful (because of a risk of aspiration).

## Treatment

Endoscopic removal of the bolus obstruction if safe to do so (□ p. 196). If this is not safe, or if passage through the GI tract poses further risk (e.g. batteries or dentures), surgical intervention is necessary. Some objects, once in the stomach, will pass through the GIT uneventfully (e.g. beads or coins); however, if left untreated, check stools and repeat abdominal X-ray to check their passage.

## Nursing management

Support and reassurance during the acute phase. Psychological support as required if the result of an abnormal behaviour pattern. For those with known strictures, advise as follows.

- Avoidance fibrous foods, steak, and so on.
- Wear dentures.
- Eat little and often.
- Chew solids well.
- Fizzy drinks with meals.

# Oesophageal rings and webs

- Schatzki ring (the main type described)—symmetrical submucosal fibrous thickening occurring in the lower third of the oesophagus and at the gastro-oesophageal junction. Seen endoscopically above the diaphragmatic indentation. Other rings associated with high-pressure zones (observed manometrically) are found in oesophageal motor disorders and diffuse oesophageal spasm (☐ p. 348).
- Oesophageal web—not circumferential, unlike rings. Occur anywhere along the oesophagus, normally in the upper third. A cervical oesophageal web is associated with iron-deficiency anaemia (Paterson–Brown–Kelly syndrome).

## Features

Often asymptomatic and of no significance. Might present with intermittent dysphagia to solids and occasionally bolus obstruction. Must exclude other causes (e.g. malignant stricture).

## Diagnosis

- Upper GI endoscopy.
- Barium swallow.
- Manometry (☐ p. 339).

## Treatment

If asymptomatic, none required. Often, diagnostic endoscopy will prove therapeutic in disrupting the web or ring. If dysphagia is persistent, oesophageal dilatation is indicated. In Paterson–Brown–Kelly syndrome, webs regress spontaneously with treatment of iron-deficiency anaemia.

### Nursing management

If symptomatic, patients might require nutritional advice (e.g. eat little and often, sit upright when eating, chew food carefully, and sip fizzy drinks to relieve obstruction), because they often become 'afraid' to eat. Reassurance and explanation regarding the nature and progression of the condition is essential.

# Oesophageal and gastric varices

Portal hypertension causes dilated collateral veins (varices) at sites of portal–systemic anastomosis. Commonly occurs at the gastro-oesophageal junction and fundus of the stomach. Veins are inelastic and become more fragile as they enlarge; they are prone to damage, resulting in severe and large haematemesis (📖 p. 704). Risk of bleed is greater with ↑ portal pressure, size of varices, and endoscopic appearance of the variceal wall (red spots).

## Causes
- Liver cirrhosis—this is the dominant cause, which is prevalent with alcohol abuse.
- Primary biliary cirrhosis.
- Chronic active hepatitis.
- Toxins (arsenic).
- Portal vein thrombosis (e.g. malignancy or pancreatitis).
- Right heart failure.
- Budd–Chiari syndrome.

## Treatment
- Resuscitation (for bleeding)—correct fluid loss and restore blood pressure.
- Pharmacological therapy—↓ portal venous pressure (e.g. β-blockers or octreotide).
- Endoscopic therapy—banding is preferential (as for haemorrhoids) or sclerotherapy (as for varicose veins).
- Sengstaken–Blakemore/Minnesota tube—in life-threatening bleeds, balloons compress varices.
- Surgery—transjugular intrahepatic porto-systemic shunt (TIPS). Shunts blood away from the portal circulation (if patient is not encephalopathic).

## Complications
- Renal failure.
- Ascites.
- Splenomegaly.
- Encephalopathy—toxins not cleared through the liver cross blood–brain barrier, leading to an altered mental state. Can be life-threatening in an acute bleed.

## Nursing management
- As for haematemesis (📖 p. 704).
- Non-judgemental support (alcoholics).
- Mental assessment (encephalopathy).
- Nutritional support.
- Involvement of appropriate agencies.

# Oesophageal diverticula

Pouches lined with one or more layers of the oesophageal wall. Occur immediately above the upper oesophageal sphincter (Zenker's diverticulum or pharyngeal pouch), near the mid-oesophagus, or immediately above the lower oesophageal (cardiac) sphincter (epiphrenic diverticulum). The pharyngeal pouch (Zenker's diverticulum) is the most important form because it can be large enough to obstruct the oesophageal lumen, causing dysphagia and aspiration of its contents (with respiratory complications).

## Causes

Unclear. It is present in intermittent dysphagia and regurgitation in the elderly, possibly as a result of abnormal motility and incoordination of sphincter relaxation. Mid-oesophageal diverticulum is more likely because of traction from inflammatory adhesions in the mediastinum.

## Symptoms

Often asymptomatic. Symptoms are related to associated motor disorders in lower oesophageal (epiphrenic) diverticulum, and dysphagia, pain, and aspiration (with respiratory complications) are associated with a pharyngeal pouch.

## Diagnosis

Upper GI endoscopy is dangerous because the endoscope could enter the false lumen and perforate the diverticulum if it is not recognized. Barium swallow and possible ENT opinion are recommended.

## Treatment

None if the patient is asymptomatic. Surgical excision (± cricopharyngeal myotomy) is the treatment of choice for symptomatic patients with pharyngeal pouch.

## Nursing management

Reassurance and support if symptomatic.

# Oesophageal spasm

A disorder of the normal peristaltic activity of the oesophagus. Diffuse oesophageal spasm can produce a characteristic 'corkscrew' appearance of the oesophagus on barium swallow.

## Symptoms

Patients complain of episodic dysphagia (📖 p. 330) and chest pain that might resemble angina. Symptoms can occur without warning, but are frequently provoked by ingestion of fluids at extreme temperatures and also by stress. Half of patients will have symptoms of GORD (📖 p. 334). Symptoms are caused by high-amplitude aperistaltic oesophageal contractions.

## Investigations

- Upper GI endoscopy—not normally helpful, although multiple simultaneous ring contractions might be seen, and other pathology can be excluded (spasm secondary to a distal obstruction).
- Barium swallow—corkscrew appearance is classic but unusual; aperistaltic contractions are common when recumbent.
- Manometry—diagnostic if positive, although negative results do not exclude the diagnosis.

## Treatment

It is not possible to relieve symptoms totally. Dilatation (📖 p. 188) is reserved for the most severe cases because the outcome is unpredictable. Drugs tried include those used for angina, amitriptyline, nifedipine, and nitrites (smooth muscle relaxants).

## Nursing management

Symptoms can be distressing and frightening. Patients need reassurance that the pain is not cardiac, especially because some drugs prescribed are also used for angina. Avoidance of extreme temperatures of fluids is advised if causative; eating little and often might help. Patients should sit upright when eating and after meals to aid movement of food down the oesophagus.

# Mallory–Weiss tears

A tear in the mucosa of the oesophagus (often at the gastro-oesophageal junction) caused by forceful vomiting and resulting in haematemesis.

## Features

History of forceful vomiting (no blood in initial vomitus); often provoked by alcohol in younger patients.

## Treatment

The majority of cases settle with conservative management. Endoscopy might not reveal the site of the tear but will exclude other diagnoses.

## Nursing management

The condition is distressing for patients and ∴ requires empathetic and reassuring management. Observation, recording, and reporting of the quantity and consistency of vomitus and vital signs if vomiting and/or haematemesis is prolonged.

# Achalasia

Motility disorder due to degeneration of the myenteric plexus (the nerves within the wall of the oesophagus); the cause is unknown. Possible autonomic neuropathy. Results in ↑ lower oesophageal sphincter pressure and failure to relax during swallowing, absent peristaltic action of oesophagus, dilatation, and accumulation of undigested food in lower oesophagus.

## Features
- Occurs at any age.
- Slow progressive dysphagia (📖 p. 330).
- Weight loss.
- Regurgitation (undigested food) and aspiration (pneumonia).
- Pain (often severe and retrosternal).
- Mega-oesophagus (with ↑ risk of cancer).

## Investigation
Exclude other diagnoses, especially oesophageal carcinoma, or diffuse spasm using the following investigations:
- Chest X-ray—will show oesophageal fluid level and fibrosis.
- Barium swallow—will show oesophageal dilatation, smooth, tapered distal narrowing, food debris, and absence of peristalsis.
- Upper GI endoscopy—to exclude stricture and examine the mucosa for cancer.
- Manometry—to exclude spasm.

## Treatment
Degeneration of the nerves cannot be corrected, so treatment is directed at symptom control and preventing complications. Balloon dilatation under X-ray screening is effective but could require frequent repeats (with a risk of perforation). Surgery is indicated if dilatation is ineffectual, frequent, or at the patient's request. Oral smooth muscle relaxants include nitrates and nifedipine; generally ineffective. Injection with botulinum toxin may help, especially in the elderly.

### Nursing management
Symptoms are difficult to resolve; treatment might worsen symptoms (e.g. relaxation might cause reflux and pain), leading to anxiety. Management is aimed at reassurance, explanation, and education. Nutritional support, with dietetic referral, if appropriate. Observe, record, and report symptoms, including regurgitation and signs of aspiration.

# Nausea and vomiting

Seen as a protective mechanism, nausea deters ingestion of offending substances and vomiting forcefully expels them. Nausea precedes vomiting but either can occur in isolation. The causes are numerous, including neurological, psychological, chemical, and mechanical causes (Table 9.1). Treatment is focused on the underlying cause.

## Mechanism

The vomiting centre in the medulla oblongata is the main site of neural control of vomiting. It receives and coordinates signals from a number of other centres and orchestrates a series of events that result in nausea, retching, or vomiting. Intrinsic muscles of stomach and oesophagus relax and the gastric contents are propelled upwards (reverse peristalsis). Muscle contraction ↑ intra-abdominal and intrathoracic pressure, aiding expulsion.

## Consequences

- Anorexia, weight loss, and fluid and electrolyte imbalance.
- Aspiration of vomitus with asphyxiation, chemical inflammation, or bacterial infection (inebriated or unconscious patients).
- Tear in oesophageal mucosa, e.g. Mallory–Weiss tear (📖 p. 349), causing haematemesis.
- Chronic vomiting (e.g. bulimia nervosa) can cause acid damage to teeth.

## Treatment

Dependent on the underlying cause, but includes appropriate anti-emetic therapy (Table 9.2)—use with caution, as prolonged use may disguise severity of symptoms and thus delay diagnosis—correction of fluid and electrolyte imbalance, endoscopy (if vomiting is prolonged), and a pregnancy test.

## Nursing management

- Record and report the volume and consistency of vomit—colour, blood, bile, and content.
- Observe for signs and symptoms of dehydration, i.e. ↓ urine output and dry tongue.
- Observe for signs and symptoms of malnutrition, monitor weight, and get dietetic input.
- Reassure and provide empathetic support—especially in chronic vomiting.

**Table 9.1** Common causes of nausea and vomiting

**Abdominal**

Gastroenteritis, peptic ulceration, pyloric stenosis, intestinal obstruction, pancreatitis, cholecystitis, appendicitis, malignancy ileus, constipation

**Irritation**

Bacterial/viral infection, food poisoning, gastric manipulation (surgery)

**Metabolic**

Diabetic ketoacidosis, hypercalcaemia, hyponatraemia, uraemia

**Drugs**

Opiates, chemotherapy, anaesthetic agents, antibiotics, many others

**Cerebral**

↑ intracranial pressure, migraine

**Vestibular**

Motion sickness, Ménière's disease

**Endocrine**

Pregnancy, Addison's disease

**Non-organic**

Severe pain, non-ulcer dyspepsia, bulimia, self-induced, memory association, unpleasant smells, offensive sights, anxiety

**Table 9.2** Anti-emetic drugs and their uses

| Drug classification | Example | Use |
| --- | --- | --- |
| Antihistamines | Cyclizine | Motion sickness, Ménière's disease |
| Phenothiazines | Chlorpromazine | Terminal illness, emesis caused by anaesthetics and opioids |
| Dopamine antagonist | Metoclopramide | Post-operative, GI disorders, migraine, cytotoxic drug therapies |
| | Domperidone | Cytotoxic drug therapies |
| Serotonin (5-HT₃) antagonists | Granisetron | Post-operative, cytotoxic drug therapies |
| Anticholinergics | Hyoscine hydrobromide | Motion sickness |
| Cannabinoid | Nabilone | Cytotoxic drug therapies unresponsive to conventional anti-emetics |

# Hiatus hernia

Occurs when the proximal stomach herniates through the diaphragm and into the thorax.

## Types

See Fig. 9.5.

- Sliding (80%)—the gastro-oesophageal junction slides up into the chest.
- Rolling or para-oesophageal (20%)—the gastro-oesophageal junction remains in the abdomen, but a portion of stomach herniates up into the chest alongside the oesophagus.

## Clinical features

Hiatus hernia is common, more so in obese patients. Half of all patients will have symptoms of gastro-oesophageal reflux (📖 p. 334).

## Investigations

Barium swallow is the best diagnostic test to ascertain the type and size of hiatus hernia. Often diagnosed incidentally on upper GI endoscopy in patients with gastro-oesophageal reflux or symptoms of dyspepsia (📖 p. 332).

## Management

Treatment and management of reflux symptoms (📖 p. 334), including weight loss. Surgery indicated if patient's symptoms are unmanageable and radiological, and pH monitoring (📖 p. 340) confirms severe reflux, or there is a para-oesophageal component and risk of strangulation.

## Nursing intervention

- Education and reassurance regarding the following:
  - The nature of hiatus hernia.
  - The treatment of hiatus hernia.
  - The rationale behind lifestyle changes to manage reflux symptoms (📖 p. 335).
- Support in making changes, including referral to appropriate agencies, e.g. smoking cessation and weight-loss programmes.

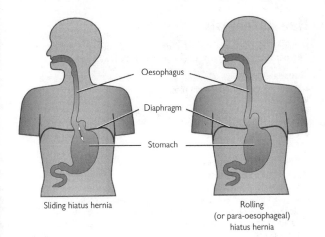

Oesophagus

Diaphragm

Stomach

Sliding hiatus hernia

Rolling
(or para-oesophageal)
hiatus hernia

**Fig. 9.5** Types of hiatus hernia. Reproduced with kind permission © Burdett Institute 2008.

# Haematemesis

Vomiting of fresh or altered (coffee-ground) blood. Commonest of gastroenterology emergencies (📖 p. 704). Risk ↑ with age.

## Causes
- Peptic (gastric or duodenal) ulcers.
- NSAIDs.
- Oesophageal and gastric varices (📖 p. 346).
- Mallory–Weiss tear (📖 p. 349).
- Oesophagitis (📖 p. 336).
- Gastric cancer (📖 p. 367).
- Angiodysplasia.

## Treatment approach
- Resuscitate and then fluid replacement.
- Assess cause and severity—obtain history, including NSAID and alcohol use, and observe vomitus.
- Establish the site of bleed—upper GI endoscopy by experienced endoscopist.
- Assess risk of re-bleed and death—Rockall risk score (📖 p. 706).
- Treat—endoscopic therapy to halt bleeding, drugs (i.e. PPI ± eradication therapy).
- Prevention—stop NSAIDs.
- Surgery—dependent on the severity of bleed or re-bleed.

## Nursing management
Haematemesis is distressing for patients and ∴ requires empathetic and reassuring management. Observation, recording, and reporting of the quantity and consistency of vomitus and vital signs if vomiting and/or haematemesis is prolonged.

# Gastroenteritis

Ingestion of bacteria, viruses, or toxins resulting in diarrhoea, vomiting, and abdominal pain of acute onset and short duration. Commonly caused by food poisoning (a notifiable disease in the UK), but often no specific cause is found (50%). Elderly or very young, immunocompromised, or hyposplenic patients are among those most susceptible to gastroenteritis.

## Causes

Possible causes are listed in Table 9.3. Symptoms from excess alcohol intake can mimic infective causes.

## Features

- History of travel.
- Eating unusual or known susceptible food types (e.g. seafood, chicken, reheated food, or take-aways).
- Excessive antibiotic use.
- More than one person affected (e.g. families, schools, or institutions).
- History of swimming or other water sport.
- Bloody diarrhoea.
- Abdominal cramps.
- Fever.
- Aching joints.
- Headaches.
- Speedy resolution.

## Investigation and treatment

Treatment is dependent on the cause, although the illness might not need investigation if uncomplicated and quickly resolved. Stool specimens for microscopy, culture, and sensitivity (MC&S) and *Clostridium difficile* toxin should be obtained. If an outbreak is suspected (e.g. in a school), food-sample analysis is recommended. If diarrhoea is persistent or associated with bleeding, refer to a gastroenterologist for endoscopic assessment. Anti-diarrhoeal and anti-emetic agents should be used with caution if symptom control is required (they could mask other conditions). In-patients should be isolated until an infective cause is excluded.

## Nursing management

### Prevention

Education on basic hygiene (e.g. hand-washing and food preparation) and precautionary measures when abroad (e.g. bottled water, avoiding ice cubes, avoiding salads, and peeling fruit).

### Acute attack

Ensure adequate fluid intake (oral rehydration fluids if diarrhoea is severe and IV fluids if the patient is dehydrated) and meticulous hygiene (e.g. hand-washing and clean eating utensils). Maintain privacy and dignity (e.g. toilet access, air fresheners, and clean laundry).

**Table 9.3** Possible causes of gastroenteritis

| Organism or source | Incubation period | Features | Associated food |
|---|---|---|---|
| Staphylococcus aureus | 1–6 h | Diarrhoea & vomiting (D&V), pain, hypotension | Meat |
| Bacillus cereus | 1–5 h | D&V | Rice |
| Red beans | 1–3 h | D&V | |
| Heavy metals (zinc) | 5 min to 2 h | Vomiting, pain (zinc) ± flu-like symptoms | |
| Scrombotoxin | 10–60 min | Diarrhoea, flushing, sweating, hot mouth | Fish |
| Mushrooms | 15 min to 24 h | D&V, abdominal pain, fits, coma, hepatic and renal failure | Mushrooms |
| Salmonella spp | 12–48 h | D&V, fever, septicaemia | Meat, eggs, poultry |
| Clostridium perfingens | 8–24 h | Diarrhoea, pain | Meat |
| Clostridium botulinum | 12–36 h | Vomiting, paralysis | Processed food |
| Clostridium difficile | 1–7 days | Bloody diarrhoea, diarrhoea, pain | |
| Vibrio parahaemolyticus | 12–24 h | Profuse diarrhoea, pain, vomiting | Seafood |
| Vibrio cholerae | 5 h to 10 days | Profuse diarrhoea, fever, vomiting, rapid dehydration | Water |
| Campylobacter spp Listeria spp | 2–5 days | Bloody diarrhoea, pain, fever, meningoencephalitis, flu-like symptoms, miscarriage | Milk, poultry, water, cheese, paté |
| Small round structured viruses | 36–72 h | D&V, fever, malaise | Any food |
| Escherichia coli type 0157 | 12–72 h | Cholera/ typhoid-like symptoms | |
| Yersinia enterocolitica | 24–36 h | Diarrhoea, pain, fever | Milk |

**Table 9.3** (Contd.)

| Organism or source | Incubation period | Features | Transmission |
|---|---|---|---|
| Cryptosporidium spp | 4–12 days | Diarrhoea in HIV | Cow/ water/man |
| Giardia lamblia | 1–4 weeks | Might be asymptomatic, lassitude, bloating, weight loss, explosive diarrhoea | Water |
| Entamoeba histolytica | 1–4 weeks | Slow onset, profuse and bloody diarrhoea | Food or water borne |
| Rotaviruses | 1–7 days | D&V, fever, malaise | Food or water borne |
| Shigella spp | 2–3 days | Bloody diarrhoea, pain, fever | Any food |

# Gastritis

Inflammation of the stomach (gastric) mucosa, as a response to injury. Mainly classified as 'acute' or 'chronic', although there are rarer special forms. Can be isolated to one area of the stomach (e.g. antrum, body, or fundus) or affect all of the stomach as 'pan' (total) gastritis.

## Causes

- Drugs (mainly NSAIDs).
- Alcohol.
- Severe stress (e.g. major surgery, trauma, or burns).
- Infection (e.g. *Helicobacter pylori*).
- Post-gastrectomy (bile reflux: alkaline toxicity).
- Crohn's disease (rare).
- HIV/AIDS.
- Parasitic infection.
- Connective tissue disorders.
- Autoimmune atrophic (antibodies attack healthy mucosa, with resultant gradual thinning of mucosa and destruction of glands). Can lead to interference with production of vitamin $B_{12}$ and pernicious anaemia.
- Chronic inflammation is common in developing countries or individuals of low socio-economic status (association with *H. pylori*); prevalence ↑ with age.

## Presentation

- Often asymptomatic, but might present with symptoms of dyspepsia (📖 p. 332), retching, or haematemesis (erosive gastritis).
- Chronic dull pain.
- Early satiety (fullness).
- Anorexia.
- Chronic inflammation (in the presence of intestinal metaplasia) could precede early gastric cancer but is not, in itself, a premalignant condition.

## Investigation

- Upper GI endoscopy—to exclude other causes.
- Histology—confirms inflammation, activity, atrophy, intestinal metaplasia, and *H. pylori*, which might not reflect either endoscopic appearance or symptoms.

## Treatment

- Not required if asymptomatic.
- If symptomatic, treat the underlying cause.
- Avoid risk factors (e.g. NSAIDs and alcohol).
- *H. pylori* eradication and appropriate drug treatment (📖 p. 364).
- Bile reflux post-gastrectomy: sucralfate 1 g four times a day; rarely, Roux-en-Y surgery is needed.
- Treat symptoms if a specific cause is not identified.

## Nursing management

Dependent on the severity of symptoms and the underlying cause.

# Gastric ulceration

*Helicobacter pylori* infection is the cause of 70–80% of gastric ulcers (📖 p. 364). Other risk factors include NSAIDS, corticosteroids, chronic antral gastritis, smoking, heavy alcohol use, and environmental stress (e.g. intensive care setting or burns).

### Incidence

Less common than duodenal ulcers; more common in the elderly. Affects ♂ and ♀ equally. Identification and eradication of *H. pylori* has led to a sharp ↓ in acute hospital admissions from ulcer disease.

### Clinical features

- Pain—related to meals and relieved by antacids.
- Vomiting.
- Weight loss.
- Some patients might be asymptomatic—drug-induced or iron-deficiency ulcers.

### Complications

Bleeding—haematemesis (📖 p. 704) and melaena—or perforation is a presenting feature in one-third of patients. Carcinoma should be excluded in the first instance and suspected if there is a failure to heal despite compliance with treatment.

### Investigations

Upper GI endoscopy to identify the ulcer and enable accurate histological assessment. Repeat 8 weeks after treatment to confirm healing (chronic gastric ulceration = higher risk carcinoma) or if there is a symptom relapse. A barium meal will show the ulcer crater, but still needs endoscopic assessment.

### Treatment and nursing management

- Stop NSAIDs.
- Treat the ulcer, including *H. pylori* eradication therapy if present.
- Stop smoking.
- ↓ alcohol intake.
- Dietary advice—avoid foods exacerbating symptoms, good nutritional intake, and regular meals.

# *Helicobacter pylori*

Spiral bacterium that colonizes mainly in the antrum of the stomach. It is the causal agent in 90–95% of duodenal ulcers and 70–80% of gastric ulcers. Listed as a grade 1 carcinogen, because gastric cancer can occur if infection leads to gastritis, atrophy, and metaplasia. Infection is strongly linked to social deprivation in childhood and is higher in insanitary overcrowded conditions. Various strains of *H. pylori* exist; host factors and the bacterial strain determine the outcome of infection (the patient could remain asymptomatic).

## Identification

- Serology—a blood test will detect antibodies; routinely performed by GPs. There is a test-and-treat strategy in dyspepsia,[1] which is useful only in detection of infection.
- Urease breath test—$^{13}$C-labelled urea taken orally. Resulting $^{13}CO_2$ is released by the urease enzyme and measured in the breath. Used to confirm success of treatment.
- Histologically—urease enzyme can be detected using simple colorimetric (CLO) test from a mucosal sample taken on endoscopy; the result is ready within 1 h.

## Treatment

Eradication therapy, combined therapy with a PPI (📖 p. 337) and a combination of antibiotics (Table 9.4); the regimen is dependent on the sensitivity and/or resistance to individual drugs. Most standard regimens are successful in up to 90% of cases. Successful eradication should be confirmed (by urease breath test) if symptoms are continued or recurrent in ulceration with history of bleeding.

---

1 National Institute for Health and Clinical Excellence (2004). *Dyspepsia: Managing Adults with Dyspepsia in Primary Care*. http://guidance.nice.org.uk/CG17/ (accessed 14.05.07).

**Table 9.4** Recommended regimens for *Helicobacter pylori* eradication

| Acid suppressant | Amoxicillin | Clarithromycin | Metronidazole |
|---|---|---|---|
| Esomeprazole, 20 mg twice daily | 1 g twice daily | 500 mg twice daily | Nil |
| | Nil | 250 mg twice daily | 400 mg twice daily |
| Lansoprazole, 30 mg twice daily | 1 g twice daily | 500 mg twice daily | Nil |
| | 1 g twice daily | Nil | 400 mg twice daily |
| | Nil | 250 mg twice daily | 400 mg twice daily |
| Omeprazole, 20 mg twice daily | 1 g twice daily | 500 mg twice daily | Nil |
| | 500 mg three times daily | Nil | 400 mg three times daily |
| | Nil | 250 mg twice daily | 400 mg twice daily |
| Pantoprazole, 40 mg twice daily | 1 g twice daily | 500 mg twice daily | Nil |
| | Nil | 250 mg twice daily | 400 mg twice daily |
| Rabeprazole, 20 mg twice daily | 1 g twice daily | 500 mg twice daily | Nil |
| | Nil | 250 mg twice daily | 400 mg twice daily |

# Pyloric stenosis

Often called 'infantile hypertrophic pyloric stenosis'. It comprises hypertrophy and hyperplasia of the pyloric sphincter during the neonatal period, mainly affecting the circular muscles of the pylorus, causing it to become elongated and thickened. Results in gastric outflow obstruction, with vomiting (projectile) and dehydration. Affects ♂ and ♀ in a ratio of 4:1, with a strong genetic factor.

## Clinical presentation

Normally presents between 3 weeks and 6 weeks of age, although late presentation (6 months) can occur. Rapidly progressive vomiting (projectile), with a palpable mass in the right upper quadrant of the stomach during feeding. Dehydration is a prominent feature; the child is hungry immediately after vomiting feed. Electrolyte imbalance results.

## Diagnosis

Confirmed on abdominal ultrasound.

## Treatment

- Correct dehydration.
- Nasogastric tube—relieve pressure.
- Surgery—pyloromyotomy.

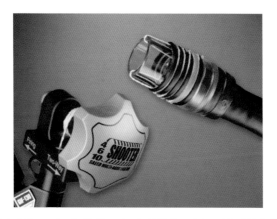

**Plate 1** Shooter banding kit. Reproduced with kind permission of Cook Medical.

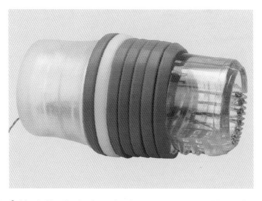

**Plate 2** Head of banding kit. Reproduced with kind permission of Boston Scientific.

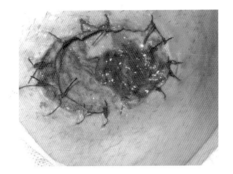

**Plate 3** Mucosal separation.

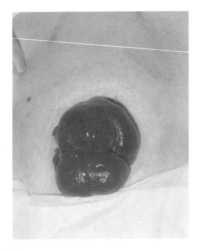

**Plate 4** Necrosis.

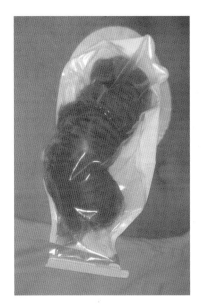

**Plate 5** Prolapse.

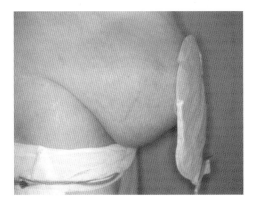

**Plate 6** Parastomal hernia.

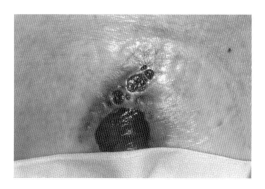

**Plate 7** Pyoderma gangrenosum.

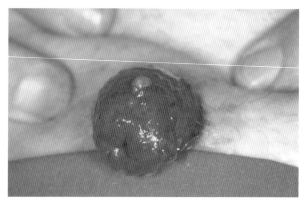

**Plate 8** Peristomal granuloma.

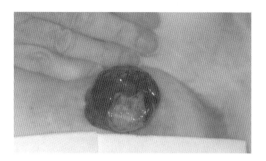

**Plate 9** Recurrent adenocarcinoma.

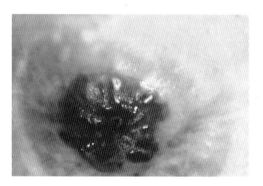

**Plate 10** Stenosis.

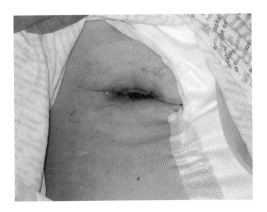

**Plate 11** Retracted stoma.

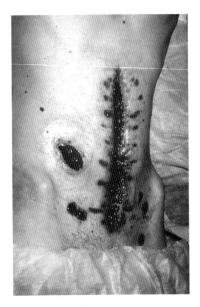

**Plate 12** Simple enterocutaneous fistula.

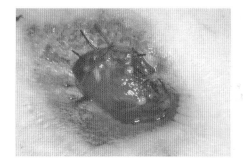

**Plate 13** Skin excoriation.

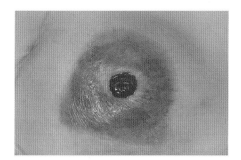

**Plate 14** Stoma allergy.

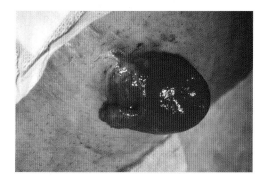

**Plate 15** Stoma trauma.

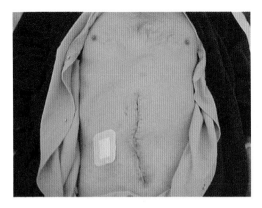

**Plate 16** Laparotomy wound. Reproduced with kind permission of the Burdett Institute of Gastrointestinal Nursing and St. Mark's Hospital, Harrow.

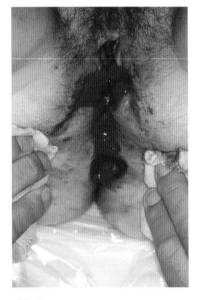

**Plate 17** Perianal fistula.

# Gastric cancer

Incidence ↓ worldwide. Includes all adenocarcinomas, apart from lymphoma (rare). Risk factors include the following:
- Chronic gastritis (📖 p. 361).
- *Helicobacter pylori* (📖 p. 364).
- Chronic gastric ulcers (📖 p. 362).
- Diet (e.g. salty or pickled/smoked foods).
- Previous gastric surgery.
- Gastric adenomatous polyps (📖 p. 369).
- Family history.
- Low socio-economic status.

## Clinical features
- Abdominal pain.
- Dyspepsia.
- Iron-deficiency anaemia.
- Anorexia and weight loss.
- Overt or occult bleeding (haematemesis, melaena, and positive faecal occult blood).

## Diagnosis
- Upper GI endoscopy and biopsy (confirms diagnosis).
- Barium meal.
- CT scan ± laparoscopy (assess resectability).

## Treatment
- Early disease can be cured (gastrectomy/partial gastrectomy).
- Palliative surgery indicated for obstruction, pain, and excessive bleeding.
- Chemotherapy or radiotherapy can be used as adjunct therapy (it is of limited use otherwise).
- Drugs (PPI and $H_2$ receptor antagonists) are effective for pain relief.

## Nursing management
Must be coordinated through specialist multidisciplinary teams and a key worker (normally a specialist nurse). Dietetic input is essential, because the cancer site inhibits adequate nutrition and post-operatively altered anatomy affects nutritional intake. Early support (psychosocial and symptomatic) is needed from relevant agencies (e.g. Macmillan nurses). Post-operative management includes prevention, identification, and management of dumping syndrome (📖 p. 368).

# Gastric dumping syndrome

Rapid gastric emptying occurs when the lower end of the small intestine (jejunum) fills too quickly with undigested food from the stomach. Defined as either 'early' dumping, occurring within 30 min of eating, or 'late' dumping, occurring 2–3 h after eating. Many patients have both forms of the syndrome.

## Causes

Occurs following some types of gastric surgery (e.g. gastrectomy and gastric bypass surgery), whereby the stomach empties more rapidly. Also seen and in patients with gastrin-secreting tumours in the pancreas. Early dumping occurs as a result of rapid hypertonic load in the small intestine. Late dumping occurs as a result of rapid carbohydrate absorption, which stimulates the pancreas to release excessive amounts of insulin into the bloodstream, causing hypoglycaemia.

## Symptoms

- Nausea.
- Vomiting.
- Bloating.
- Cramp.
- Diarrhoea.
- Sweating.
- Dizziness.
- Fatigue.
- Palpitations.

The timing of symptoms is the main difference between early and late dumping.

## Nursing management

Ensure that patients are aware of the risk of dumping syndrome; it can be frightening, especially following gastric surgery. With regard to diet, advise patients to ↓ osmotic load and slow gastric emptying as follows:
- Eat smaller, more frequent meals.
- ↓ carbohydrate intake (especially simple carbohydrates).
- ↑ fibre intake.
- Drink before or after meals, rather than during meals.

Changes to diet are not always easy in a hospital environment, so consider snacks between meals and involve a dietitian. Eating might relieve symptoms of late dumping; surgical revision is a last resort.

# Gastric polyps

Often an incidental finding on endoscopy. The most common polyps (70%) are hyperplastic (regenerative) and of no consequence. Adenomatous polyps in the stomach are unusual but have the same malignant potential as colonic adenomatous polyps.

## Symptoms

The majority of patients are asymptomatic. Occasionally, polyps can bleed and present as haematemesis (📖 p. 704) or melaena. Rarely, large pedunculated polyps can obstruct the pylorus, leading to nausea, abdominal bloating, and vomiting (± projectile).

## Investigation

Upper GI endoscopy is indicated, if symptoms exist, to elicit the cause. Histological assessment of all polyps is essential because early gastric cancers can look insignificant.

## Treatment

Treat symptoms; this could include removal of the polyp (polypectomy). Removal or resection of adenomatous polyps is essential (also consider colonic assessment).

## Nursing management

Provide reassurance regarding natural history and progression.

# Small bowel

Structure and function  372
Malabsorption  374
Coeliac disease (gluten-sensitive enteropathy)  375
Bacterial overgrowth and lactase deficiency  376
Small bowel infection  378
Short bowel syndrome  380
Vitamin $B_{12}$ deficiency  381
Duodenal ulcers  382
Meckel's diverticulum  383
Small bowel tumours  384
Intestinal failure: overview  386
Intestinal failure: definition and classification  387
Intestinal failure: pathogenesis  388
Intestinal failure: assessment and planning  390
Intestinal failure: treatment  392
Intestinal failure: psychological and social considerations  394

# Structure and function

The length of the small intestine, measured from the duodeno-jejunal flexure, is variable and ranges from 2.75 m to 8.50 m. The surface is deeply folded and covered with villi and micro-villi to maximize surface area. After a surgical resection, it is more important to know the length of bowel remaining than the length removed so as to predict if patients may need nutrition support. The small bowel consists of three sections: duodenum, jejunum, and ileum (Fig. 10.1).

### Duodenum: 20 cm long

In the duodenum, large polypeptides, polysaccharides, and triglycerides are broken down to peptides, monosaccharides, disaccharides, glycerol, and free fatty acids by pancreatic enzymes. Lipid is made soluble by bile (essentially a soap), which forms micelles. The pancreatic and biliary secretions amount to ~1.5 L/day.

▶ Note that molecules are not broken down to single amino acids and sugars here, because the osmolality of the small bowel contents would be high and cause water to diffuse into the lumen if they were.

### Jejunum

At the brush boarder of the small intestine, diglycerides, triglycerides, dipeptides, and tripeptides are hydrolysed to single sugar and amino acid molecules immediately before absorption. Sugars and amino acids are absorbed mainly from the jejunum, whereas lipids are absorbed over the whole length of small intestine. Within the enterocytes, long-chain triglycerides are formed into chylomicrons, which enter the lymphatic system, whereas medium-chain triglycerides enter the portal blood.

### Ileum

2–4 m long. There is no definite demarcation between the jejunum and the ileum. Continues digestion and absorption, particularly vitamin $B_{12}$ in the terminal ileum. pH neutral to alkaline. Ends at ileo-caecal valve.

### Motility

Most meals empty from the stomach within 2–3 h. Liquid empties faster than solid. Most food residue has passed into the colon within 6 h. In the fasting state, a wave of contraction occurs every 90 min (the migrating myoelectric complex) and passes from the stomach to the ileum. During this wave, the pylorus opens wide (>1 cm) so that any debris in the upper gut is cleared and passed into the colon.

### Specific absorption functions

Bile acids are mainly absorbed from the last 100 cm of ileum. If this has been resected, the bile salt pool might be depleted and unabsorbed bile salts could cause diarrhoea, partly because they cause salt and water secretion in the colon.

Vitamin $B_{12}$ is consumed in meat (especially liver). A protein (intrinsic factor) binds to vitamin $B_{12}$ within the stomach and this complex is absorbed in alkaline conditions, with calcium, in the terminal 60 cm of ileum.

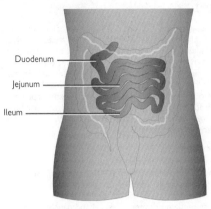

**Fig. 10.1** Duodenum, jejunum, and ileum. Reproduced with kind permission © Burdett Institute 2008.

# Malabsorption

Malabsorption is characterized by a failure of macronutrient absorption. Malabsorption of lipid is the most obvious form clinically because it gives rise to diarrhoea with malodorous stool that is pale and floats (steatorrhoea) and the patient might notice an oily layer in the toilet water. Steatorrhoea might be due to pancreatic disease (severe malabsorption) or intestinal disease (milder malabsorption). In pancreatic malabsorption, diabetes mellitus might occur before the malabsorption becomes apparent. Patients with malabsorption present with weight loss, fatigue, diarrhoea (steatorrhoea), and often deficiencies of fat-soluble vitamins (A, D, E, and K), iron, and folic acid (rarely vitamin $B_{12}$).

## Tests for malabsorption

The traditional test for fat malabsorption is 3-day faecal fat collection (<20 mmol/day is normal for consumption of 60–100 g fat/day). However, this test is unpleasant for laboratory workers, so other indirect tests might be used, such as the butter fat or $^{14}C$-triolein breath test. A number of tests are available to differentiate between intestinal and pancreatic causes of malabsorption. Malabsorption of the sugar xylose is commonly used to test intestinal absorption (25 g of the sugar is consumed and then urine is collected for the next 5 h: <4 g (16%) of xylose in the urine indicates intestinal malabsorption). The tests commonly used to demonstrate a pancreatic cause of malabsorption rely on pancreatic enzymes cleaving a molecule to produce a metabolite that is then absorbed and measured in the urine or blood (e.g. the para-amino benzoic acid (PABA) or pancreolauryl test).

# Coeliac disease (gluten-sensitive enteropathy)

Coeliac disease is a common (about 1% of the population) inflammatory disorder of the small intestine induced by the gliadins of wheat, hordeins of barley, and secalins of rye. The inflammation is associated with a loss of villous height and crypt hypertrophy, and leads to malabsorption. Coeliac disease gets better after the exclusion of gluten from the diet (and recurs if re-challenged). Rarely, coeliac disease can be complicated by the development of a small bowel T-cell lymphoma, which is more likely to occur in patients with untreated disease or those who do not rigidly follow the diet. Coeliac disease might present as a typical malabsorption problem or, owing to the simplicity of performing serological tests, it might be diagnosed in people presenting with anaemia, infertility, amenorrhoea, osteoporosis, ataxia, or peripheral neuropathy, or ↓ growth (in children).

The diagnosis is made according to a duodenal or jejunal biopsy showing a loss of villi and an inflammatory cell infiltrate. Blood tests are now >90% sensitive and specific and call into doubt the need for a histological diagnosis. Anti-endomysial and anti-tissue transglutaminase antibodies have largely replaced tests for IgA antigliadin antibodies.

The diagnosis is confirmed by a rapid favourable response to a gluten-free diet, and, if this occurs, a re-biopsy of the small bowel and a re-challenge with gluten are unnecessary.

## Nursing implications

Patients are advised to join the Coeliac UK[1] charity, which gives up-to-date recommendations about foods and recipes. Essentially, the diet involves avoiding wheat, rye, and barley and using rice, corn, buckwheat, potato, soybean, or tapioca flours. Oats are usually avoided because the same machinery that harvests wheat is also usually used to harvest oats and ∴ cross-contamination of the oats might be enough to reactivate coeliac disease. If a patient is accidentally exposed to gluten, lesions in the mucosa will develop within 8–12 h of exposure.

Some dietary products are available on prescription in the UK. Patients may need support to adhere to the diet, which may impose social restrictions.

---

1 Coeliac UK. http://www.coeliac.co.uk (accessed 14.05.07).

# Bacterial overgrowth and lactase deficiency

Bacterial overgrowth is said to occur if the flora in the upper small bowel resembles that found in the colon. These micro-organisms (mainly anaerobes—bacteroides, lactobacilli, and coliforms) compete for nutrients and might injure the enterocytes. Bacterial overgrowth can occur if there is no gastric acid or the small bowel has diverticulae, blind loops (out-of-circuit loops of bowel, e.g. jejuno-ileal bypass), or abnormal motility (which might be a lack of the migrating myoelectric complex (MMC), e.g. with scleroderma, amyloid myopathy, visceral neuropathy or myopathy, diabetic autonomic neuropathy, or chronic bowel obstruction). Other causes include a lack of pancreatic enzymes (chronic pancreatitis), immunodeficiency syndromes (e.g. common variable immunodeficiency, combined immunodeficiency diseases, or HIV infection), and cirrhosis.

Bacterial overgrowth may present with bloating and diarrhoea. In more severe forms it is characterized by weight loss, steatorrhoea, vitamin $B_{12}$ deficiency (folate deficiency is rare), and, often, hypoproteinaemia. The significant steatorrhoea that occurs with bacterial overgrowth might be due to the bacteria both deconjugating bile salts and inactivating pancreatic enzymes.

Ideally, the diagnosis of bacterial overgrowth can be confirmed by aspirating the upper small bowel contents at endoscopy. A positive result is the finding of $>10^5$ organisms/ml. Neither breath tests using glucose, lactulose, or C14 xylose nor urinary indicators are specific or sensitive tests. Often, a trial of antibiotics is used and the diagnosis is confirmed if the symptoms improve.

Treatment is with long courses of antibiotics (some clinicians rotate these agents every 6 weeks). Classically, tetracycline or metronidazole is used. If they are ineffective, co-amoxiclav, ciprofloxacin, cefoxime, or chloramphenicol might be used.

## Lactase deficiency and lactose-tolerance tests

Lactase deficiency is a cause of osmotic diarrhoea. Lactase is found on the small bowel and colon brush border and it hydrolyses the disaccharide lactose to glucose and galactose. The levels of lactase are high at birth but ↓ with age. It is absent in some adults, especially those of Asian or African Caribbean origin; however, lactase activity is usually present in >75% of white Caucasians. Secondary lactase deficiency often complicates small intestinal infection and inflammatory diseases. Diarrhoea results rapidly after ingestion of milk. Lactase deficiency can be diagnosed by measuring a rise in the level of hydrogen in the breath after drinking 50 g of lactose (if there is no lactase, bacteria metabolize the lactose that arrives in the colon to produce hydrogen, which is detected in breath samples).

## Nursing implications

These patients are advised to avoid milk products. This may have implications particularly for children (protein and calorie intake) and post-menopausal women (calcium intake), and advice is needed on alternative sources of nutrients.

# Small bowel infection

The organisms causing infection that involves primarily the small bowel are different in adults, children, and immunocompromised patients. In children, viral causes of gastroenteritis are common and include rotavirus, calcivirus, enteric adenovirus, and astrovirus. In previously healthy adults, bacterial causes might include *Salmonella* spp, *Escherichia coli*, *Vibrio cholerae*, or *Vibrio parahaemolyticus*. Even a change in bacterial flora, as might occur with travelling or taking antibiotics, can cause diarrhoea. Infection of the small bowel rarely causes blood in the stool and, unlike in inflammatory bowel disease, there is not usually an ↑ in the platelet count. Diagnosis usually depends on stool microscopy and culture. A small bowel biopsy and/or aspirate might be needed, especially in the immunocompromised. Many of the organisms that cause diarrhoea mainly affect the large bowel and are discussed elsewhere (📖 p. 462). Generally, the treatment is to withhold food for 24–48 h but maintain hydration and then gently reintroduce foods.

Other organisms that can infect the gut include tuberculosis and *Yersinia* spp, which can both affect the terminal ileum and be confused with Crohn's disease.

## Giardiasis

A specific cause of acute or chronic diarrhoea is infection with the protozoa *Giardia duodenalis* (previously called *Giardia lamblia*), which is acquired from drinking water contaminated with its cysts or by direct faeco-oral contact. The trophozoites colonize the upper small bowel and cause malabsorption. The condition is diagnosed by duodenal aspiration (occasionally biopsy) and the trophozoites or cysts can be found in the stool. Treatment is with at least 5 days of oral metronidazole (400 mg three times daily.)

## Small bowel infection in immunocompromised patients

In immunocompromised patients, many organisms can infect the small bowel, including *Candida* spp, *Mycobacterium avium intracellulare*, *Cryptosporidium* spp, *Microsporidium* spp, *Isospora* spp, and cytomegalovirus (CMV). There is also an enteropathy specific to patients with HIV.

## Whipple's disease (intestinal lipodystrophy)

Whipple's disease is an uncommon systemic disorder which may start with arthropathy or arthritis but develops into a systemic illness characterized by intestinal malabsorption, skin pigmentation, generalized lymphadenopathy, arthritis, fevers, and possibly cardiac and cerebral involvement. The serum albumin level might be low.

It is caused by a Gram-positive, PAS-positive, but not acid-fast, bacterium called *Tropheryma whippelii*. The diagnosis is made from duodenal biopsies that show large glycoprotein-containing macrophages and the presence of the organism in the lamina propria.

Many antibiotic combinations (e.g. tetracycline, penicillin, erythromycin, and cephalosporins) treat this illness, which used to be fatal. However, trimethoprim and sulfamethoxazole are generally given in combination for 6–12 months. Sometimes IV penicillin is given for 2 weeks after the diagnosis has been made. Relapses are common (~35%) and nervous system effects might develop after treatment. It is wise to re-biopsy the small bowel to check that the organisms have disappeared.

## Short bowel syndrome

If <200 cm small bowel remains, patients might develop problems of malabsorption, leading to undernutrition and salt, water, and magnesium depletion, and consequently dehydration (□ p. 386 for intestinal failure). There are two clinical types of patient with a short bowel: those with jejunum anastomosed to colon, usually because of mesenteric infarction or Crohn's disease, and those with an end jejunostomy, usually because of Crohn's disease (Fig. 10.2). Patients with jejunum–colon mainly have problems with undernutrition, renal calcium oxalate stones, and gallstones; with adaptation, they show an improvement in intestinal absorption with time. Patients with a jejunostomy have major problems with water and sodium loss from their stoma and loose 100 mmol of sodium per litre of stomal output; they also have problems with hypomagnesaemia, undernutrition, and gallstones. Their stomal output does not ↓ with time.

Depending on the severity of the resulting intestinal failure, oral or IV nutrition, fluid, or drugs might be given to slow motility and/or ↓ secretions (□ p. 392). In general, a patient with <50 cm of jejunum remaining and a functioning colon in continuity is likely to need parenteral nutrition. A patient with <100 cm of jejunum ending in a jejunostomy is likely to need long-term parenteral saline and nutritional support. If stomal output exceeds 2 L/day, a patient is likely to have problems of salt and water depletion.

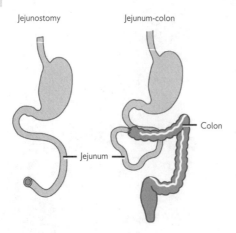

**Fig. 10.2** Patients with short bowel. Reproduced with kind permission © Burdett Institute 2008.

# Vitamin B$_{12}$ deficiency

The common causes of vitamin B$_{12}$ deficiency are dietary, gastric, or terminal ileal disease and bacterial overgrowth. Rare causes include pancreatic disease (less calcium, which is needed for B$_{12}$ absorption) or infestation with the fish tapeworm (*Diphyllobothrium latum*). People who are vegans, and ∴ consume no meat or dairy products. might develop vitamin B$_{12}$ deficiency. Patients with pernicious anaemia (who make antibodies to gastric parietal cells and/or intrinsic factor) or who have had their gastric antrum removed can develop vitamin B$_{12}$ deficiency. Because the last 60 cm of terminal ileum is responsible for the absorption of vitamin B$_{12}$, disease (e.g. Crohn's disease) or resection of this area might cause vitamin B$_{12}$ deficiency. The stores of vitamin B$_{12}$ in a healthy person last for 3–7 years, so it takes a long time for a macrocytic anaemia to develop.

### Shilling test

A Shilling test can be performed to determine where vitamin B$_{12}$ malabsorption is occurring. After a large intramuscular dose of vitamin B$_{12}$ has been given, $^{57}$Co-cyanocobalamin is given alone and urine is collected for 24 h; the amount of radioactivity in the urine is determined. Then, on another occasion, $^{57}$Co-cyanocobalamin is given with intrinsic factor and the results compared.

### Treatment

A course of intramuscular hydroxocobalamin is given to replenish the stores (largely hepatic) and then a maintenance dose is given (1 mg of hydroxocobalamin every 3 months). Give calcium or bicarbonate if pancreatic calcium deficiency. A rise in the reticulocyte count after 7 days indicates a response.

### Nursing implications

Patients need dietary advice and education about the importance of regular therapy in chronic deficiency. As anaemia may develop slowly, patients may stop therapy and feel well for long periods before symptoms develop.

# Duodenal ulcers

Ulceration in the first part of the duodenum is most commonly caused by *Helicobacter pylori*, a spiral-shaped bacterium, which inhabits the mucus layer of the gastric antrum. *H. pylori* produces an enzyme, urease, which catalyses the reaction that converts urea to ammonia and carbon dioxide. This reaction is not only the basis of the indirect tests for *H. pylori*, but also might be responsible for the pathogenic role of *H. pylori*. The bacteria produce ammonia locally in the mucosa of the gastric antrum, thereby causing an alkaline environment. The antrum responds to this by secreting ↑ gastrin, which causes the gastric fundus to secrete supraphysiological amounts of gastric acid and pepsinogen. This ↑ in the levels of acid and pepsinogen is thought to cause gastric metaplasia in the duodenum, and it might be these areas that ulcerate, possibly owing to further colonization by *H. pylori* (📖 p. 364).

*H. pylori* infection can be diagnosed by a breath test or gastric antral biopsy. The $^{14}$C-urea and $^{13}$C-urea breath tests involve consuming radio-labelled urea; if *H. pylori* is present, urease degrades the urea to $^{14}$C-carbon dioxide or $^{13}$C-carbon dioxide and ammonia. The radio-labelled carbon dioxide is excreted in the breath and thus can be measured. Gastric antral pinch biopsies can be taken during an upper gastrointestinal endoscopy.

*H. pylori* can be seen on normal H&E (haematoxylin and eosin) staining of the biopsy by an experienced histopathologist or a silver stain can be used. Most commonly, the biopsy is put into an agar gel that contains urea and a pH-sensitive indicator; this is called a campylobacter-like organism (CLO) test, which is what *Helicobacter* was first called. The urease from *H. pylori*, if present, causes the agar to become alkaline (by producing ammonia) and thus the indicator changes colour, usually to a deep red–pink colour. There are also serological tests available that detect IgG antibodies to *H. pylori*.

The treatment of *H. pylori* involves taking a combination of antibiotics for 1–2 weeks, in addition to a proton-pump inhibitor (PPI). Amoxicillin (1 g twice daily) and clarithromycin (500 mg twice daily), with omeprazole (20 mg twice daily) or lansoprazole (30 mg twice daily), are most commonly used. Metronidazole (400 mg twice daily) was used until recently instead of clarithromycin, but metronidazole resistance has become common. Tetracycline and bismuth preparations are rarely used.

Other causes of duodenal ulceration include the ingestion of NSAIDs, Crohn's disease (of the upper small intestine), or, rarely, a gastrinoma.

# Meckel's diverticulum

This is found in 1–3% of the population and is the most common congenital abnormality of the GIT. It occurs as a vestigial remnant of the vitello-intestinal duct, which was attached to the mid-gut when it was extruded into the extra-embryonic coelom during fetal development. It is present ~1 m from the ileo-caecal valve on the anti-mesenteric border, has its own blood supply, and has gastric mucosa within it. The condition is usually asymptomatic. Complications, which are more common in ♂, can occur and include inflammation, giving rise to a pain similar to appendicitis, lower GI bleeding (especially common in young children), ulceration (can be infected with *H. pylori*), perforation, and obstruction. Although often diagnosed at laparotomy, it might also be diagnosed using a $^{99m}$Tc pertechnetate scintigraphic scan. If detected and causing problems such as recurrent GI bleeding, it is wise for it to be surgically removed.

# Small bowel tumours

They might be benign, hamartomatous, intermediate, or malignant. The majority of small bowel tumours are malignant in adults.

## Benign tumours

Benign tumours of the small bowel are uncommon and include the following:

- Adenomas.
- Hamartomas.
- Fibromas.
- Haemangiomas.
- Leomyomas.
- Lipomas.

Peri-ampullary duodenal adenomas are common in patients with familial adenomatous polyposis. Hamartomas occur in juvenile polyposis, Peutz–Jegher's syndrome, and Cronkhite–Canada syndrome.

### Peutz–Jegher syndrome

Peutz–Jegher syndrome is an autosomal dominant inherited condition of mucocutaneous pigmentation (mouth, lips, dorsum of hands, and feet) and gastrointestinal polyposis. The gastrointestinal polyps ↑ in size with time and may cause small bowel obstruction, intussusception, or bleeding. There is ↑ recognition that the polyps, which are most common in the jejunum, can undergo adenomatous and malignant transformation. In addition, these patients have an ↑ risk of ovarian, breast, or testicular tumours. Regular screening of the small bowel, with polyp removal, is justified (🕮 p. 485).

## Malignant tumours

Cancers affecting the small bowel are rare. In the UK, ~750 people are diagnosed with a small bowel cancer each year. There are four main types of malignant tumour:

- Adenocarcinoma—the most common type of small bowel cancer, which usually appears within the duodenum. Can develop from adenomatous polyps and can rarely occur in patients with coeliac disease.
- Sarcoma—can develop in the supportive tissues of the body, e.g. Kaposi's sarcoma. Leiomyosarcomas grow in the muscle wall of the ileum. A gastrointestinal stromal tumour (GIST) can develop in any part of the small bowel.
- Carcinoid (usually in terminal ileum).
- Lymphoma—usually a non-Hodgkin lymphoma (NHL). Tumours can be primary or secondary.

More rarely fibrosarcoma, leiomyosarcoma, or metastatic tumours may occur.

The cause is often unknown, although patients with Crohn's disease, coeliac disease, and Peutz–Jegher syndrome might be at ↑ risk.

## Presentation
The symptoms are often vague and difficult to diagnose.[1] They might include any of the following:
• Altered blood in the stools (melaena).
• Vague crampy abdominal pain.
• Weight loss.
• Diarrhoea.

The patient might present with malignant bowel obstruction giving rise to intermittent colicky abdominal pain. 50% of tumours occur in the duodenum, 30% occur in the jejunum, and 20% occur in the ileum.

## Diagnosis
• Endoscopy or colonoscopy.
• Barium X-rays.
• CT scans.
• Ultrasound scans.

## Treatment
Surgery is the main treatment and can be a curative resection or palliative bypass, depending on the site of origin and extent of the tumour. Radiotherapy and/or chemotherapy are occasionally used. Chemotherapy drugs include fluorouracil alone or combination with various other drugs. Interferon can be used for carcinoid tumours and imatinib can be used to treat a GIST.

## Nursing advice
Patients might have experienced a delay in diagnosis and express a range of reactions, including shock and uncertainty to be diagnosed with this rare type of cancer. Also, a definitive prognosis can be hard to give.

Patients who have surgery might require a special diet, supplements, or medicines, depending on the extent of resection.

1 Moertel CG (1987). Karnofsky Memorial Lecture: an odyssey in the land of small tumours. *Journal of Clinical Oncology* **5**, 1503–22.

# Intestinal failure: overview

'Intestinal failure' (IF) is a term that describes patients who require specialized replacement regimens to compensate for an inability to maintain health through normal absorption of sufficient nutrients or electrolytes from food and drink.

Often still referred to as 'short-bowel syndrome', IF is one of the most difficult gastrointestinal conditions to manage because, in addition to malabsorption of food and drink, reabsorption of gastrointestinal secretions can be impaired, resulting in large quantities of water and electrolytes being lost through a stoma or the rectum, if the intestine is in continuity. The term 'short-bowel syndrome' has been highlighted as misleading because it could suggest an intestine that has actually been shortened through resection.
▶ Note that symptoms can occur not only following massive resection of the small intestine, but also in the presence of extensive inflammation or motility disorders in an intact intestine or an intestine of sufficient length.[1] It is now recognized that the term 'intestinal failure' provides a more accurate description.

National Specialist Commissioning Advisory Group (NSCAG) funding for the Severe Intestinal Failure Service for England has been designated to the Hope Hospital (Salford, UK) and St Mark's Hospital (London, UK). The contract proposes that only the most complex cases of IF should be referred to the national centres, so that their difficult medical, surgical, radiological, and nursing needs can be efficiently managed using a multiprofessional approach.

1 Wood S (1996). Nutrition and the short bowel. In: Myers C (ed.) *Stoma Care Nursing*. Arnold, London.

# Intestinal failure: definition and classification

Nightingale defined IF as '... decreased intestinal absorption so that macronutrient and/or water and electrolyte supplements are needed to maintain health and/or growth. Undernutrition and/or dehydration result if no treatment is given or if compensatory mechanisms do not occur'.[1]

IF can be graded in severity by the requirement and route for supportive nutrition/fluid[1] (Table 10.1).

▶ Recognize that an individual with IF might alter in their severity classification over a period of time. Compensatory mechanisms, such as intestinal adaptation after massive intestinal resection, restorative surgery, and the individual's ability to cope with the enormous physiological and psychological changes that IF has brought about, can all improve the extent to which IF affects them and the degree of support that is required. The key determinant is whether a patient can maintain a positive fluid or nutritional balance.

**Table 10.1** Classification of intestinal failure[1]

| | |
|---|---|
| Mild IF | Can be managed with oral nutrition ± oral rehydration solution (glucose/saline) |
| Moderate IF | Enteral tube is used for nutrient administration ± rehydration solution |
| Severe IF | Must have parental nutrition/fluids to survive because unable to maintain health by enteral absorption alone |

1 Nightingale J (2001). *Intestinal Failure*. Greenwich Medical Media, London.

# Intestinal failure: pathogenesis

## Aetiology of IF

Fig. 10.3 shows the aetiology of patients referred to the National Intestinal Failure Service in 2005/2006 (Hope & St. Mark's Hospitals). Several of these underlying conditions have led to massive intestinal resection (📖 p. 380), whereas others involve extensive intestinal disease or inflammation. The causes are changing over time, with less Crohn's disease (possibly due to the use of biological agents in treatment) and more mesenteric vascular disease.

▶ Note that several of these conditions, e.g. Crohn's disease, might lead to both massive intestinal resection and continuing disease within the remaining bowel.

## How much intestine is enough?

If the small intestine is in continuity with the colon, ~50 cm of functioning jejunum is required for survival without parenteral supplementation. Without continuity, ~100 cm of functioning jejunum is required.

▶ Note that these figures are merely a guide and that the individual's ability to maintain health will vary and also be dependent on the level of ongoing compliance with the IF management regimen.

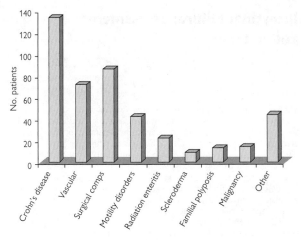

**Fig. 10.3** Aetiology of referrals to the Intestinal Failure Service in 2005–2006.

# Intestinal failure: assessment and planning

The broad aims of treatment in this complex group of patients are:
• To maintain a fluid and electrolyte balance.
• To maintain an adequate nutritional status.
• To enable the individual to achieve an acceptable quality of life.

The key elements of assessment are shown in Table 10.2.

Large intestinal losses can lead to life-threatening metabolic instability, so accurate monitoring and appropriate management of the fluid and electrolyte balance is the priority.[1] In terms of nutritional status, a multidisciplinary patient-focused approach is essential to work on the longer-term goals of achieving a body weight and BMI that are not only within healthy parameters, but also acceptable to the individual. Long-term rehabilitation can be difficult for many because they struggle to come to terms with the, often catastrophic, life-changing events that have taken place. Patients and their families need clear and easily understandable information regarding the physiological changes that have taken place so that they can begin to understand the rationale behind the treatment plan, ultimately aiding compliance.

▶ The multidisciplinary team must be on hand for support and can make referrals for additional help (e.g. counsellor, medical social worker, psychologist, or occupational therapist), if appropriate.

1 Wood S (1996). Nutrition and the short bowel. In: Myers C (ed) *Stoma Care Nursing*. Arnold, London.

**Table 10.2** Assessment of intestinal failure

| | |
|---|---|
| Length of residual intestine | Surgical measurement—the length, anatomy, and condition of the remaining intestine should be recorded |
| | Radiological measurement—if surgical details are unavailable or felt to be inaccurate, contrast follow-through examination is useful |
| Intestinal motility | The movement of food and fluid through the intestine and length of time taken for food to appear in effluent |
| Fluid and electrolyte balance | Accurate fluid-balance records |
| | Daily body weight at a regular time |
| | Blood urea and serum electrolytes |
| | Serum magnesium |
| | Random urine sodium concentration |
| Nutritional status | Body weight—taking into account any dehydration or oedema |
| | Presence of fat stores/muscle mass |
| | Symptoms of deficiencies in particular nutrients |
| | Serum albumin and total protein |
| | Calcium, phosphate, and alkaline phosphate |
| | Haemoglobin and mean corpuscular volume |
| | Vitamin $B_{12}$ and folate |
| | Serum ferritin |
| Psychosocial considerations | Overall mood |
| | Stamina |
| | Anxiety and depression score |

# Intestinal failure: treatment

To devise a treatment plan that will maximize the patient's potential for a good recovery and rehabilitation, it is essential that there is rigorous assessment of physiological and psychological factors. Table 10.2 provides a framework for assessing the patient with intestinal failure on which to base the treatment plan. Table 10.3 gives an outline treatment plan.[1]

**Table 10.3** Treatment plan for intestinal failure

**Stage 1. Establishing physiological stability**

Oral fluid restriction (500 ml to 1 L daily)

Reliable venous access

IV sodium chloride (0.9%) until random urine sodium >20 mmol/l

Accurate fluid-balance record to inform fluid and electrolyte replacement

Fluid: calculated from the previous day's output and daily body weight (1 kg = 1 L)

Sodium: 100 mmol for each litre of output plus 80 mmol for insensible losses

Potassium: 60–80 mmol daily

Magnesium: 8–14 mmol daily

Calories, protein, vitamins, and trace elements if unable to absorb through the enteral route

**Stage 2. Introducing an oral intake**

Continue IV therapy

Begin low-fibre diet and anti-diarrhoeal medication 30–60 min before eating. Separate food and fluids, and discourage drinking with meals

Limit non-electrolyte drinks to 1 L daily. Give oral rehydration solution (📖 p. 393)

Encourage energy-dense and sodium-rich snacks

Give gastric antisecretory medication and magnesium oxide capsules (may not be generally available) (12–16 mmol daily)

Aim to withdraw IV therapy gradually

**Stage 3. Rehabilitation and long-term care**

Educate the patient and family so that there is a good understanding of bowel function and how that has changed. This should aid compliance with the regimen

Referral to appropriate services in primary care, e.g. district nurses or stoma care

Referral to a social worker for information on entitlement to benefits

If the patient requires long-term IV support at home, a comprehensive programme of education and training should be started to facilitate discharge

After discharge there should be regular monitoring of the patient, correcting abnormalities and replacing particular nutrients, as required

1 Wood S (1996). Nutrition and the short bowel. In: Myers C (ed) *Stoma Care Nursing*. Arnold, London.

## Oral rehydration solution

Restricting oral hypotonic fluids, sipping a glucose–saline solution (sodium concentration 90–120 mmol/l), and taking anti-diarrhoeal or anti-secretory drugs ↓ the high output from the jejunum. With nothing commercially available, the team at St Mark's Hospital devised their own formula (Table 10.4).

The electrolyte mix can be kept in the fridge and served chilled. Small amounts of flavourings (e.g. fruit cordial or lemon juice) can be added to aid palatability.

▶ The electrolyte mix should be presented as an essential part of treatment, rather than an optional drink.

**Table 10.4** Electrolyte mix

| | |
|---|---|
| Glucose | 20 g |
| Sodium chloride | 3.5 g (dissolved in 1 L of tap water) |
| Sodium bicarbonate | 2.5 g |

# Intestinal failure: psychological and social considerations

Many IF patients will have undergone numerous investigative procedures and multiple operations, requiring lengthy hospital admissions (of months rather than weeks). Those referred to specialist centres might find themselves vast distances from home, family, and friends. It is ∴ unsurprising that many patients experience psychosocial difficulties, such as depression, from feelings of isolation, loneliness, and low morale. Patients have often faced major surgery, life-threatening illness, and long periods in hospital. Many will be underweight long term or have scars or a stoma and must adjust to a new body image. Some must adapt to a life without eating, with all the social and psychological impacts this implies.

A multidisciplinary team approach, offering support and counselling, is essential to patient recovery and rehabilitation. This will encourage the patient to gradually gain confidence in the team and begin to form relationships that will be effective for recovery and the attainment of goals.

# Liver

Structure and function  396
Viral hepatitis  398
Non-viral hepatitis  400
Cirrhosis: background and causes  401
Cirrhosis: symptoms and management  402
Complications of cirrhosis  404
Haemochromatosis (inherited)  408
Non-alcoholic fatty liver disease
    and non-alcoholic steatohepatitis  410
Other liver disorders  412
Liver disease in pregnancy  414
Liver cancer: primary  416
Liver cancer: secondary  418
Liver transplant  420
Investigations and findings  422
Blood tests relating to liver disease  424

# Structure and function

The liver is essential for life. It is a large smooth convex organ contained within a fibrous capsule in the right-hand upper quadrant of the abdominal cavity, under the diaphragm and protected by ribs. The organ moves during respiration. It comprises right and left lobes, with eight segments (Fig. 11.1).

The liver weighs approximately 1800 g in ♂ and 1400 g in ♀. Cords of hepatocytes (polyhedral cells with central spherical nuclei, which are arranged in hexagonal lobules) radiate in spokes from a central vein; capillaries (sinusoids) are located between the cells. The cells have surface villi, which provide an ↑ surface area for transfer of substances from the blood. Bile canniculi drain bile via the bile ducts towards the gall bladder. Liver tissue has a huge regenerative potential following acute damage, and the organ can regrow up to two-thirds of its weight.

The liver has >500 functions, but the main physiological functions its include the following:

- Metabolism and storage of carbohydrates, proteins, and fats.
- Glucose homeostasis—conversion of blood glucose to glycogen after meals, storage, and conversion of glycogen back to glucose during periods of fasting. Ensures the availability of energy to the body and keeps the blood sugar level even in feast and famine. Controls glucose availability and fat storage and mobilization.
- Drug and hormone metabolism—three phases: oxidation, conjugation, and elimination through secretion of bile or via the kidneys.
- Detoxification of micro-organisms and toxic substances absorbed through the gut—prevents them entering the general circulation.
- Vitamin storage—fat-soluble vitamins A, D, E, and K, in addition to vitamin $B_{12}$. Minerals are also stored.
- Bile formation and secretion—enables the liver to eliminate substances and emulsify fat.
- Manufacture of substances necessary for blood coagulation and other proteins.
- Cholesterol excretion.
- Destruction of worn-out red blood cells.

## Blood supply

The portal circulation enables nutrients and other substances absorbed through the gut to pass through the liver before entering the systemic circulation. Portal veins carry 70% of the blood supply to the liver directly from the small intestine; this blood supply is nutrient rich. There are three hepatic veins, which drain into the vena cava. There are also multiple collateral veins (which are dilated in cirrhosis—varices).

The hepatic artery carries 30% of the blood supply to the liver; 25% of cardiac output goes to the liver.

## Liver disease

This is a leading cause of morbidity and mortality: it is one of the 10 leading causes of death. There has been a threefold ↑ in deaths from liver disease in the past 30 years. Many patients with liver disease are <65 years. Diseases of the liver and pancreas account for three-quarters of GI hospital admissions.

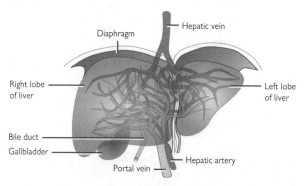

**Fig. 11.1** Liver structures. Reproduced with kind permission © Burdett Institute 2008.

# Viral hepatitis

Hepatitis is characterized by inflammation of liver. Chronic hepatitis can lead to fibrosis and eventually cirrhosis (usually over the course of many years).

## Viral hepatitis

Different viruses have different routes of transmission and effects. Viral hepatitis may rarely develop into fulminant hepatitis, which is sudden and severe; encephalopathy develops within 2–3 weeks.

### Hepatitis A virus (HAV)

HAV is transmitted by contaminated water and food and excreted in faeces. The viral incubation period is 2–6 weeks, after which flu-like symptoms develop, with nausea and diarrhoea. Jaundice can develop 1 week later. A blood test will be positive for the virus. There is no specific treatment, but the patient usually makes a complete recovery after a few weeks or months (the patient must avoid alcohol). No long-term damage is suffered and immunity develops following recovery. The disease is occasionally severe in vulnerable people. Vaccination lasts up to 10 years.

### Hepatitis B virus (HBV)

HBV is spread by contact with body fluids, including blood (most usual), but also semen, vaginal secretions, and breast milk. In the UK, 1 out of 1000 individuals are carriers. The disease is often transmitted by immigrants, infected parents to their children, or IV drug users; some cases are sexually transmitted. The virus has an incubation period of 1–6 months. A blood test can detect viral antibodies. Mild disease presents with flu-like symptoms, with nausea and vomiting. HBV infection may be acute or chronic. Occasionally, acute disease is severe and a liver transplant might be needed. Patients can become carriers, with a risk of cirrhosis and primary liver cancer. Test the whole family. To prevent the spread of the virus, vaccinate the whole family and educate about transmission routes (be careful with body fluids). There is currently no available treatment for acute disease. In chronic disease, most patients recover and are clear from the virus without treatment. 10–20% remain infected or become carriers. Interferon, lamivudine, adefovir dipivoxil, or antivirals can be given (drug side effects can be severe). The patient should maintain a balanced diet, with minimal alcohol intake. Vaccination against the virus includes three doses over a period of 3 months, with a booster every 5 years.

### Hepatitis C virus (HCV)

HCV is usually blood borne, spread by IV transmission (at least 50% of patients with HCV are IV drug users), from mother to baby, or sexually (rare). Before 1991 also via blood transfusion. Between 0.02% and 0.04% of the UK population are infected. Vague flu-like symptoms may develop, with nausea, pain, a lack of concentration, and anxiety. Symptoms can mimic chronic fatigue syndrome. There are many genotypes of virus, but a blood test will detect antibodies from exposure (which might not be present immediately) and hepatitis C polymerase chain reaction (PCR) test for active viral replication (need for treatment).

20% of patients with HCV infection, recover, 80% become chronic carriers, and 60% have chronic hepatitis. The risk of cirrhosis is 20% (could take at least 20–30 years to develop), and there is also a risk of liver carcinoma (2–3%) and non-Hodgkin lymphoma.[1] Cirrhosis develops sooner (within 10 years) in ♂ and if the patient drinks alcohol regularly or excessively. A proportion (20%) of patients also have HIV infection.

First-choice treatment is usually pegylated interferon and ribavirin. This combination therapy resolves around 50% of cases, although different genotypes of the virus respond to medication differently. Combination therapy can have serious side effects (e.g. malaise, depression, anaemia, neutropenia, and thrombocytopenia), which can limit tolerance. A balanced diet with minimal alcohol intake is also required, in addition to long-term specialist care. The survival rate is 90% at 5 years and 80% at 10 years. Careful counselling regarding the implications of chronic infection is needed. HCV infection can be slowly progressive. The patient should be advised to avoid blood donation, that there is a small risk of sexual transmission, and not to share needles, razors, or toothbrushes.

### Hepatitis D virus (HDV)

HDV infection occurs only in conjunction with hepatitis B (the virus needs the hepatitis B virus to reproduce). HDV infection is most common in developing countries; however, in the UK, the virus is prevalent in IV drug users (75% of cases) and patients receiving frequent blood transfusions (especially before 1991—less common now because all blood is tested before transfusion). HBV and HDV co-infection has a higher risk of cirrhosis than HBV infection alone. HDV is transmitted in the same ways as HBV (i.e. through contact with body fluids and blood) and IV transmission is common. The virus has an incubation period of 3–12 weeks. A blood test can be used to detect positive antibodies. There is no vaccination against HDV, but vaccination against HBV will prevent infection. Most infection is self-limiting. Severe cases: treatment may be with interferon.

### Hepatitis E virus (HEV)

Most cases of infection are reported in developing countries, in which epidemics can occur. Faeco-oral transmission is common (rather than transmission through contact with blood or body fluids). The virus has an incubation period of 2–12 weeks. HEV infection is an acute self-limiting illness, without a risk of chronic infection or long-term damage, except during the last trimester of pregnancy. Pregnant ♀ who become infected have a one in five risk of fatality and a high risk of miscarriage. No vaccine is available against the HEV.

1 Giordano TP, Hendersan L, Landgren O, et al. (2007). Risk of non-Hodgkin lymphoma and lymphoproliferative precursor disease in US veterans with Hepatitis C virus. *Journal of the American Medical Association* **297**, 2010–17.

# Non-viral hepatitis

## Alcoholic hepatitis

A high concentration of alcohol damages cells and they swell. Ballooning hepatocytes retain protein and water. Filaments (Mallory bodies) develop in hepatocytes. Neutrophils, macrophages, and lymphocytes accumulate, followed by cell necrosis and collagen deposition. Eventually, fatty liver develops, with 10% of patients developing cirrhosis ( p. 401). The Department of Health recommends a maximum of 3–4 units (10 ml pure alcohol = 1 unit) per day for men, 2–3 units for women, to prevent adverse effects from alcohol consumption.

## Autoimmune hepatitis

Most common in young ♀, especially those with other autoimmune diseases. The cause is unknown and diagnosis is made by exclusion of other causes of hepatitis. Patients are either asymptomatic, presenting with fatigue, or symptomatic with acute jaundice. Patients often take up to 2 years to respond to treatment with steroids and immunosuppressants. Treatment is successful in 90% of patients, but continuous treatment might be required. If the disease is uncontrolled after approximately 4 years, liver transplantation may be necessary in some cases.

## Further reading

Department of Health (2007). *Alcohol and health.* http://www.dh.gov.uk/en/policyandguidance/healthandsocialtopics/alcoholmisuse/(accessed 14.05.07).

# Cirrhosis: background and causes

The liver has a great capacity for repair and regeneration. Chronic (or occasionally severe acute) inflammation and scarring leads to diffuse damage/necrosis of hepatocytes. Nodules may develop and fibrotic tissue replaces the normal cell architecture, hardening this tissue and causing irreversible scarring of the liver (cirrhosis). Cirrhosis can result in derangement of the portal circulation—which impedes blood flow. May eventually lead to:

• Functional failure.
• Hepatocellular carcinoma.

In the UK, there are 3000 deaths from cirrhosis annually, of which 1200 are alcohol related.

## Pathophysiology

Hepatocytes become necrosed and are replaced by useless fibrous nodules and scar tissue. The normal delicate architecture of the liver is lost, with two major results:

• Derangement of the portal circulation, which impedes blood flow.
• Functional failure.

There are three major aetiological types of cirrhosis.

Alcoholic cirrhosis—resulting from increased consumption of alcohol. Prevalence increased in the UK (and other countries). Can be a chronic condition or related to binge-drinking. Susceptible individuals develop progressive liver disease from alcoholic hepatitis (📖 p. 400) and eventual cirrhosis. The disease can progress from a large fatty liver to a small shrunken liver with fibrous nodules and an impeded blood flow. Cirrhosis is more probable if the patient also has HCV infection (📖 p. 398) or any other liver condition. Hepatocellular carcinoma eventually develops in 15–20% of patients with cirrhosis.

Primary biliary cirrhosis (PBC)—the cause is unknown (?autoimmune), but the disease results in the destruction of bile ducts, leading to an accumulation of bile in the liver and inflammation. Commonly occurs in 5 (9 out of 10 cases). The disease runs in families, commonly occurs in the middle-aged, and patients could also have other autoimmune disorders. Infection can trigger cirrhosis in predisposed individuals. Antimitochondrial antibody (AMA) is found using a blood test. Patients could have xanthelasma (deposits of cholesterol-laden macrophages) around their eyes.

Post-necrotic cirrhosis—after acute fulminant hepatitis or chronic viral hepatitis.

In liver cirrhosis, many vital functions of the liver are lost to a greater or lesser degree. The main causes are as follows:

• Alcohol abuse—50% of cases.
• Any form of chronic hepatitis.
• Primary biliary cirrhosis.
• Primary sclerosing cholangitis.
• Haemochromatosis.
• AMA.
• Wilson's disease—a congenital failure to excrete copper, leading to deposition of copper in the liver and brain.

# Cirrhosis: symptoms and management

## Symptoms
- May be completely asymptomatic until advanced.
- Fatigue.
- Itching.
- Right upper quadrant discomfort.
- Fever.
- Anorexia.
- Nausea.
- Arthritis.
- Palmar erythema.
- Dry eyes.
- Diarrhoea.
- Dark urine.
- Jaundice.

Cirrhosis can remain compensated for many years before symptoms develop. 'Decompensated' cirrhosis results from the liver being unable to compensate for loss of function: portal hypertension and hepatic insufficiency result. Jaundice, variceal haemorrhage, ascites, or encephalopathy may signal decompensation.

## Investigations
A series of biochemical tests (liver function tests) on a blood sample are used to investigate hepatic disease:
- ↑ aminotransferase suggests hepatocellular disease.
- A predominant ↑ in alkaline phosphatase indicates cholestatic or biliary tract problems.

Additionally, ultrasound and biopsy of the liver are used as diagnostic tools or to assess the extent of liver damage. See liver investigations (📖 p. 422).

## Management
Cirrhosis is by definition irreversible. Antiviral therapy can sometimes halt progression of cirrhotic damage in viral hepatitis, and primary biliary cholangitis is treated with ursodeoxycholic acid and immunosuppressants. However, management of cirrhosis focuses primarily on treating its complications (📖 p. 404), as follows:
- Treat alcohol dependence (e.g. naltrexone).
- Colestyramine—itching.
- Moisturize—dry skin.
- Tear replacement—dry eyes.
- Dietary restrictions are generally not required in uncomplicated cirrhosis, although ↓ fat intake can help in steatorrhoea and patients with oedema should avoid salt in their diet.
- Avoid alcohol.
- Diuretics—↓ fluid accumulation.
- Vitamin supplements—malabsorption.
- Monitor osteoporosis.

- Warn patients with clotting disorders, e.g. take extra care with dental treatment.
- Portal hypertension with bleeding varices is a serious complication of cirrhosis that can be treated by primary or secondary prophylaxsis: Primary, banding to eradicate varices; secondary, β- blockers.
- Patients with complications, e.g. resistant ascites, are candidates for a shunt procedure or liver transplant.

## Further reading

Patient information can be obtained from britishlivertrust.org.uk (accessed 22 May 2008).

# Complications of cirrhosis

The effects and complications of liver cirrhosis are many and varied (Box 11.1).

## Portal hypertension

↑ pressure in the portal vein results from cirrhosis (↑ resistance to blood flow) or a blood clot. Normal pressure 1–5 mmHg; 12 mmHg ≥ risk of oesophageal or gastric bleeding (see below).

### Symptoms

It can be asymptomatic, but signs and symptoms are as follows:

- Enlarged spleen.
- Collateral vessels may develop.
- Varices.
- Ascites.
- Haemorrhoids.
- Caput medusae—dilated veins around the umbilicus.
- Rarely, a result of parasitic disease (common in developing countries) or pancreatic disease.

### Management

Non-selective β- blockers (e.g. propranolol) may prevent development of varices. Endoscopic screening for varices at 1–3 year intervals. Alcohol abstinence. Or targeted at managing secondary effects of varices and ascites.[1]

## Oesophageal/gastric varices

Varices are caused by dilation of the collateral veins and formation of new veins in the upper stomach and oesophagus. 30 – 50% of patients with portal hypertension 30%–50% will develop bleeding varices. Varices are progressive over time; if they are alcohol-related, they can regress if the patient avoids alcohol.

### Symptoms

Although varices can be detected by endoscopy, they can be asymptomatic unless they bleed. Bleeding may be triggered by bacterial infection. A slow oozing bleed can present as anaemia, whereas a large bleed can present as haematemesis or melaena which is an emergency (📖 p. 704). A significant bleed requires >2 units of blood, systolic blood pressure <100 mmHg, or pulse >100 beats/min.

### Management

The mortality rate is 50% from the first major bleed in high-risk patients. Treatment is with blood and fluid replacement. The risk of re-bleeding is assessed using the Childs–Pugh score (Table 11.1): class A ≈ 5% risk of re-bleeding within 1 year and class C ≈ 50% risk of re-bleeding within 1 year.

---

1 Samonakis D *et al* (2004). Management of portal hypertension. *Postgraduate Medical Journal* **80**, 634–41.

The acute control of bleeding varices is outlined in more detail on 📖 p. 194. Protect the patient's airway and resuscitate. Variceal band ligation or sclerotherapy can be used, but if they are not available, terlipressin can be used instead. If bleeding is difficult to control, use a Sengstaken tube. A transjugular intra-hepatic portosystemic shunt (TIPS) or surgery is used for repeated bleeds. Propanolol can be used to prevent bleeding or re-bleeding.

Because of the high mortality rate, all patients with diagnosed cirrhosis should undergo endoscopy. Patients without varices should undergo endoscopy again after 3–4 years. Patients with grade I varices should undergo endoscopy again after 1 year. Patients with grade II or III varices should receive propranolol or band ligation of varices as a preventive measure.

## Box 11.1 The effects and complications of liver cirrhosis

- Portal hypertension and collateral circulation.
- Oesophageal or gastric varices (bleeding).
- Ascites.
- Circulatory changes.
- Pulmonary changes.
- Jaundice.
- Tissue loss.
- Changes in nitrogen metabolism.
- Disordered blood coagulation.
- Fetor hepaticus.
- Skin changes, e.g. spider naevi.
- Hepatic encephalopathy.
- Osteoporosis.
- Endocrine changes, e.g. gynaecomastia.
- Hepatitis—HAV, HBV, HCV, HDV, and HEV.

**Table 11.1** Childs–Pugh score for assessment of the severity of cirrhosis

| Category | 1 | 2 | 3 |
|---|---|---|---|
| Encephalopathy | 0 | I/II | III/IV |
| Ascites | Absent | Mild/moderate | Severe |
| Bilirubin (µmol/L) | <34 | 34–51 | >51 |
| Albumin (g/L) | >35 | 28–35 | <28 |
| International Normalized Ratio (prothrombin time) | <1.3 | 1.3–1.5 | >1.5 |

Class A: score 6 or less.
Class B: score 7–9.
Class C: score 10 or more.

### Ascites

Ascites is the collection of fluid in the peritoneal cavity (between the layers of the peritoneum). Mild ascites can be diagnosed using ultrasound. Moderate ascites cause some abdominal distension. Severe ascites causes marked abdominal distension.

Portal hypertension causes fluid to accumulate in the peritoneum. If the level of protein in the blood is ↓, the osmotic gradient is disturbed, leading to salt and water retention. Lymphatic secondary tumours can block lymph drainage. Ascites can be a response to secondary tumours in the peritoneum.

75% of patients with ascites, have cirrhosis; 50% of patients with cirrhosis for at least 10 years develop ascites. The mortality rate for ascites is 50% at 2 years. Consider whether a liver transplant is appropriate in such patients.

#### Symptoms
- Abdominal distension.
- Shifting dullness on percussion.
- Pain.
- Peripheral oedema.

#### Management
- First line: diuretics—spironolactone or furosemide.
- ↓ salt intake.
- Bedrest is not helpful.

#### Paracentesis

If treatment fails to control ascites, use paracentesis to drain. Explain procedure to patient and reassure. Informed consent. Ultrasound to check pre-procedure. Commercial kits available. Clean skin and sterile drapes. Insert needle 15 cm lateral to the umbilicus. Up to 10 L of fluid can be removed over of period of 1–6 h; turn the patient to ensure efficient drainage. Monitor for hypotension and hypovolaemic shock, haematoma, leakage from drain site (might require a suture), and perforation (rare). Usually need albumin infusion if large volume (3–4 L) removed (1 unit of 20% human albumin solution to every 3 L of ascites removed). Send sample for laboratory analysis. Rarely, a peritoneo-venous shunt is required. TIPS is rarely used as it is prone to complications. Liver transplant may be considered.

#### Complications of ascites in cirrhosis

Spontaneous bacterial peritonitis is common and has a 20% mortality rate. Treat with antibiotics (cephalosporins) and provide long-term prophylaxis with norfloxacin.

### Hepatic encephalopathy

A reaction to toxins inadequately managed by the failing liver (exact mechanism is uncertain).

*Symptoms*

Brain oedema is common. Because nitrogen products can mimic neuro-transmitters, a range of neurological symptoms can present. Ammonia and electrolyte disturbances have a variable effect on the level of consciousness, from slight confusion to coma and death.

*Management*

Treatment is with lactulose (to limit the production of ammonia by colonic bacteria). Restrict the amount of protein in the diet. Good nutrition is very important in recovery.

## Hepato-renal syndrome

The syndrome is characterized by combined severe liver and renal failure. Usually fatal. The exact mechanism is unclear.

*Symptoms*

- ↓ renal blood flow.
- ↓ glomerular filtration rate.
- ↓ urine output.
- Sodium retention.
- Disorders of the renin–angiotensin pathway.
- Affects levels of aldosterone, norepinephrine, and vasopressin.

*Management*

Vasoconstrictor medication (e.g. terlipressin which also increases renal blood flow and filtration). Plasma volume expansion with albumin infusion. Dialysis (haemo or peritoneal) may be used.

## Further reading

British Society of Gastroenterology (2006) *Guideline on Management of Ascites in Cirrhosis*. http://www.bsg.org.uk/pdf_word_docs/ascites_cirrhosis.pdf (accessed 14.05.07).

# Haemochromatosis (inherited)

An inherited (recessive) condition related to the HFE gene, which is also called genetic haemochromatosis, GH, and iron-overload disorder. It is the most common genetic disorder in Caucasians, affecting 1 out of 400 individuals in the UK. In addition, 10% of the population are carriers. The disease is characterized by the body absorbing too much iron from food, which is deposited in liver, pancreas, heart, endocrine glands, and other organs. Iron levels can be 20-fold greater than normal. A normal healthy adult absorbs 1–2 mg iron/day, which can ↑ to 3–6 mg/day in haemochromatosis. Occasionally, the disease results from repeated blood transfusions, chronic liver disease, or thalassaemia. If identified before cirrhosis and diabetes develop, life expectancy remains normal. Haemochromatosis may also be acquired, e.g. due to repeated blood transfusion, cirrhosis (uncontrolled iron uptake), or excessive dietary iron intake (uptake increased by alcohol and vitamin C).

## Signs and symptoms

Patients are often asymptomatic. The disease is usually diagnosed in adults >40 years as part of investigation for abnormal liver function tests, investigation for other conditions (e.g. joint pain in diabetes), or on routine blood test or screening of affected family members. Common symptoms, if present:

• Fatigue, mood swings, and depression.
• Abdominal pains.
• Bronze skin pigmentation ('bronze diabetes').
• Diabetes mellitus in two-thirds of patients (damaged pancreas produces insufficient insulin).
• Arthritis (especially in the first two finger joints).
• Heart arrhythmias.
• ♀ might be asymptomatic because they lose iron during menstrual bleeding—early menopause is common.
• In ♂, the genital organs shrink and there is a loss of libido (pituitary effect).
• Liver enlargement and cirrhosis eventually.
• Eventually, liver failure and primary liver carcinoma.

## Diagnosis

• ↑ blood ferritin levels (consider transferritin saturation levels).
• The presence of the HFE gene (blood test).
• Enlarged liver.
• Liver biopsy—if liver damage is suspected.

## Treatment

Venesection once or twice a week until iron levels are normalized (~500 ml of blood is removed each time (~250 mg of iron)). Treatment for up to 2 years could be necessary. The body can store 10–20 g excess iron. Following successful treatment, venesection is performed several times a year to maintain a normal iron level. The venesection service is often nurse-led. Venesection is contraindicated in patients with anaemia or cardiac disease. In these patients, use desferrioxamine, which binds to iron and enables its excretion (efficacy limited). Cirrhosis and diabetes cannot be reversed. The patient will have a normal life expectancy if they are treated before severe complications develop. The patient may develop cirrhosis and all its complications (📖 p. 402) Occasionally, for severe liver damage, a liver transplant is required.

## Nursing care

Patients need a significant amount of support and counselling on the genetic implications. Test siblings and children. Avoid red meat and offal (high in iron), alcohol (promotes iron absorption and affects the liver), vitamin C (encourages iron deposition), vitamin supplements, and cereals with added iron. Tea and milk can ↓ iron absorption. Some centres advise that diet change (except restricted alcohol) is not needed if undergoing venesection.

The Haemochromatosis Society (http://www.ghsoc.org) can provide patient support.

## Further reading

Yen AW, Fancher TL, Bowlus L (2006). Revisiting hereditary hemochromatosis: current concepts and progress. *American Journal of Medicine*, **119**, 391–9.

# Non-alcoholic fatty liver disease and non-alcoholic steatohepatitis

## Non-alcoholic fatty liver disease (NAFLD)

Cause unclear. May be similar in presentation to alcoholic hepatitis (i.e. inflammation and scar tissue), with fatty deposits, but not related to alcohol consumption. Associated with metabolic syndrome (obesity, hypertension, diabetes mellitus, high cholesterol) and some medications, particularly steroid use. May present at any age (including children), but most often in middle age. Patients develop fatty liver, but the condition seldom progresses to cirrhosis. About 10% have cirrhosis and its complications. A routine blood test commonly detects abnormal liver function, but patients can be asymptomatic, or present with fatigue, malaise, and right-hand upper abdominal pain and an enlarged liver. Once cirrhosis is established, the symptoms will be the same (☐ p. 402) The prevalence is ↑ and the disease might affect up to 10–20% of the population in affluent countries. Treatment includes weight loss (not too rapid), exercise, control of diabetes, a low-fat diet, cholesterol lowering medication and limiting alcohol intake. May progress to NASH (see below).

## Non-alcoholic steatohepatitis (NASH)

Risk factors: as for NAFLD. Potentially mores serious and progressive than NAFLD, with hepatic fatty deposits, inflammation, and ultimately cirrhosis, but may be asymptomatic, or stable and non-progressive, for many years. Often found on routine blood tests. May present with fatigue and discomfort. Distinguish from NAFLD by liver biopsy. May be triggered by insulin resistance. Treatment is with weight loss, diabetes control, diet and exercise, alcohol avoidance. Medications to treat are under investigation. If cirrhosis has developed, liver will be scarred and hardened. May need transplant if severe.

# Other liver disorders

## Gilbert's syndrome

An inherited (recessive) condition in which an ↑ level of bilirubin is incompletely broken down by liver because of a lack of an enzyme that conjugates it. The syndrome is not harmful, except that the patient can develop jaundice when they are unwell or fasting (raised levels of unconjugated bilirubin). It affects 2–5% of the population. Treatment is not usually required. Patients can join an official support group (http://www.gilbertssyndrome.org.uk).

## Wilson's disease

- A rare inherited (recessive) disorder of copper metabolism, affecting 1 in 30 000 individuals. Affected individuals cannot excrete copper (which is essential for cell metabolism), leading to an accumulation of copper in liver cells and subsequently necrosis of the cells. Copper can also build up in the brain causing variable psychiatric symptoms. The disease usually presents in adolescents and young adults, with varied vague symptoms. It can be misdiagnosed as adolescent mood swings, although the liver is enlarged. Patients might have brown rings in their eyes under the cornea (Kayser–Fleischer rings). The following symptoms can develop later:
- Jaundice and ascites.
- Liver failure.
- Progressive fatal neurological disorders.

Diagnosis is made using a blood test for copper levels or caeruloplasmin (a copper-binding protein) or liver biopsy. The disease can progress to cirrhosis or acute or chronic hepatitis; if untreated, it can be fatal. Treatment is with penicillamine (for life), which binds copper; however, one-third of patients develop troublesome side effects. Trientine or tetrathiomolybdate (available on a named patient basis in the UK) can also be used. Avoid shellfish, nuts, chocolate, and mushrooms (which are high in copper). The patient might need a liver transplant if diagnosed late (transplant is curative). First-degree relatives should have copper levels checked. No specific genetic test yet available. Patients can join an official support group (http://www.wilsonsdisease.org.uk)

## Paracetamol overdose

Paracetamol has a narrow therapeutic index (there is a small dose between therapeutic and toxic levels). Deliberate or accidental overdose is common. The patient might not realize harm is caused because they are awake and feel well. Acute overdose is characterized by renal failure, ↑ intracranial pressure, coma, multi-organ failure, and systemic sepsis. Paracetamol overdose is the primary cause of acute liver failure; 0.4% overdoses are fatal. N-acetylcysteine is an antidote. Acute transplant may be needed. If the patient survives, a complete recovery, with no residual damage, is common.

## Drug reactions

Because the liver has a major role in detoxifying drugs, a variety of other idiosyncratic drug reactions (e.g. to tetracycline, NSAIDs, and ecstasy) is possible and can be severe.

## Porphyria

An inherited disorder of haem synthesis. Often presents with neurological symptoms or psychosis.

# Liver disease in pregnancy

## Normal pregnancy

Liver function tests often altered (e.g. raised plasma volume leads to lowered serum albumen). Interpret blood tests with caution in pregnant women. Some pregnancy symptoms can mimic liver disease (spider naevi, palmar erythema, due to high oestrogen levels). Gallstones: increased risk in pregnancy (6% of pregnancies); slowed gall bladder emptying + hormonal—can treat as non-pregnant (📖 p. 443) but avoid surgery in last trimester. Rarely, choledocholithiasis leads to pancreatitis, which can be serious (📖 p. 430) Pregnancy can lead to symptom exacerbation in women with pre-existing liver disease (e.g. bleeding varices).

## Viral hepatitis

Most common cause of jaundice in pregnancy. Mothers with hepatitis B and C risk infection of baby at delivery unless prophylaxis and immunization given. Developing countries: hepatitis E and herpes simplex virus (HSV) infections: high risk of infant and mother mortality.

## Obstetric cholestasis

1:10 000 pregnancies. Characterized by ↓ flow of bile from the liver, usually in the last trimester. The cause is unknown (?accumulation of hormones). Itching (pruritus) is common (80%) and can be severe, often at night; nausea, dark urine, and pale stools or jaundice (20%) may occur. The syndrome disappears spontaneously after birth. Racial and genetic predisposition (often family history). It can be serious for the baby, possibly causing prematurity or stillbirth. ∴ it is important to recognize and treat the syndrome. Treat with ursodeoxycholic acid or similar. Colestyramine may help itching. Induce delivery at 37–38 weeks' gestation. Resolves after delivery. Risk recurrence in future pregnancy.

## Pre-eclampsia and eclampsia

May involve liver as a complication, with hepatocellular necrosis in severe forms. HELLP (haemolysis, elevated liver enzymes, low platelet count) may be associated with severe pre-eclampsia. Pain, weight gain, nausea, oedema, and malaise. Prompt delivery crucial. 2% maternal mortality; 30% fetal mortality. Very rarely hepatic rupture and infarction associated with pre-eclampsia.

## Acute fatty liver of pregnancy (AFLP)

Rarely (1: 13 000 deliveries), obstetric fatty liver also develops in the third trimester, which is serious and accompanied by nausea, vomiting, pain, and jaundice. Or can present as fulminant liver failure and encephalopathy. Associated with pre-eclampsia and twins. 20% mortality of mother and baby. Deliver the baby urgently and manage liver failure.

## Further reading

Knox TA and Olans LB (1996). Liver disease in pregnancy. New *England Journal of Medicine* **335**, 569–76.

# Liver cancer: primary

The majority of cases of liver cancer in developed countries are secondary to a primary tumour elsewhere in the body. Often, symptoms present late in both primary and secondary liver cancers. Imaging diagnoses most cases.

## Primary liver tumours

2500 new cases per year in UK. The ratio of prevalence in ♂:♀ is 2:1.

## Hepatocellular carcinoma (hepatoma or HCC)

A primary tumour of hepatocytes, which is a complication of many liver diseases, particularly alcoholic liver disease, hepatitis C infection, hepatitis B infection, and haemochromatosis, especially if cirrhosis present. High-risk patients should be screened regularly (every 6 months) using ultrasound and a blood test to detect ↑ level of α-fetoprotein (AFP)—not totally reliable alone. Screen all cirrhotic patients to detect complications early. HCC is only potentially curable if it is detected when small.

Developing counties: associated with aflatoxin from mouldy grain and peanuts.

Often, there are no early symptoms, with the exception of discomfort if the liver is enlarged. A referred pain might be felt in the shoulder. Later, patients present with loss of appetite, weight loss, nausea, lethargy, jaundice, and ascites.

The tumour has a doubling time of 4 months. Transplant is possible, if a single tumour <5 cm or 2–3 tumours <3 cm each. Stages are shown in Table 11.2.

### Treatment

Depends on the size and stage of the tumour, in addition to the presence of comorbidities and the patient's general health. Small single tumours <5 cm or up to three small tumours <3 cm can be resected surgically or removed by a lobectomy (partial liver resection) or liver transplant. If the tumour is inoperable, ablation can be performed using percutaneous ethanol or injection of acetic acid. In addition, laser or radiofrequency ablation can destroy the tumour using heat or cryotherapy can freeze the tumour. Chemoembolization (via an artery in the groin under X-ray guidance) may restrict blood supply and thus growth of the tumour and/or deliver chemotherapy agents directly to the tumour.

Chemotherapy or radiotherapy can be used for larger/multiple/spread tumours (efficacy limited).

## Cholangiocarcinoma

A rare and aggressive primary tumour of the bile ducts. The prevalence is ↑ (the reason is unknown) and cholangiocarcinoma now accounts for 1000 deaths/year in the UK. The prevalence in ♂ and ♀ is equal. The disease usually presents with jaundice and weight loss when already advanced. The disease is linked to sclerosing cholangitis (📖 p. 625), ulcerative colitis, smoking, chronic gallstones, and parasitic infection (in developing countries). Surgery is the only potential cure, but the prognosis is poor. Radiotherapy and chemotherapy have little benefit; further trials are required. Cholangiocarcinoma is difficult to treat, but a biliary stent can relieve obstructive jaundice. The survival rate at 5 years is <15%.

**Table 11.2** Stages of hepatocellular cancinoma

| Stage | Description |
| --- | --- |
| 1 | <2 cm, with no spread |
| 2 | Affecting the hepatic blood vessels or more than one tumour |
| 3A | >5 cm or spread to local blood vessels |
| 3B | Spread to adjacent organs (e.g. bowel or stomach) but not lymph nodes |
| 3C | Spread to local lymph nodes |
| 4 | Remote spread (e.g. lung) |

# Liver cancer: secondary

Almost all primary tumours can spread to the liver. The following primary tumours most commonly produce secondary tumours in the liver:

- Bowel.
- Breast.
- Stomach.
- Lung.
- Ovary.
- Skin.
- Pancreas.

The tumour spreads through the bloodstream. Occasionally, the primary site is undetected. Treatment depends on the primary site, extent of the tumour, and the patient's general health. Chemotherapy is the mainstay of therapy, especially if it was successful in treating the primary tumour.

Radiotherapy is palliative only (relieves discomfort and nausea).

## Colorectal secondary tumours

At diagnosis, 20–25% of patients with colorectal cancer have secondary liver tumours; this figure ↑ to 40–50% 3 years after diagnosis. In the UK, 33000 new cases of colorectal cancer are diagnosed each year. In patients with a primary bowel tumour, surgery can resect a limited secondary liver tumour if no other secondary tumours are found. CT should be performed on diagnosis of colorectal cancer to assess the liver. A blood test should also be performed to detect the serum level of carcinoembryonic antigen (CEA). It is now considered unethical not to offer surgery for resectable tumours. Aim for clear resection margins, because this technique is potentially curative. Up to two-thirds of the liver can be removed without harm to the patient. The survival rate after surgery is 25–44% at 5 years. Chemotherapy can shrink liver metastases before surgery. Ablation can also be used. Ensure multidisciplinary discussion (between patient, physician, surgeon, radiologist, oncologist, and nurse specialist) to ensure opimal decision-making.

## Neuroendocrine secondary tumours

Often, symptoms of hormone overproduction can indicate a tumour. A neuroendocrine secondary tumour is the only type of liver tumour for which liver transplant is considered.

# Liver transplant

Liver transplantation is increasingly routine, although it remains major surgery. In the UK, ~650 liver transplants are performed each year (seven specialist units; a team approach is crucial). A cadaver donor is usual; there is a shortage of donors, so the patient could wait months or years on the transplant waiting list. The blood group and body size must be matched. In children, a live donor can donate a lobe. Patients experience great anxiety and uncertainty while on the waiting list; support is needed. An in-patient pre-operative assessment lasting 1–2 weeks is necessary.

## Indications

A liver transplant is only considered for end-stage irreversible liver failure for which other treatments have failed to maintain adequate liver function, e.g. acute fulminant hepatitis (15% of transplants) or chronic conditions. Transplant should be avoided in most patients with cancer or sepsis. Most liver transplants are performed because of cirrhosis secondary to primary biliary cirrhosis, primary sclerosing cholangitis, alcoholic cirrhosis (less commonly), primary liver tumours <2 cm, HCV, and paracetamol overdose. The procedure is contraindicated in patients with HIV/AIDS (except if a good CD4 lymphocyte count), a primary non-liver tumour, or cardiopulmonary disease, and those who are unable to comply with the post-operative drug regimen for life or who continue to misuse drugs or alcohol.[1] Try to plan the transplant for before the patient becomes too unwell to cope with major surgery.

## Risks and survival

There is a risk during removal of the original liver: bleeding owing to portal hypertension, varices, and clotting disorders. The operation lasts 6–10 h. There are considerable risks associated with liver transplantation, so the patient must give their informed consent to surgery. The survival rate is 90% at 1 year and 75% at 5 years (the survival rate is lower in patients >65 years and for acute transplant).

## Post-operative management

The patient remains in intensive care for 12–24 h and is ventilated at first. Central venous pressure line, nasogastric tube, and urinary catheter will be in place. Right upperquadrant wound.

Multiple drains are usual. Monitor for bleed (anatomosis + disordered clotting: 5% need transfusion; 3% re-operation for bleeding), sepsis or bile leak. 50% acute rejection: most respond to medication.

Patient will be given immunosuppressants ∴ risk infection; antibiotics; antifungal liquid (prophylaxis for mouth infections); antacid. 2–3 weeks hospitalization.

Convalescence lasts 3–6 months, after which many individuals return to a full normal life, including work.

Monitor the patient for rejection of the transplant. Most individuals need lifelong immunosuppressants, e.g. azathioprine, prednisolone, and

1 British Society of Gastroenterology (2000). *Indications for Referral and Assessment in Adult Liver Transplantation.* http://www.bsg.org.uk (accessed 14.05.07).

ciclosporin (with consequent risk of infection and side effects). Early rejection usually occurs within 5–10 days of the transplant. Signs of rejection include:

- Fever.
- Malaise.
- Hepatomegaly (inflammatory).
- Abdominal tenderness.
- Itching.
- Jaundice.

Treat rejection with immunosuppressants. Late rejection occurs 1–9 months after transplant, with symptoms that include fever, fatigue, jaundice, and itching. Pregnancy is well tolerated once the acute phase is over.

▶ Medication and monitoring is required for life. ∴ teamwork between specialist centres, the local hospital, and primary care is also crucial.

Patients can experience sleep disturbance, anxiety, or depression. In addition, they are at risk of new-onset diabetes, hypertension, and high cholesterol levels.

## Further reading

Killenberg PG and Clavien PA (2006). *Medical Care of the Liver Transplant Patient*. Blackwell Oxford.

Prasad KR and Lodge JP (2001). Transplantation of the liver and pancreas. *British Medical Journal* 322, 845–7.

# Investigations and findings

## History

History-taking is the same as for any general health history. Make a special note of drug/alcohol/substance use and misuse (important not to pre-judge or stigmatize). Take a family history. Ask about diet and any symptoms of infection.

## Physical examination

The liver may be enlarged or small in chronic alcoholic liver disease. In primary biliary cirrhosis it may be enlarged. An enlarged spleen is common in chronic liver disease. Look for skin discoloration or jaundice; sclera indicate jaundice.

## Jaundice

- Diagnose on examination and blood tests.
- Usually develops if bilirubin >45 µmol/L of blood.
- Pre-hepatic—haemolytic conditions.
- Hepatic—liver damage.
- Post-hepatic—obstruction of the flow of bile.

## Stigmata of chronic liver disease

Classic findings, usually associated with cirrhosis, are as follows:
- Palmar erythema—red discoloration of the palms of the hands.
- Finger clubbing (rare).
- Spider naevi.
- White nails (leuconychia).
- Skin pigmentation (jaundice or haemochromatosis).

## Blood tests relating to liver disease

📖 p. 424.

## Imaging

- Endoscopy.
- Ultrasound—fast and clear fluids only for 4–6 h before imaging.
- CT/MRI.
- Laparoscopy.
- Hepatic angiogram.

## Liver biopsy

Taking a sample of liver tissue to determine the extent of liver damage. May be percutaneous, ultrasound, CT or MRI guided, or transjugular. A fine hollow needle is used to biopsy the liver under local anaesthetic. The patient must be able to expire and hold their breath. Anxious patients might need midazolam sedation. Before the procedure:
- Obtain informed consent.
- Measure the prothrombin time and platelet count.
- Determine the patient's blood group.
- Save plasma.

- Give vitamin K to patients with clotting disorders.
- Give prophylactic antibiotics to patients at risk of bacteraemia
  (e.g. those with heart valve disease).

The biopsy track might be plugged (with gelatin) after the procedure. Biopsy can be painful, so give analgesia as indicated. The patient should have bedrest for 6–8 h after the procedure because of the risk of intraperitoneal haemorrhage or leakage of bile. Observe the patient's vital signs every 15 min for 2 h, then every 30 min for 2 h, and finally every hour for 2 h. Most complications (61%) present within first 2 h following biopsy. Day case (usual) or overnight observation if high risk of bleed (clotting disorders).

### Risks

The mortality rate is 0.01%. Morbidity can result from pain, hypotension, vasovagal episodes (might require atropine), puncture to other organs (rare), or a significant bleed (1 out of 500 patients). There is a small risk of spreading the tumour along the needle track in suspected cancer, so laparoscopy might be preferable to needle biopsy.

### Patient information given on discharge

Take painkillers if needed at home; rarely, can bleed up to 5 days later; monitor signs.

# Blood tests relating to liver disease

A variety of blood tests can indicate abnormal liver function (Table 11.3). A full blood count (FBC), virology screen, and urinalysis are also useful.

**Table 11.3** Blood tests for liver damage and disorders

|  | Normal range | Likely abnormality in liver disease | Reason |
|---|---|---|---|
| Albumin | 35–50 g/L | ↓ | Synthesized in the liver |
| Bilirubin | 3–17 μmol/L | ↑ | The liver conjugates and excretes in bile |
| Aminotransferases (AST, ALT) | 5–35 IU/L | ↑ | Leakage from damaged hepatocytes into plasma |
| Alkaline phosphatase | 30–300 IU/L | ↑ | Leakage from damaged hepatocytes into plasma. ↑ production in PBC and secondary cancer |
| Auto-antibodies, e.g. AMA, ANA, ASMA | Various | ↑ in auto-immune liver disorders | PBC and auto-immune hepatitis: inflammation in response to circulating antibodies |
| Hepatitis A, B, C | No antibodies | Antibodies may be present | Antibodies produced in reaction to infection (past or active) |
| Alpha-1 antitrypsin | 1.5–3.5 g/L | Deficiency | Genetic deficiency (Caucasians) of this protease inhibitor which controls inflammation can lead to liver damage |
| G-GT | 0–0.5 μkat/L | ↑ | ↑ after alcohol ingestion |

**Table 11.3** (*Contd.*)

|  | Normal range | Likely abnormality in liver disease | Reason |
|---|---|---|---|
| Prothrombin time | 10–14 s | Prolonged (or vitamin K deficiency) | Made in the liver. Vitamin K-dependent. No production or biliary obstruction. Bile salts needed for absorption |
| Immunoglobulins |  | ↑ | Formed in the liver |
| α-fetoprotein | <10 kU/L | ↑ | Especially in hepatocellular cancer or hepatitis |
| Copper | 11–22 μmol/L | ↑ in Wilson's disease | Unable to excrete copper |
| Ferritin | 150–200 mcg/L | ↑ in haemo-chromatosis | Increased iron absorption |
| Iron saturation (total iron binding capacity) | 30–50% saturated | ↑ in haemo-chromatosis and hepatitis | Increased iron absorption |

AST, aspartate aminotransferase; ALT, alanine aminotransferase; AMA, anti-mitochondrial antibodies; ANA, antinuclear antibodies; ASMA, anti-smooth-muscle antibodies; PBC, primary biliary cirrhosis; G-GT, gamma-glutamyltransferase.

# Pancreas

Structure and function  *428*
Acute pancreatitis  *430*
Chronic pancreatitis  *432*
Malignancies and tumours  *434*
Cystic fibrosis  *436*
Other pancreatic disorders  *437*

# Structure and function

## Introduction
The pancreas has several functions and thus abnormalities or diseases can cause a variety of complications. Curing some pancreatic diseases might not be possible.

## Structure
The pancreas lies horizontally below the stomach and comprises the body, head and tail, with a central pancreatic duct. It is a large gland, comprising exocrine and endocrine tissue, and is ~12.5 cm in length and 2.5 cm thick; the tail is situated by the spleen and the head encircles the duodenum (☐ Fig 13.1, p. 441). The main pancreatic duct joins the common bile duct, before opening into the duodenum at the ampulla of Vater.

## Function
The pancreas performs two distinct functions: endocrine and exocrine.

### Endocrine function
The pancreas secretes the hormones insulin and glucagon from the Islets of Langerhans (scattered throughout the pancreas) into the bloodstream to control blood sugar levels. Insulin secretion is stimulated mainly by an ↑ in the blood glucose concentration. Glucagon secretion is stimulated by hypoglycaemia. Hormones such as epinephrine also have an effect on pancreatic secretion. The exocrine function of the pancreas is not considered further in this volume.

### Exocrine function
The pancreas has an exocrine function as an accessory digestive organ, producing digestive enzymes that are synthesized and stored. Secretion is stimulated by hormonal signals when food enters the duodenum. The pancreas secretes ~1500 ml/day of enzyme-rich fluid (clear colourless pancreatic juice) into the duodenum. Secretions help neutralize acidic chyme (bicarbonate), which enters the duodenum from the stomach. The enzymes are used to digest fats (pancreatic lipase), proteins (trypsin and chymotrypsin), and carbohydrates (amylase). Pancreatic juice is highly irritant to skin (implications for high output stoma).

## Further reading
Keshav S (2004). *The Gastrointestinal System at a Glance*. Blackwell Science, Oxford.

# Acute pancreatitis

Acute pancreatitis is a relatively common acute inflammatory process. The incidence of acute pancreatitis is approximately 2 per 100 000 individuals per year in the UK.[1]

## Causes

The causes of acute pancreatitis are as follows.
• Obstructive—common-bile-duct stone or obstructing tumour.
• Toxic—alcohol abuse (especially after a heavy binge).
• Drug-related.
• Infection (usually viral).
• Metabolic.

Acute pancreatitis is predominantly associated with alcohol or gallstones (80%), although in up to 10% of patients there is no identifiable cause. Digestive enzymes become activated in the pancreas and start to 'digest' pancreatic tissue.

## Symptoms

Although clinical presentations vary, acute pancreatitis should be considered in patients presenting with acute abdominal pain. Symptoms often include the following.
• Epigastric pain, radiating to the back.
• Acutely unwell.
• Often, nausea or vomiting.
• Possibly abdominal distension.

Symptoms usually resolve completely over a few days. Can be very severe inflammation and necrosis (1 in 5 cases). Leak of pancreatic enzymes to other organs with renal and respiratory complications. Occasionally fatal.

## Investigations

• Blood amylase and lipase (will be raised).
• Blood sugar monitoring (inflammation can disturb endocrine function).
• Plain X-ray of the chest and abdomen to exclude other causes of the symptoms.
• Ultrasound can detect gallstones, but is not as useful for visualizing the pancreas.
• A computerized tomography (CT) scan can exclude pancreatic tumours and necrosis or infected necrosis—the latter requires surgery.
• Endoscopic ultrasound may be used to identify patients that require a therapeutic endoscopic retrograde cholangiopancreatography (ERCP).

1 Long RG and Scott BB (2005). *Gastroenterology and Liver Disease*. Elsevier Mosby, London.

## Management

Treatment is usually hospitalization for IV fluids and strong analgesia; a nasogastric tube can be useful to control vomiting. Recovery is usually spontaneous within 2–4 days. For those with severe pancreatitis, intensive care therapy could be required, and giving prophylactic antibiotics might prevent septic complications. Early ERCP with 24–72 h of admission can ↓ morbidity and mortality in patients where gallstones are impacted and causing the pancreatitis. Surgical debridement might be required if there is infected necrosis. Reverse any underlying cause if found (gallstone surgery, limit alcohol intake).

# Chronic pancreatis

Chronic pancreatitis is a progressive inflammatory disease of the pancreas. The patient reports severe, recurrent episodes of abdominal pain associated with an inflamed pancreas. The cause of chronic pancreatitis is often alcohol abuse and the incidence is probably ↑ as alcohol intake increases.

## Causes
- Hereditary.
- Cystic fibrosis.
- Tropical pancreatitis.
- Congenital abnormalities.
- Auto-immune.
- Some drugs.
- High blood fats.
- Alcohol abuse.
- Hyperparathyroidism.
- Following acute pancreatitis which fails to resolve completely (may be repeated episodes).

Often, the first attack occurs following an episode of binge drinking, with attacks becoming more frequent until the pain is more persistent and severe. Diabetes develops in one-third of patients.

## Signs and symptoms
- Severe dull epigastric pain—radiating to the back.
- Nausea and vomiting.
- Weight loss.
- Pain on eating.
- Steatorrhoea—pale, malodorous faeces, with a high fat content.

## Treatment
Chronic pancreatitis is treated by controlling symptoms or the cause of pancreatitis if possible.
- Pain (often intractable)—caution is often required with opioids; patches can be useful.
- Diabetes—oral hypoglycaemic drugs.
- Fat malabsorption and/or steatorrhoea: low fat/high carbohydrate diet or pancreatic enzyme replacement.
- Abstinence from alcohol.

Surgery is not usually necessary, but following procedures are occasionally indicated:
- Beger procedure—duodenal resection, preserving pancreatic head.
- Frey's procedure—extended lateral pancreaticojejunostomy.
- Whipple's procedure—( 📖 p. 434).

Complications associated with chronic pancreatitis include formation of pseudocysts, biliary stricture, and gastroduodenal obstruction.

## Pancreatic rupture

Following a severe force to the abdomen, the pancreas can rupture. If pancreatic juice escapes, it can painfully digest tissues and the pancreas. Emergency surgery is required.

## Further reading

Long RG and Scott BB (2005). *Gastroenterology and Liver Disease*. Elsevier Mosby, London.

# Malignancies and tumours

Neoplasms of the pancreas can originate from either exocrine or endocrine cells and can be benign or malignant.[1] Carcinoma of the pancreas has become more common in Western countries during the past 30 years. In the UK, it is the tenth most common cause of cancer death, with a median survival after diagnosis of only 6 months, despite chemotherapy and other oncological therapy. Risk factors: chronic pancreatitis, diabetes, smoking, diet (↑ in high fat, sugar, and red meat diets).

Cancer of the pancreatic head accounts for two-thirds of pancreatic cancers and can present as follows:
- Pruritus—caused by high bilirubin levels; non-responsive to antihistamines.
- Back pain—a poor prognostic factor.
- Severe cachexia.
- Jaundice.
- Dark urine and pale stools—because of jaundice.

▶ Because prognosis is poor, do not set unrealistic expectations. It is also of limited benefit to undertake too many investigations or treatments to try and improve the quality of life for the patient. Referral for palliative care is recommended.

Whipple's procedure, which is the only hope of cure, can resect <15% of tumours. Radiotherapy and chemotherapy are not generally effective, and the survival rate is low. Stenting can be useful for carefully assessed patients, and may relieve jaundice symptoms. Treatment can include pain control using NSAIDs, paracetamol, or opioid analgesia. Nutritional support can help those with cachexia. Macmillan support is useful.

## Whipple's procedure

Whipple's procedure was named after Dr A Whipple and is also called 'Whipple's pancreaticoduodenectomy'.

Whipple's procedure is the standard surgical option for cancer of the head of the pancreas. However, resection is not justified if there is portal vein involvement. Involvement of the splenic artery and vein is not a contraindication for surgery.

The procedure basically removes the following *en bloc*:
- Distal stomach (antrum).
- Duodenum.
- Proximal jejunum.
- Complete of the head of pancreas (or possibly the entire pancreas).
- Distal common bile duct.
- Gall bladder.
- Possibly the spleen (if there is localized cancer of the pancreas body and tail).

---

1 Bornman PC and Beckingham IJ (2001). Pancreatic tumours. In: Beckingham IJ (ed) *ABC of Liver, Pancreas and Gall Bladder*. BMJ Books, London.

It is necessary to remove the head of the pancreas and the duodenum because they share the same arterial blood supply. Reconstruction is achieved by attaching the stomach, pancreas, and common bile duct to the jejunum. The procedure might include preservation of the pylorus.

The rate of resection of pancreatic cancer is ~20%. The 5-year survival rate after Whipple's procedure is only ~10%. Surgical results are variable but improving, although the results from centres at which the surgery is performed differ drastically.

## Patient information

Further information for patients with pancreatic cancer is available from http://www.cancerhelp.org.uk/default.asp?page=2795

## Further reading

Long RG and Scott BB (2005). *Gastroenterology and Liver Disease*. Elsevier Mosby, London.

# Cystic fibrosis

Cystic fibrosis is a hereditary disease affecting exocrine glands. In Caucasians, cystic fibrosis affects ~1 in every 2500 children. Lack of a specific gene controlling salt transport produces thick mucus. Cystic fibrosis predominantly affects the lungs and digestive system, including the pancreas.

Diagnosis is often made soon after birth, but a few people are diagnosed much later. Diagnosis as a baby could be due to lack of growth. This is because the pancreas does not produce enzymes to digest the fat in food properly. Pancreatic insufficiency results in malabsorption and a failure to thrive, and could lead to chronic pancreatitis. Because fat is not absorbed, stools contain excess fat, have a greasy appearance, and are malodourous.

In adulthood, if not properly treated, cystic fibrosis can continue to present with steatorrhoea and possibly also abdominal pain and constipation.

The treatment for cystic fibrosis problems related to the pancreas is to take pancreatic enzymes with meals to aid digestion. Vigorous daily physiotherapy is required to loosen sticky lung mucus and aid breathing. There is also an ↑ risk of complications if chest infection occurs, necessitating prompt antibiotic therapy. Life expectancy is ↑; now patients commonly live into their late 40s.

# Other pancreatic disorders

## Whipple's disease

! Note: distinguish from Whipple's procedure (surgery for pancreatic cancer (📖 p. 434)). More details on 📖 p. 378 (small bowel infection).

Whipple's disease is uncommon, affecting predominantly older Caucasian ♂. An infection with the bacterium *Tropheryma whipplei* causes malabsorption of fat, diarrhoea, and joint disease in the majority of cases. Presentation is as follows:

- Diarrhoea.
- Arthropathy.
- Malaise.
- Fever.
- Weight loss.
- Anaemia.
- Skin plaques.
- Hypoproteinaemia.
- Oedema.

Almost any system can be affected, including the cardiovascular system. Often need >1 year antibiotics. If untreated with antibiotics, it can be fatal.

## Diabetes mellitus

Diabetes mellitus is the most common medical condition resulting from pancreatic abnormality. However, management does not directly relate to the pancreas.

## Congenital abnormalities

Congenital pancreatic abnormalities can include an annular pancreas or pancreas divisum. Individuals could present with chronic pancreatitis.

## Further reading

Long RG and Scott BB (2005). *Gastroenterology and Liver Disease*. Elsevier Mosby, London.

# Gall bladder and biliary system

Structure and function  440
Gallstones: cholelithiasis  442
Gallstones: cholecystectomy  444
Other biliary conditions  446

# Structure and function

## Gall bladder

Small pear-shaped sac (3 × 7 cm) tucked beneath the liver, with a capacity of 30–50 ml. The function of this organ is to store and concentrate (up to 10×) the bile produced by the liver. The gall bladder comprises the fundus, body, and neck. The surface of the gall bladder is covered by columnar epithelium arranged in rugae (folds); there is no submucosal layer. Layer of smooth muscle. Contraction of the smooth muscle of the gall bladder pushes bile into the common bile duct.

## Bile

Bile is produced by the liver. It is secreted from hepatocytes within the liver and is made from waste products from the breakdown of red blood cells and excess cholesterol. It passes into the bile canaliculi (small canals), ductules, and ducts, which merge into the right and left hepatic ducts and then unite as the common hepatic duct which joins the cystic duct from the gall bladder to form the common bile duct (Fig. 13.1). The common bile duct unites with the pancreatic duct at the ampulla of Vater, and empties into the duodenum via the sphincter of Oddi. The function of the bile ducts is to convey bile from the liver and gall bladder to the small intestine. The liver contains >2 km of bile ducts.

Bile is a green-brown syrupy liquid which is made up of 97% water, 0.7% bile salts (acids manufactured in the liver from cholesterol), 0.2% bile pigments, mostly bilirubin (from the breakdown of red blood cells), and excess cholesterol excreted from the body. Between 0.5 and 1 L of bile is synthesized per day. Bile has a pH of 7.6–8.0. It does not contain any digestive enzymes, but bile salts (sodium and potassium salts, such as chenodeoxycholic acid and cholic acid) have an important role in emulsifying fats (they have a detergent-like action on fats, enabling them to be dispersed in water, and activate lipase, which also emulsifies fats) and also enable absorption of fat-soluble vitamins (e.g. vitamins A, D, E, and K) and iron. Bile deodorizes faeces and colours it brown (with stercobilin from the breakdown of bilirubin). Bile is released in response to food, especially fat, in the duodenum.

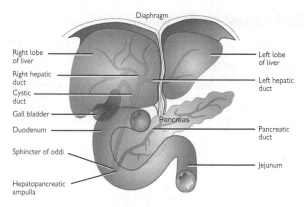

**Fig. 13.1** Structure of the biliary system. Reproduced with kind permission © Burdett Institute 2008.

# Gallstones: cholelithiasis

Cholelithiasis is defined as the presence of gallstones in the gall bladder or bile ducts. Gallstones are usually small (pea-sized) but can fill the whole gall bladder; multiple stones might be present.

Cholesterol stones are usually yellow-green and are made primarily of hardened cholesterol. They account for 75% of gallstones. The remainder (25%) are pigment stones (black or brown; calcium, salts, and pigment).

Gallstones are common: they occur in 10% of adults. The incidence ↑ with age, occurring in 30% of ♀ >50 years, and has a ratio of ♀:♂ of 2:1. There is a familial link, and the condition is more prevalent in Caucasians.

The following patient groups are predisposed to gallstones:
- High cholesterol content in bile.
- Previously been pregnant.
- Overweight or rapid weight loss.
- Patients with high oestrogen levels.
- People on lipid-lowering drugs.
- Crohn's disease (loss of bile acid receptors in the terminal ileum leads to excessive bile salt secretion).

## Symptoms

More than 80% of patients with gallstones are asymptomatic. Gallstones can be diagnosed by a chance finding on imaging for another problem. However, the following symptoms can occur:
- Pale stools.
- Jaundice.
- Colicky shooting abdominal pain, usually with or after eating (especially high-fat meals).
- Pain below the ribs on the right-hand side, possibly referred to the back or shoulder.

If symptoms are severe, 'biliary colic' may also present with fever, nausea, and vomiting. Severe pain can be caused by the stone passing along the bile duct or secondary to inflammation (cholecystitis).

## Complications

- Cholecystitis (inflammation).
- Infection of the bile duct.
- Obstruction of bile duct (choledocholithiasis).
- Rarely, ascending cholangitis, erosion, and carcinoma of the gall bladder or biliary ducts.

## Investigation

- 95% of gallstones are diagnosed by ultrasound scan.
- Cholangiography—IV contrast X-ray to visualize the bile ducts.
- MRI or CT scan.
- Endoscopic retrograde cholangio-pancreatography (ERCP)—a catheter is endoscopically introduced into the bile ducts (📖 p. 206).

## Choledocholithiasis

The presence of stones in the common bile duct or hepatic duct. A lodged stone prevents flow of bile into the duodenum. The condition can be asymptomatic or present with right upper quadrant abdominal pain, biliary colic, and obstructive jaundice (signs are pigmented sclera of eyes and skin, dark urine, and pale stools). Life-threatening cholangitis or acute pancreatitis may also occur. Therapeutic ERCP to remove the stone/s is the preferred method of medical treatment. Unlike stones in the gall bladder, choledocholithiasis is usually treated, even if it is asymptomatic, because of the serious potential complications.

## Management of gallstones

Asymptomatic gallstones require no treatment. However, symptomatic gallstones should be treated according to the severity and frequency of pain, as follows:

- Low-fat diet—can control the worst symptoms, but changes will not reverse stone formation.
- Painkillers.
- Cholesterol stones can occasionally be dissolved by medication.
- Laparoscopic cholecystectomy ( p. 444).
- Dissolution therapy and lithotripsy—ultrasonic shock waves are used to break up the stones and the pieces are passed in the faeces.

## Acute cholecystitis

Usually the result of a gallstone obstructing the bile duct. Acute onset of pain and low-grade fever. May vomit. Right subcostal pain with Murphy's sign (deep inspiration exacerbates pain during RUQ palpation). Usually subsides in 2–3 days. Often requires hospital admission, with IV fluids and analgesia. Nil by mouth; possibly antibiotics. Will often need subsequent cholecystectomy.

## Further reading

Beckingham IJ (2001). ABC of diseases of the liver, pancreas and biliary system. Gallstone disease. *British Medical Journal* **322**, 91–4.

# Gallstones: cholecystectomy

This is the most common abdominal operation. It is an elective procedure, which is seldom performed acutely, except if perforation is suspected or seems imminent. If the patient is asymptomatic, surgery is usually only performed if stones are located in the bile duct. The vast majority of surgery is laparoscopic. The procedure is safe, even in elderly and infirm patients, except if cirrhosis is also present. There is a very low rate of bile duct injury and the conversion rate from laparoscopic to open surgery is <5%. Open surgery is rarely performed. Cholangiography might be performed during surgery to image and confirm the bile duct anatomy and presence of stones in the ducts.

## Surgical complications

The main risk is injury to the bile ducts, with subsequent stricture (Fig 13.2). Injury is often not noticed during surgery. If the bile ducts are completely occluded, the patient presents with jaundice; less than complete occlusion of the bile ducts results in pain. Treatment of occlusion is usually with endoscopic balloon dilatation, endoscopic stent placement, or surgical reconstruction (e.g. Roux-en-Y choledochojejunostomy).

## Post-cholecystectomy syndrome

Patients with post-cholecystectomy syndrome may experience a variety of abdominal symptoms (often unchanged from those experienced peri-operatively), including pain, bloating, nausea, and dyspepsia.

## Cancer

There is possibly a slight ↑ in the risk of colorectal (especially right-sided colon) cancer in patients after cholecystectomy (which could be the effect of the gallstones rather than surgery). This is still debatable.

## Recurrence

The bile acid ursodeoxycholic acid can be given as medication after completing therapy, to stop gallstones recurring, but up to 25% of patients could have recurring symptoms 1 year after stopping therapy. May cause diarrhoea.

## Nursing care

Cholecystectomy is performed with increasingly short hospital stays. Minimal care is needed. Most patients recover and return to normal activity (including work) within 1 week. Use the opportunity for patient education on modifying cholesterol intake and general health advice.

## Patient information

Information about gallstones. http://www.corecharity.org.uk (accessed 14.05.07).

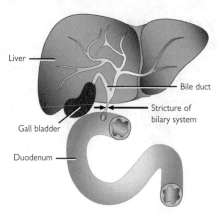

**Fig. 13.2** Post-cholecystectomy stricture of the bile duct.

# Other biliary conditions

## Primary sclerosing cholangitis

Diffuse inflammation and fibrosis of the biliary system, often resulting in strictures and leading to occlusion of the bile ducts, biliary cirrhosis, and, eventually, cirrhosis. The cause is unknown.

The condition can be primary or associated with inflammatory bowel disease (IBD) or other autoimmune diseases, such as systemic lupus erythematosus, systemic sclerosis, or type 1 diabetes mellitus.

Primary: mostly young adult males with IBD.

### Symptoms
- Jaundice.
- Pruritus (skin itching).
- Abdominal pain.
- Possibly weight loss and fatigue.
- Fat malabsorption leading to steatorrhoea.
- Deficiency of fat-soluble vitamins.

In IBD, the condition could progress to cholangiocarcinoma.

### Tests
- ↑ alkaline phosphatase.
- Imaging by ERCP.
- Liver biopsy.

### Treatment
Treatment is mostly targeted at avoiding complications:
- Correct nutritional deficiencies.
- Treat pruritus.
- Avoid infection.

Dilatation or stenting might be possible. Antibiotics should be given if bacterial infection is present. The patient might need liver transplantation in end-stage liver failure.

## Biliary malignancies

Surgery is indicated for adenocarcinoma of the gall bladder secondary to chronic cholecystitis. Tumours of the bile ducts or ampulla (usually adenocarcinoma) also occur; survival is often poor. Surgery for a tumour in the ampulla is called 'Whipple's procedure' (□ p. 434).

# Colon

Structure and function  448
Appendix  449
Abdominal bloating  450
Paralytic ileus  451
Laparotomy: nursing care  452
Laparoscopic abdominal surgery: nursing care  454
Ischaemic colitis  456
Pseudomembranous colitis  458
Radiation enteritis and colitis (radiation enteropathy)  460
Infectious colitis  462
Pseudo-obstruction  470
Colonic decompression  472
Flatus and its disorders  474
Diverticular disease  476
Colorectal cancer  478
Screening for colorectal cancer  482
Intestinal polyposis syndromes: overview  483
Intestinal polyposis syndromes: familial
    adenomatous polyposis  484
Intestinal polyposis syndromes:
    Peutz–Jeghers syndrome  485
Intestinal polyposis syndromes: juvenile polyposis  486
Intestinal polyposis syndromes:
    MYH-associated polyposis  487
Hereditary non-polyposis colorectal cancer  488
Chemotherapy for cancer of the colon and rectum  490
Surgical management of colon cancer  492
Malignant bowel obstruction  494
Partial and total colectomy  496
Megacolon and megarectum  497
Toxic megacolon  498
Chronic abdominal pain  500
Irritable bowel syndrome  502

# Structure and function

## Structure

The colon is a tubular structure of ~30–40 cm in length at birth, reaching 1.5 m in length in the adult. It starts at the ileocaecal valve and caecum and ends distally at the anal verge. The nerve supply to the colon is a complex interaction of intrinsic nerves (enteric nervous system) and extrinsic nerves (autonomic nervous system), which modulate colonic motility, secretion, blood flow, and submucosal immune function.

There are four layers in the intestinal wall:

- Serosa—a single layer of mesothelial cells, which encases the intestine to form its outermost layer.
- Muscularis—the outer longitudinal and inner circular layers of smooth muscle fibres.
- Submucosa—a heterogeneous population of cells, including lymphocytes, plasma cells, macrophages, eosinophils, fibroblasts, and mast cells embedded in dense connective tissue.
- Mucosa—this is divided into a further three layers:
  - Muscularis mucosae—a thin layer of smooth muscle, forming the border between the mucosa and submucosa.
  - Lamina propria—the narrow region between the muscularis mucosae and the surface epithelial cells with their glands.
  - Intestinal epithelium—an inner layer of highly specialized cells, which absorbs sodium and water and secretes mucus.

The colonic epithelium, unlike that of the small intestine, lacks villi; the colonic mucosa consists of tightly packed crypts, lined primarily by goblet cells with intervening flat epithelial surfaces covered by absorptive cells. The average lifespan of a colonocyte is 3–5 days.

## Function

The colon has three important functions:

- Concentration of faeces through water and electrolyte absorption.
- Storage and controlled evacuation of faeces.
- Digestion and absorption of undigested food.

The caecum and ascending colon have a major role in water and electrolyte absorption and fermentation of undigested sugars, and the left colon (descending colon, sigmoid colon, and rectum) is predominantly involved in storage and evacuation of stool.

# Appendix

The appendix is a thin tubular structure with a closed end that attaches to the caecum. It ranges from 2 to 20 cm in length, and is ~8 mm in diameter. The inner lining of the appendix produces a small amount of mucus that flows through the appendix and into the caecum. The wall contains lymphatic tissue that forms part of the immune system. The appendix does not have a role in the digestive process in humans.

## Appendicitis

This is inflammation of the appendix, which occurs if the opening of the appendix becomes blocked by a build-up of mucus from the caecum. This blockage causes an ↑ in bacterial activity which, in turn, leads to inflammation/infection. This inflammation/infection can spread and cause the appendix to rupture, leading to peritonitis.

### Signs and symptoms
- Abdominal pain/tenderness—classic sign of patient guarding.
- Pyrexia.
- Nausea.
- Vomiting.

### Diagnosis
- FBC—↑ white blood cell count.
- Urinalysis.
- Abdominal X-ray.
- Ultrasound.
- Barium enema.
- CT scan.
- Laparoscopy—if the appendix is inflamed, it is removed at the same time.

### Treatment
- Appendectomy, with antibiotic cover.

### Complications
- Perforation.
- Peritonitis.
- Sepsis.
- Wound infection.

## Appendix and inflammatory bowel disease (IBD)

It is unclear whether the appendix has an important role in older children and adults. It has been noted that previous appendicectomy is protective against, or is associated with, a protective factor against ulcerative colitis.

## Acute abdomen

This is described as the acute onset of abdominal pain and is a potential emergency. An acute abdomen could reflect a major problem in the organs of the abdomen, such as the appendix (appendicitis), gall bladder (cholecystitis), intestine (perforation), or spleen (ruptured). The term 'acute abdomen' is used to reflect the current medical situation (📖 p. 708).

# Abdominal bloating

## Classification

Abdominal bloating and distension are terms that are often used interchangeably. However, it has been suggested that the term 'distension' should be reserved for an actual change in girth, whereas the term 'bloating' should be used for the subjective symptom of abdominal enlargement. The prevalence of bloating does not change with age, but it is more common in ♀. Abdominal distension is a cardinal feature of certain organic dysfunctions, such as intestinal obstruction, megacolon, faecal loading, or ascites. Bloating can also be a feature of coeliac disease or pancreatic disorders. More commonly, the complaint of abdominal bloating or distension is part of a functional disorder, and the typical history in such cases is that there is a diurnal pattern to the complaint (being worse in the mornings and after meals). Up to 75% of patients with irritable bowel syndrome (IBS) and 90% of patients with constipation report bloating. In patients with IBS, abdominal bloating is usually associated with a measurable degree of distension—in other words, although psychological factors might influence how the symptom is reported, the complaints of bloating and distension are not purely psychogenic. In fact, the degree of distension is associated with the reported severity of bloating. By contrast, the complaint of bloating without distension is thought to be related to perceptual abnormalities, and, indeed, such patients demonstrate visceral hypersensitivity to distension of a balloon in the gut.

## Pathophysiology

There is no excess of abdominal gas in patients with bloating—the normal volume of intestinal gas is 200 ml. Furthermore, antibiotics and probiotics (which alter gut flora and ∴ modify intestinal gas production) and lactulose (which ↑ bacterial gas production) do not seem to alter the complaint of bloating. Rather, although gas volumes might be normal, several experiments have suggested that the defect might lie in the way in which gas is handled by the intestine. Following a meal, there is a relaxation of the abdominal wall to 'accommodate' the meal and it is possible that distension might occur in patients who have an exaggeration of this reflex.

## Treatment

The first step in management is to ensure that an organic cause has been excluded, without over-investigating the patient. Patients often consume excessive quantities of fibre, and ∴ ↓ fibre intake can be beneficial. Additionally, limiting intake of fizzy drinks, artificial sweeteners, and fat might help. Drugs aimed at altering gas volumes (e.g. charcoal, simeticone, antibiotics, probiotics, and neostigmine) have not been reliably shown to help. Anti-spasmodics and anti-depressants might help improve symptoms generally in patients with IBS and, as a result, improve bloating. Hypnotherapy for IBS does seem to specifically improve bloating.

# Paralytic ileus

Known as paralysis of the intestine. To be termed paralytic ileus, the intestinal paralysis does not need to be complete but must be sufficient to prohibit the passage of food through the intestine and lead to a blockage. It is a functional blockage (obstruction) most commonly seen following abdominal surgery but also associated with certain drugs and various other injuries and illnesses. The small bowel becomes distended throughout its length. Absorption of fluid, electrolytes, and nutrition is impaired. Significant amounts of fluid may be lost from the extracellular compartment.

## Causes
- Trauma (e.g. surgical).
- Intestinal ischaemia.
- Sepsis.

## Clinical features
- Usually history of recent abdominal surgery or trauma.
- Abdominal distension is often apparent.
- Pain is often not a prominent feature.
- Vomiting may occur.
- No flatus evident.
- Auscultation will reveal absence of bowel sounds.

## Investigation
- Plain abdominal X-ray—highlighting loops of bowel.
- Gas may be present in large bowel.
- Water-soluble contrast maybe useful if unclear as to whether obstruction is mechanical or functional.

## Management
- Prevention is better than cure.
- Treat conservatively.
- Bowel should be handled as little as possible.
- Fluid and electrolyte replacement.
- Source of sepsis should be eradicated.

Established paralytic ileus should be managed with:
- Nasogastric tube.
- Fluid and electrolyte replacement.
- No drugs are available to reverse the condition.

Paralytic ileus usually resolves spontaneously after 4 or 5 days.

## Further reading
Luckey A, Livingstone E and Tache Y (2003). Mechanisms and treatment of post-operative ileus. *Archives of Surgery* **138**, 206–14.

# Laparotomy: nursing care

A laparotomy is a surgical incision into the abdomen, which is used as an exploratory procedure to identify and repair a problem or a planned procedure to gain open access to the internal organs. A large single cut is made through the muscle layer, to reveal internal organs. Once complete, the muscles and skin layer are resewn or staples are used (Plate 16).

## Pre-operative nursing care for laparotomy and laparoscopic abdominal surgery

Both physical and psychological methods of care are essential in ensuring that the patient feels relaxed and prepared for the forthcoming procedure. It helps to establish a good rapport with the patient and family, and aids the process of discharge planning. Explanation, using appropriate language, will help to allay anxiety and ↓ fear:

- Introduce the ward environment.
- Explain the procedure and general anaesthetic.
- Discuss pain relief.
- Discuss the length of stay—with the current trend in using 'accelerated/enhanced recovery after surgery' (ERAS), in which the aim is to discharge the patient much more quickly.
- Bloods.
- Baseline observations.
- Anti-embolic stockings.
- Nil by mouth.
- Bowel preparation—if appropriate.
- Nameband, notes, X-ray, consent form, and blood label.
- Operation site marked—if appropriate.
- Referral to a stoma care nurse—if appropriate.

## Post-operative management

- Assess vital signs regularly—at 30 min, 1 h, 2 h, 4 h, and 6 h. Check pulse, BP, and oximetry.
- Assess for haemorrhage or hypovolaemic shock—this would be evident in ↓ BP and ↑ pulse. Also look for pale, cold, and clammy skin.
- Check the need for nasal/masked oxygen.
- Monitor pain—use epidural/Venflon patient-controlled analgesia (PCA). PCA is usually needed for 2–4 days post-operatively.
- Observe the wound, drains, and stoma for signs of leakage—↑ in blood loss from drains might indicate bleeding internally and result in shock. A stoma, if present, should be observed for viability in blood supply and output.
- Nutrition—reintroduce diet and fluids according to surgical instruction because practice now varies owing to ERAS. Consider referral to a dietitian, if appropriate.
- Accurate fluid-balance chart for input and output—a urethral/suprapubic catheter might be used. Urine output should be at least 30 ml/h.
- Check IV sites regularly.
- Mouth care.

- Pressure area care—especially during the first 24 h post-operatively.
- Check calves regularly for signs of thrombosis—redness, swelling, and heat. Mobilize the patient on day 1 post-operatively.
- Psychological care—dependent on clinical findings and the presence of a stoma, for example.

## Possible complications

- Bleeding.
- Infection.
- Anastamotic leak—occurs in 5–15% of colonic anastomoses.
- Adhesions (scar tissue).
- Obstruction.
- Incisional hernia.

## General post-operative advice

- Follow-up usually at 6 weeks by the surgeon, unless otherwise specified.
- No driving for ~6 weeks post-operatively.
- Give advice about avoiding heavy lifting and returning to work—this is dependent on the occupation and general state of health, but varies between 2 and 3 months.
- Provide a clip remover, if appropriate, for the practice nurse.
- Sick certificate.
- The patient having a laparotomy could be discharged in 3–10 days.

# Laparoscopic abdominal surgery: nursing care

Sometimes known as 'keyhole surgery' or 'minimally invasive surgery' (MIS). A laparoscope is inserted into the abdomen or pelvic cavity and the image that results is viewed on a screen in the operating theatre. This procedure produces ↓ trauma to the abdominal wall than open surgery; it is performed through a series of small incisions (<1 cm in diameter), which quickly heal. Usually, the patient will have three port-hole scars on their abdomen. The peritoneum is usually expanded with $CO_2$ so that the surgeon can achieve a good view.

## Benefits
- Better cosmetic result.
- Patients tend to recover quickly.
- ↓ pain experienced.
- ↓ risk of herniation.
- ↓ risk of adhesions.

## Pre-operative nursing care
📖 p. 452.

## Post-operative management
- Assess vital signs regularly—every 30 min, 1 h, 2 h, 4 h, and 6 h. Check pulse, BP, and oximetry.
- Assess for haemorrhage or hypovolaemic shock.
- Check need for nasal/masked oxygen.
- Monitor pain—use epidural/Venflon PCA. PCA is usually needed for 2–4 days post-operatively.
- Observe the wound, drains, and stoma for signs of leakage—↑ in blood loss from drains might indicate bleeding internally and result in shock. A stoma, if present, should be observed for viability in blood supply and output.
- Nutrition—reintroduce diet and fluids according to surgical instruction because practice now varies owing to ERAS. Consider referral to a dietitian, if appropriate.
- Accurate fluid-balance chart for input and output—a urethral/suprapubic catheter might be used. Urine output should be at least 30 ml/h.
- Check IV sites regularly.
- Mouth care.
- Pressure area care—especially during the first 24 h post-operatively.
- Check calves regularly for signs of thrombosis—redness, swelling, and heat. Mobilize the patient on day 1 post-operatively.
- Psychological care—dependent on clinical findings and the presence of a stoma, for example.

## Possible complications
- Bleeding.
- Infection.

- Anastamotic leak—occurs in 5–15% of colonic anastomoses.
- Adhesions (scar tissue).
- Obstruction.
- Incisional hernia.

## General post-operative advice

- Follow-up usually at ~2 weeks by the surgeon, unless otherwise specified.
- No driving for 6 weeks post-operatively.
- Give advice about avoiding heavy lifting and returning to work—this is dependent on the occupation and general state of health, but varies between 2 and 3 months.
- Sick certificate.
- If the patient suffers undue pain, they should be seen by surgical team without delay.
- The patient having laparoscopic surgery could be discharged in 3–5 days.

## Further reading

Dunn D and Rawlinson N (1998). *Dunn's Surgical Diagnosis and Management: A Guide to General Surgical Care* (3rd edn). Cambridge University Press.

# Ischaemic colitis

An inflammation of the colon where the blood supply has been compromised due to colonic ischaemia.

## Incidence
● Uncommon.

## Predisposing factors
● Thrombosis—inferior mesenteric artery thrombosis.
● Emboli—mesenteric arterial emboli, cholesterol emboli.
● Decreased cardiac output, arrhythmias, or atrial fibrillation.
● Shock—sepsis, haemorrhage, hypovolaemia.
● Trauma.
● Strangulated hernia or volvulus.
● Drugs—oestrogens, immunosuppressive agents, psychotropic agents.
● Surgery.
● Vasculitis.
● Disorders of coagulation.
● Colonoscopy.
● Barium enema.
● Idiopathic.

## Signs and symptoms
● Left iliac fossa pain.
● Nausea and vomiting.
● Loose motion often containing dark blood.
● Marked tenderness in left iliac fossa.

## Differential diagnosis
● Dysentery.
● Acute diverticular disease.
● Acute IBD.
● Perforation.
● Pancreatitis.

## Investigations
● Endoscopy—may show blue swollen mucosa not showing contact bleeding and sparing the rectum.
● Plain abdominal X-ray—outline segment gas.
● Barium enema—shows 'thumb printing' in early phase.

## Management
● Medical—IV therapy with systemic broad-spectrum antibiotics.
● Surgical—only if evidence of perforation, sepsis, haemorrhage, ischaemic stricture, segmental colitis, continuation of symptoms for more than 2 weeks.

## Complications
In up to one-third of patients, a stricture develops—usually asymptomatic and does not usually need to be resected.

## Further reading

Sreenarasimhaiah J (2003). Diagnosis and management of intestinal ischaemic disorders. *British Medical Journal* **326**, 1372–6.

# Pseudomembranous colitis

Pseudomembranous colitis (PMC) is a severe colonic inflammation secondary to overgrowth of *Clostridium difficile*, with production of toxins A and B. PMC usually occurs in the setting of antibiotic therapy, but sporadic cases can occur.

*C.difficile* is a Gram-positive anaerobic spore-forming bacillus, which is the leading cause of enteric nosocomal infection in hospitals. The prevalence of PMC ranges from 0.1% to 10.1% of in-patients receiving penicillins or cephalosporins. The incubation period is long, ranging from 1–5 days after starting antibiotic therapy to 1–5 weeks after stopping antibiotics.

## Transmission

Patient-to-patient transmission is the major mode of the spread of infection, but transient carriage on healthcare workers' hands, stethoscopes, and clothing has also been documented, in addition to contamination of commodes, neonatal bathing tubs, telephones, and rectal thermometers.

## Risk factors

These include advanced age and exposure to antibiotics. Almost all antibiotics have been implicated in *C.difficile*-associated diarrhoea, but the most frequent agents include cephalosporins, ampicillin, amoxicillin, and clindamycin.

## Clinical presentation

- Watery diarrhoea.
- Abdominal cramps.
- Anorexia.
- Fever.

In severe cases, marked leucocytosis and hypoalbuminaemia occurs in up to 25% of patients. Complications include:
- Fulminant colitis—2–3% of patients.
- Colonic perforation.
- Toxic megacolon.
- Hypotension.
- Electrolyte disturbances.
- Prolonged ileus.
- Death.

## Differential diagnosis

- Antibiotic-associated diarrhoea.
- Ischaemic colitis.
- Diarrhoea caused by other enteric pathogens.
- Adverse reactions to medications.

## Diagnostic methods

Stool samples should be sent to the laboratory for the detection of *C.difficile* toxins. Most pathogenic strains of *C.difficile* produce toxins A and B, which are easily detected. Endoscopy is not necessary, unless the diagnosis remains in doubt or rapid diagnosis is necessary. At endoscopy, pseudomembranes can be seen on the surface of the colon, which are almost pathognomic of PMC.

## Prevention and treatment

Prevention is directly related to the mode of transmission and involves the use of disposable gloves and single-use disposable rectal thermometers, washing using chlorhexidine, and disinfection of the patient's environment.

In cases of PMC, the relevant antibiotic should be stopped if this has not already been done. Metronidazole and vancomycin are equally effective in treating this infection, but metronidazole is the drug of choice, with vancomycin being used as second-line treatment. Patients who are not tolerating oral therapy can be treated with IV metronidazole, although this is much less effective.

## Prognosis ± treatment

Patients who are diagnosed while taking antibiotics usually recover within 7 days. If the diagnosis is delayed and antibiotics are continued, the condition can last up to 3 weeks. The mortality rate can be as great as 75% without treatment.

# Radiation enteritis and colitis (radiation enteropathy)

Caused by acute or chronic injury to the gut from exposure to therapeutic or supra-therapeutic levels of ionizing radiation.

## Risk factors

- Concomitant chemotherapy.
- High-dose radiation therapy.
- Uraemia or diabetes mellitus.
- Pelvic inflammatory disease.
- Hypertension.
- Thin-body habitus.
- Abdominal or pelvic surgery.
- Accelerated fractionation regimens for delivering radiotherapy.

## Pathogenesis

### Acute radiation enteropathy

Caused by radiation-induced cell death (apoptosis). Stem cells located at the base of crypts are particularly vulnerable. It results in denuding of the intestinal mucosa and lasts for the duration of therapy, subsiding 10–15 days after radiation therapy has stopped. Intestinal permeability to bacteria and other antigens is ↑ and diarrhoea results from ↑ fluid and electrolyte loss. It occurs soon after the onset of radiotherapy.

### Chronic radiation enteropathy

Caused by a progressive occlusive vasculitis, which might affect all layers of the bowel wall. Tissue hypoxia and ischaemia occur, resulting in mucosal atrophy and ulceration, in addition to fibrosis of the muscularis and thickening of the serosa. Stricturing might ensue.

## Clinical presentation

### Acute radiation colitis

- Diarrhoea.
- Abdominal discomfort.
- Tenesmus.
- Rectal bleeding.

### Chronic radiation colitis

- Constipation.
- Altered motility.
- Diarrhoea.
- Abdominal discomfort.
- Tenesmus.
- Rectal bleeding.
- Adhesions.
- Perforation.
- Secondary cancer.
- Fistula formation.

Radiation proctitis is also associated with internal anal sphincter damage, resulting in faecal incontinence. Rectal bleeding is also more common.

## Diagnosis

- Colonoscopy—demonstrates changes of mucosal or transmural inflammation.
- Biopsies—might be inconclusive.
- Barium investigations—might be normal or show ulceration, submucosal thickening, single or multiple strictures, adhesions or fistulae, or simply a loss of the normal haustral pattern.
- Capsule endoscopy—demonstrates mucosal changes.

## Treatment

- Antidiarrhoea drugs, e.g. loperamide and codeine phosphate.
- Biofeedback.
- Sucralfate enemas.
- Oral metronidazole.
- Corticosteroid and salicylate enemas.
- Low-dose antidepressants.
- Fentanyl patches.
- Gabapentin.

Bleeding that fails to respond to medical therapy may be treated by direct endoscopic ablative therapy (laser, heater probe, or argon plasma beam).

▶ Exclude constipation and faecal loading as the cause of pain.

# Infectious colitis

This is an acute disease of the large colon caused by micro-organisms. Infectious colitis is classified into three groups: bacterial, viral, and parasitic. The various micro-organisms, associated features and recommended treatments are shown in Table 14.1.

Infectious colitis remains a major cause of morbidity and mortality across the world. New pathogens are identified and old ones re-emerge, leading to a constant battle against the development of resistance to many treatments currently available. As resistance to antibiotics varies please check local antibiotic policies.

**Table 14.1** Infectious colitis

| Micro-organism | Aetiology/epidemiology | Pathophysiology | Signs/symptoms | Diagnosis | Treatment |
|---|---|---|---|---|---|
| **Bacterial** | | | | | |
| Aeromonas | Live in fresh water Infection occurs by drinking, swimming, or bathing in contaminated water | Produce toxins that damage the colon | Watery diarrhoea Fever Vomiting | Via stool culture | Aggressive rehydration Drug therapy such as tetracycline |
| Campylobacter | Infection of GI tract or blood. Common strain of bacteria that causes sudden gastroenteritis Infection occurs by eating contaminated food or contact with faecal matter from an infected animal or person | Incubation period 1–7 days Invades lining of the intestines and secretes toxins | Cramping abdominal pain Diarrhoea Malaise Fever Blood in stool Tenesmus Faecal urgency | Via stool culture | Aggressive rehydration Drug therapy such as erythromycin |
| Clostridium difficile | Prolonged use of antibiotics leading to overgrowth of the bacterium | Produces two toxins which damage lining of bowel wall | Diarrhoea Abdominal pain Cramps Tenderness | Via stool culture | Stop any antibiotic therapy |

**Table 14.1** (Contd.)

| Micro-organism | Aetiology/epidemiology | Pathophysiology | Signs/symptoms | Diagnosis | Treatment |
|---|---|---|---|---|---|
| Clostridium difficile (continued) | Older and younger people more susceptible | | Fever<br>Stools may contain blood, pus, and mucus<br>If untreated can lead to toxic megacolon | | Symptoms should subside after 12 days; if not commence metronidazole or vancomycin |
| Escherichia coli | Commonly found in human intestine generally causing no problems<br>Five strains | Certain strains produce toxins that damage lining of the bowel wall | Non-bloody diarrhoea<br>Severe abdominal pain | Via stool culture | Rehydration |
| Salmonella | Spread by eating contaminated foods | Secretes cytotoxins and penetrates the epithelial cells of the intestine.<br>Can invade bloodstream<br>Incubation period 6–72 h | Headache<br>Joint pain<br>Sore throat<br>Constipation<br>Loss of appetite<br>Diarrhoea<br>Abdominal cramps<br>Tenderness<br>Fever | Via stool, blood, or urine culture | Ampillicin or amoxicillin |

| | | | | |
|---|---|---|---|---|
| Shigella | Similar to E.coli Found in human intestines and spread from one contaminated person to another | Incubation period 1–4 days. Penetrates the epithelial cells of the intestine and bloodstream | Fever Irritability Drowsiness Loss of appetite Nausea Vomiting Diarrhoea Abdominal pain Bloating Increased urge to defecate | Via stool, blood, or urine culture | Ciprofloxacin Rehydration therapy |
| Vibrio spp | Infect small intestine leading to cholera | Produce toxins causing small bowel to produce large amounts of fluid. Incubation period 1–3 days | Sudden onset Painless watery diarrhoea Vomiting Severe thirst Muscle cramps Weakness | Via stool culture or rectal swab | Aggressive oral and IV rehydration therapy |
| Yersinia | Also known as the Black Death Spread through flea bites | Incubation period 4–6 days | Fever Diarrhoea Rash Abdominal symptoms | Via blood, peritoneal fluid, and throat swabs | Cefotaxime and tetracycline both effective treatments |

**Table 14.1** (Contd.)

| Micro-organism | Aetiology/ epidemiology | Pathophysiology | Signs/symptoms | Diagnosis | Treatment |
|---|---|---|---|---|---|
| **Viral** | | | | | |
| Astroviruses | Commonly occurs in young children  Little known about mechanism of infection | Incubation period 3–4 days  Once infected an immunity develops to subsequent infections | Abdominal pain  Diarrhoea  Vomiting  Nausea  Fever  Malaise | Via stool culture | Fluid replacement therapy |
| Caliciviruses | Also known as viral gastroenteritis, usually faecal to oral transmission but can be respiratory | Incubation period 12 h to 4 days.  Causes damage to lining of the bowel wall | Diarrhoea  Vomiting  Fever  Headache  Malaise  Generalized muscular pain  Abdominal cramps | Via stool culture | Replacement of fluid, symptomatic therapy, and anti-diarrhoeal drugs |
| Enteroviruses (non-polio) | Usually faecal to oral transmission but can be respiratory, affecting mainly children | Incubation period 3–6 days | Vomiting  Diarrhoea  Abdominal pain  Sometimes hepatitis | Via stool culture | Replacement of fluid, symptomatic therapy, and anti-diarrhoeal drugs |

| | | | | |
|---|---|---|---|---|
| Rotavirus | Most common cause of gastroenteritis in children worldwide | Incubation period 1-3 days | Diarrhoea | Enzyme immuno-assay |
| | | Less pronounced inflammation of the mucosa when compared with other infectious causes | Fever | or latex |
| | Major cause of dehydration and death in children in the developing world | | Vomiting | agglutination to detect virus |
| | | | Abdominal pain | |
| | | | Profound dehydration leading to shock in small infants | Rapid and aggressive fluid and electrolyte replacement |

**Parasitic**

| | | | | |
|---|---|---|---|---|
| *Cryptosporidium* | If immune system weakened these parasites thrive and can cause infectious colitis that can prove fatal | Incubation period 2-14 days | Watery diarrhoea | Via stool culture |
| | | Found in the epithelial cells but how it causes severe diarrhoea is not understood | Abdominal cramps | |
| | Most common source of infection is drinking contaminated water | | Nausea | |
| | | Severe watery diarrhoea can inhibit treatment especially in HIV patients | Vomiting | Rapid and aggressive fluid and electrolyte replacement |
| | Transmitted from farm animals or pets to humans | | Fever | |

**Table 14.1** (Contd.)

| Micro-organism | Aetiology/ epidemiology | Pathophysiology | Signs/symptoms | Diagnosis | Treatment |
|---|---|---|---|---|---|
| *Cyclospora cayetanensis* | Transmitted through food | Incubation period 1–2 days but can be weeks<br><br>Some patients can be ill for as long as weeks without a confirmed diagnosis.<br><br>Shortens and widens the intestinal villi, causing diffuse oedema leading to severe watery diarrhoea. | May be asymptomatic for a period of time<br>Watery diarrhoea<br>Flu-like symptoms<br>Flatulence<br>Burping<br>Weight loss<br>Abdominal discomfort<br>Bloating<br>Nausea | Via stool culture | Trimethoprim-sulfamethoxazole |
| *Entamoeba histolytica* | Transmitted via stool of infected patient in the form of cysts<br><br>Common sources of infection are contaminated food, water, and enema equipment | Incubation period 1–4 weeks<br><br>Can be carried without harm but if invades epithelial lining of the colon ulcers occur | Symptoms vary in severity<br>Abdominal distention<br>Flatulence<br>Constipation<br>Loose stool<br>Fever<br>Tenderness around liver | Via stool culture<br>Liver CT scan or ultrasound | Oral amoebicide drugs or luminal amoebicide depending on severity |

| | | | | | |
|---|---|---|---|---|---|
| *Giardia lamblia* | Single cell parasite that attaches to the lining of the intestinal wall<br>Transmission via contaminated water or food | Incubation period 1–4 weeks | May be asymptomatic initially<br>Unable to tolerate fats<br>Flatulence<br>Steatorrhoea<br>Abdominal pain | Antigen detection 'stool test' | Trimethoprim-sulfamethoxazole |
| *Isospora belli* | Related to poor sanitation | Incubation period 8–14 days | Fever<br>Watery diarrhoea<br>Anorexia<br>Weight loss<br>Abdominal pain | Via stool culture | Trimethoprim-sulfamethoxazole |
| *Strongyloides stercoralis* | Intestinal parasitic threadworms<br>Transmitted in poor sanitation areas | Occurs from drinking contaminated water<br>Passes through intestinal mucosa to bloodstream | Diarrhoea<br>Abdominal pain<br>Skin rashes<br>Fever | Identification of worm larvae in stool | Tiabendazole effective therapy (unlicensed in the UK)<br>Secondary bacterial sepsis can prove fatal |

# Pseudo-obstruction

This is a clinical syndrome characterized by the symptoms and signs of intestinal obstruction in the absence of an occluding lesion of the intestinal lumen. The intestinal walls cannot contract sufficiently to generate peristaltic motion. It is caused by disorders of the smooth muscle (visceral myopathy), myenteric plexus, or extraintestinal nervous system (visceral neuropathy).

Chronic intestinal pseudo-obstruction might be primary or secondary to systemic illnesses. Chronic idiopathic intestinal pseudo-obstruction is now recognized as a heterogeneous syndrome, but it has multiple causes.

## Clinical manifestations

- Intestinal pseudo-obstruction.
- Abdominal pain (rarely).
- Distension.
- Vomiting.
- Weight loss.
- Steatorrhoea (chronic only).
- Diarrhoea.

Predominant colonic involvement usually results in constipation or megacolon, or both. Many patients have involvement of the oesophagus, which might be asymptomatic or cause dysphagia, chest pain, regurgitation, reflux, and heartburn. Gastric involvement produces gastroparesis.

## Investigations

The laboratory abnormalities reflect the degree of malabsorption and malnutrition, in addition to the presence of underlying disorders. Patients with diarrhoea usually have steatorrhoea owing to bacterial overgrowth in the small bowel, and often have vitamin $B_{12}$ malabsorption. Mucosal biopsies of the small bowel are of no value in diagnosing this condition.

Plain abdominal X-rays might resemble a paralytic ileus or mimic true mechanical obstruction. Barium contrast studies should be performed if pseudo-obstruction is suspected. About a third of patients have a distended stomach and delayed gastric emptying. The duodenum is usually, but not invariably, abnormal. A barium enema can show colonic dilatation and elongation. If extreme this is classified as a 'megacolon'.

The urinary tract should be studied to look for evidence of megacystitis or mega-ureters. If there is continuing diagnostic uncertainty, a full-thickness biopsy of the small bowel can be performed.

## Treatment

No treatment is curative or halts the natural history of any of the disorders causing intestinal pseudo-obstruction. The goals of treatment are to alleviate symptoms and restore and maintain nutrition, fluid, and the electrolyte balance. Drug therapy using metoclopramide, domperidone, erythromycin, and octreotide can be tried. Broad-spectrum antibiotics are useful in treating patients with bacterial overgrowth.

Endoscopic decompression or neostigmine may be used in acute pseudo-obstruction.

Dietary adjustments often involve frequent small meals, with a low-fat lactose-free low-fibre diet. Supplement drinks are useful, if tolerated. Vitamin and mineral supplements should be prescribed.

Surgery can be considered as a last resort and depends on the area affected. Long-term parenteral nutrition might be necessary to maintain patients nutritionally. Small intestinal transplantation has been performed in extreme cases.

# Colonic decompression

Colonic decompression is performed in one of three ways.
- Endoscopically—transanally.
- Through the anterior abdominal wall—transabdominally. The procedure is performed to remove pressure from the lumen of the colon. Such an ↑ in pressure is reported in patients with distal obstructions (e.g. those related to malignancy or sigmoid volvulus) or conditions in which there is ↑ colonic tone (e.g. pseudo-obstruction or Ogilvie's syndrome).
- Chemically—neostigmine

## Management

See Box 14.1 for management of Ogilvie's syndrome (acute pseudo-obstruction without mechanical cause). Involves reversal of whichever of the causative factors is possible, followed by bolus doses of neostigmine (to overcome the parasympathetic inhibition), if needed. If the colon remains inflated, endoscopic decompression might then be required. An unprepared colonoscopic procedure is performed, ideally with $CO_2$ rather than air, to minimize further air retention in the colon. Aspiration of colonic air is then performed, while examining to exclude any mechanical obstruction. These procedures are often relatively straightforward because the colon is grossly distended, making intubation relatively easy. Occasionally, fluoroscopic guidance might be required if the colon is too atonic, stool is profuse, or the lumen is not easily identified. A flatus tube can be left in the colon at the end of the procedure if it is felt that there might be a recurrence of pressure build-up. This enables the colon to keep decompressed, because the distal end protrudes from the patient's anus at atmospheric pressure; the obvious complication is patient discomfort, and ∴ early removal might be needed.

Chronic intestinal pseudo-obstruction is an idiopathic condition that causes recurrent episodes of non-mechanical obstruction, resulting in a clinical picture similar to Ogilvie's syndrome. Treatment is similar, but because pain can be a major feature, adequate analgesia is also often needed.

Sigmoid volvulus causes colonic obstruction because the mesentery lengthens, enabling a dilated sigmoid colon to twist over on itself, which causes a mechanical blockage. In this context, retention of a flatus tube is often helpful, both to decompress the proximal colon and to help hold the sigmoid stented in place without the formation of a recurrent volvulus.

Transabdominal decompression is a more recent procedure, performed primarily in patients with recurrent episodes of non-mechanical obstruction. It might also be performed if irrigation of the colon is desired, such as in spinal injury or, rarely, severe chronic constipation (see PEC, 📖 p. 318). A colonoscopic procedure is performed and a tube similar to a gastrostomy feeding tube is inserted (using a 'push–pull' technique) into the colon, either in the sigmoid or in the caecum. This can then be used as a conduit to instil irrigating fluid or a port through which the colon can be vented to the atmosphere and decompressed.

## Box 14.1 Ogilvie's syndrome

Occurs if there is interruption of the intra-abdominal autonomic nerves, resulting in either sympathetic excess or parasympathetic inhibition, or both.

Sympathetic excess: results in proximal small bowel and colonic ileus. Parasympathetic inhibition: results in a degree of distal spasm.

Ogilvie's syndrome occurs in the following contexts:
• Abdominal surgery or trauma.
• Retroperitoneal tumour.
• Metabolic disturbance.
• Being bedridden.
• Therapy with strong opiates. This combination is typically reported in patients in intensive care units.

# Flatus and its disorders

Healthy people pass gas from the anus on average between 10 and 20 times/day, releasing ~500–750 ml of air. This is ↑ if the diet includes large quantities of non-absorbable sugars (e.g. beans and tropical fruits). Lactulose is another non-absorbable sugar, which explains why this laxative causes excessive flatulence. Contrary to lay belief, age and gender do not influence the frequency of passing flatus. It is true that some people pass flatus more often others, and it is probable that these differences are due, in part, to different individuals' gut flora, in terms of the bacteria's ability to produce gas.

## Odourless flatus

Swallowed air accounts for 80% of flatus and the remaining 20% is derived from bacterial fermentation of ingested food. The different sources of flatus influence the composition of the wind: swallowed air accounts for a vast amount of odourless nitrogen ($N_2$), which constitutes the majority of flatus, and fermentation produces $CO_2$ and methane, which can give the odour to flatus. For every litre of liquid drunk, 1700 ml of air is swallowed into the stomach; in a 24-h period, ~2500 ml of air is swallowed in the saliva that is swallowed by an average adult. 80% of this air is burped out and the rest is passed as flatus. Thus, excessive passage of odourless flatus is usually $N_2$, resulting from excessive air swallowing (aerophagy) and/or ↓ belching. Some people aspirate air into the oesophagus in a subconscious attempt to initiate a belch. Attempting to suppress air-swallowing voluntarily is usually ineffective, and some experts recommend that patients hold an object such as a pencil between their teeth to prevent jaw closure.

▶ In recognizing that most flatus is related to air-swallowing and meal content, it is crucial to prevent the patient having unnecessary investigations and ineffective treatments predicated on the usually erroneous belief that the excessive flatus was being produced in the GIT.

## Offensive flatus

These are rare causes of excess flatus, but they must be considered. Any diarrhoeal illness can cause excess flatus owing to ↑ gut motility. In addition, small bowel causes of diarrhoea (e.g. food poisoning, lactose intolerance, or coeliac disease) and pancreatic diarrhoea (e.g. chronic pancreatitis or gallstone disease) cause persistence of undigested sugars and fats in the gut, and these can be fermented by bacteria, causing excess flatus.

Finally, irritable bowel syndrome can be associated with rectal dysfunction, which can cause excessive numbers of passages of flatus, without actually ↑ flatus volume.

# Diverticular disease

Diverticula are small herniations in the bowel wall, most frequently occurring in the sigmoid colon, particularly in patients the Western world (Fig. 14.1). Often, diverticula occur at the weakest point in the colonic wall at which the blood vessels supply the mucosa in the circular muscle layer. A diverticulum is an out-pouching of the mucosa of the lining of the bowel. These out-pouches are blind ends within the bowel wall in which undigested food particles, faecal matter, and debris can collect. This trapped detritus can lead to inflammation and diverticulitis.

## Cause

Thought to be caused by high colonic pressures, which result from chronic constipation or a low-fibre diet. Most common as a result of a refined 'Western European' diet. It is prevalent with ↑ age. Less than 20% of patients develop complications, but these can include perforation, peritonitis, fistulae, strictures, bowel obstruction, and haemorrhage.

## Symptoms

Many patients with diverticular disease are unaware that they have the disease because the majority are asymptomatic. Others might experience mild abdominal pain, altered bowel habit or stool consistency, or rectal bleeding. In an acute episode, left lower abdominal pain and tenderness on examination, with low-grade pyrexia, tachycardia, and leucocytosis are reported. Frequency and/or urgency of urine is also reported, as is the potential for septic shock in severe cases.

## Conservative management

- Dietary advice.
- ↑ water intake—2 L/day.
- Analgesia, if required.
- Advice on bowel habit.
- Health education.

## Alternative therapies/surgical management

Perforation or peritonitis might be the first indication that a patient is suffering from diverticulitis. Blood loss from a bleeding diverticulum is often significant and dramatic and occurs without warning. In acute diverticulitis, manage the patient medically for 3 days before taking the decision to operate, provided the patient's condition does not deteriorate.

For emergency surgery, the patient is unlikely to have pre-operative counselling and siting for a possible stoma. Lack of information might lead to post-operative problems in accepting a stoma.

Elective surgery usually results in a segmental colectomy without formation of a stoma.

## Investigations

- History-taking.
- Abdominal examination.
- Digital rectal examination.
- Flexible sigmoidoscopy.

- Full blood count (FBC)—including haemaglobin, erythrocyte sedimentation rate (ESR), C-reactive protein (CRP), and white blood cell count (WBC).
- Carcinoembryonic antigen (CEA)—check for concomitant cancer.
- Barium enema.
- CT.
- CT pneumocolon—enables more of the internal structure of the bowel to be seen and is less traumatic for older patients.
- Colonoscopy.

### Indications for surgery

Surgery is performed if the disease is severe and life threatening. The preferred surgical option is Hartmann's procedure. Indications for surgery:

- Infection.
- Perforation.
- Peritonitis.
- Recurrent diverticulitis.
- Paracolic or pelvic abscess.
- Sigmoid mass.
- Fistulae.
- Obstruction.
- Stricture.
- Major haemorrhage.

Although diverticular disease is common, it is still poorly understood and recent advances continue to focus on the technological side. The rates of mortality, morbidity, and formation of a stoma vary by surgeon.

### Further reading

Black P and Hyde C (2005). *Diverticular Disease*. Whurr, London.

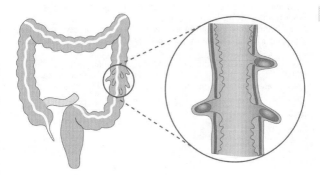

**Fig. 14.1** Diverticular disease of the colon. Reproduced with kind permission © Burdett Institute 2008.

# Colorectal cancer

## Prevalence

More than 33 000 people in the UK are diagnosed with cancer of the large bowel (colorectal cancer) each year and it accounts for 11% of all cancer deaths, the second leading cause of cancer deaths after lung cancer.[1] Overall, there is little difference in prevalence between the sexes, although there is an ↑ in later life rates for ♂. The incidence of disease ↑ with age: <5% of cases occur in the <40 age-group and >50% of colorectal cancers occur in individuals >60 years old, peaking between 70 and 80 years of age.[2] Worldwide, environmental influences affect colorectal cancer epidemiology, linking high incidence to developed industrialized countries and low incidence to less developed areas, such as Asia and many parts of Africa.

## Pathophysiology

- >90% of cases are adenocarcinomas.
- Most arise from adenomatous polyps (adenomas) (see Fig. 14.2).
- Adenomas are common. Benign tumours present in about one-third of all European and US populations; <5% of cases are thought to develop into invasive carcinomas.[3]
- The majority of colorectal cancers are sporadic.
- ~5% of colorectal cancers are inherited—the main types are familial adenomatous polyposis (FAP) and hereditary non-polyposis colorectal cancer (HNPCC); (📖 pp. 484, 488).

## Carcinogenesis (formation and development of cancer)

Sporadic colorectal cancers arise from a sequence of molecular and histopathological changes caused by genetic instability and environmental influences. This is known as the 'adenoma–carcinoma sequence' (Fig. 14.2): molecular changes include multiple acquired genetic alterations within oncogenes (promoting malignant transformation) and tumour-suppressor genes (causing loss of the inhibition of cellular proliferation).

Environmental factors linked to development of colorectal cancers are advanced age, high-red-meat diet, high-fat diet, smoking, alcohol consumption, and obesity.

A newly discovered pathway for carcinogenesis, mainly responsible for HNPCC, is now thought to also occur in ~15% of sporadic colorectal cancers, involving mutations in the genes responsible for repair of mismatched DNA base pairs (i.e. mismatch repair genes).

## Risk factors

📖 p. 480.

---

1 Office for National Statistics (2005). *Registrations of Cancer Diagnosed in 2002, England.* Series MB1 no.33. Office for National Statistics, London.

2 Rawlings B (2005). The biological basis of bowel cancer. In: Borwell B (ed) *Bowel Cancer: Foundations for Practice.* Whurr, London, pp.3–17.

3 Midgley R and Kerr D (1999). Colorectal cancer. *Lancet* **353**, 391–9.

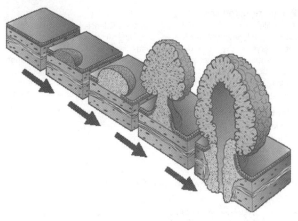

**Fig. 14.2** Adenoma–carcinoma sequence. Reproduced with kind permission
© Burdett Institute 2008.

## Prevention and screening

The political agenda, social issues, and the evidence base for colorectal cancer development have all served as driving forces for improving survival rates through the early detection and diagnosis of colorectal cancer. The identification of risk factors and implementation of health promotion and education initiatives, in addition to the development of colorectal cancer screening programmes, have contributed to the achievement of prevention, earlier detection, and, ultimately, improved outcomes for patients.

## Identification of risk factors

### Hereditary

- Personal history of adenomas or colorectal cancer.
- First-degree relative aged <60 years with adenoma or colorectal cancer or two first-degree relatives of any age with colorectal cancer.
- Inherited colorectal cancer syndromes—HNPCC and FAP.
- Long-standing ulcerative colitis and Crohn's colitis.

### Lifestyle

- Diet—a key issue in the causation and prevention of colorectal cancer. A diet high in fat is usually linked to colorectal cancer, particularly through ↑ consumption of red meat and a diet low in fish, vegetables, and fruit intake. A connection between a low intake of dietary fibre and an ↑ risk of colorectal cancer is also suggested by a link between a prolonged stool transit time, ↑ contact of carcinogens with the colorectal mucosa, and, possibly, ↓ protective fermentation activity within the bowel.
- Alcohol and smoking—possibly leading to ↑ risk of developing adenomas in addition to several forms of cancer, especially those with low levels of folate in the diet.
- Physical inactivity and obesity—individuals who are less physically active have ↑ risk of developing colorectal cancer, possibly because of prolonged stool transit time and a diet high in fat.

## Health promotion and education

The multidisciplinary approach to care, health education programmes in primary and secondary care, active collaboration between healthcare professionals and the voluntary sector, and a focus on disease prevention all contribute to the following:

- ↑ public awareness of colorectal cancer.
- Awareness of lifestyle and hereditary risk factors.
- Awareness of symptoms and their early detection.
- ↑ uptake of colorectal cancer screening programmes.

# Screening for colorectal cancer

Greater knowledge of the natural history of colorectal cancer and diagnostic procedures now offer the prospect of ↓ mortality from the disease through implementation of mass population-screening programmes. Screening tests should be simple, cost-effective, reliable, specific, and sensitive. A national programme for the UK has commenced and as from 2006 ♂ and ♀ aged 60–69 years have been invited to be screened for colorectal cancer. This is gradually being rolled out nationally.

*Screening tests*

- Faecal occult blood test (FOBT)—cheap and non-invasive, e.g. the guaiac (haemoccult) test used to detect small amounts of non-visible blood in the stool. The test can be performed at home using a small stool sample smeared onto a card containing guaiac, which is then sent for analysis. Positive results require additional screening in the form of a colonoscopy. Randomized trials have shown ↓ mortality from colorectal cancer using biennial screening in the >50 years age group. Some foods in the diet or drugs (e.g. iron or NSAIDs) can cause false-positive results; other preparations (e.g. vitamin C) and a lack of bleeding in tumours can produce false-negative results. It might be difficult for those with impaired dexterity or visual difficulties to carry out the test. It requires the support of primary care teams for information and education to assist compliance.
- Flexible sigmoidoscopy—enables the whole of the left-hand side of colonic and rectal mucosa to be examined, which is where 60% of cancers occur. It is resource intensive because training in flexible sigmoidoscopy is required. Sedation is not needed. Single-enema preparation. Infrequent testing is required because the progression through adenoma to carcinoma is usually slow (>10 years). The procedure does not examine the proximal colon and ∴ potentially 40% of adenoma/cancers remain undetected.
- Colonoscopy—follow-up to a positive FOBT. It is used as a 'gold standard' screening tool in the USA and enables the whole colonic and rectal mucosa to be examined, although it is expensive and resource intensive. Training is required for colonoscopists and continued quality assurance is required to ensure the standards of colonoscopy are met. Full bowel preparation is needed, and possibly sedation. Pain, discomfort, and anxiety threaten compliance and the procedure carries a risk of perforation. It is recommended for those with a strong family history of cancers occurring more commonly in the right-hand side of the colon.

Although not yet available as a screening tool, CT virtual colonoscopy might be used in the future. It requires full bowel preparation but is minimally invasive.

## Further reading

Borwell B (2005). Prevention, screening and early detection. In: Borwell B (ed) *Bowel Cancer: Foundations for Practice*. Whurr, London, pp.3–17.

# Intestinal polyposis syndromes: overview

The word 'polyposis' means multiple polyps. Intestinal polyposis syndromes are rare, genetic in origin, and, in addition to colorectal cancer, patients are at ↑ risk of malignancy in general. The four polyposis syndromes described here are FAP, Peutz–Jeghers syndrome (PJS), juvenile polyposis (JP), and *MYH*-associated polyposis (MAP).

Families with a history of polyposis syndromes undergo huge physical and psychological trauma and need ongoing support. Table 14.2 highlights some physical manifestations related to polyposis type.

**Table 14.2** Manifestations related to polyposis type

| Polyposis type | Features other than polyps | Cancers other than colorectal | Inheritance and gene |
|---|---|---|---|
| FAP | Epidermoid cysts, osteomas, desmoid, congenital retinal pigmentation, and abnormal dentition | ↑ risk, especially upper GI and thyroid | Autosomal dominant *APC* gene (chromosome 5) |
| PJS | Pigmented lesions on lips, buccal mucosa, fingers, and toes | ↑ risk, especially pancreas and breast | Autosomal dominant *STK11(LKB1)* gene (chromosome 19) |
| JP | Large head and hands, clubbing, and congenital abnormalities | ↑ risk | Autosomal dominant *SMAD 4* gene (chromosome 18) |
| MAP | Still under investigation | Under investigation | Recessive *MYH* gene (chromosome 1) |

# Intestinal polyposis syndromes: familial adenomatous polyposis

Previously called 'Gardner's syndrome'. FAP accounts for 80% of families with a polyposis syndrome. There is a 50% chance of inheriting the disease if one parent is affected. Therefore:

- Genetic testing or colorectal screening is advised from early teens.
- Genetic testing is possible for most, but not all, families.
- The condition is characterized by hundreds to thousands of adenomatous polyps throughout the colon and rectum.
- In asymptomatic children, bowel screening will usually reveal polyps in the teenage years.
- If symptomatic, children should be screened at a younger age.
- In the attenuated form, the polyps might not develop until late in life and the number of adenomas will be fewer.
- Treat with surgery (colectomy with ileorectal anastomosis or restorative proctocolectomy) <25 years—total proctocolectomy with ileostomy should only be performed if neither of these options is possible.
- The average age of colorectal malignancy is 39 years in untreated patients.
- Adenomas develop in the duodenum, especially around the ampulla, in most patients.
- Fundic gland polyps are found in the stomach of ~50% of cases.
- Upper GI screening, using a side-viewing endoscope, should commence at 25 years of age—at an earlier age if symptomatic.
- Surveillance of the rectum, pouch or ileostomy, and duodenum is required for life—adenomas develop at all these sites and might progress to malignancy.
- Genetic counselling when considering conception.

# Intestinal polyposis syndromes: Peutz–Jeghers syndrome

- Genetic testing is available for most families.
- Freckles on lips, buccal mucosa, fingers, and toes usually develop at ~2–3 years of age. Parents of children known to be at risk of inheriting PJS are usually watchful for these freckles.
- PJS polyps might develop anywhere throughout the GIT.
- Polyps in the small bowel can cause severe abdominal pain and intussusception if left untreated.
- Parents are advised to obtain a referral to a paediatric gastroenterologist familiar with PJS within the first 1–2 years of a new baby's life. An emergency consultation can then be arranged at any time if the parent is worried that small bowel obstruction might be occurring.
- Genetic testing of young children is advised to confirm the diagnosis.
- In young children, regular bowel screening is not advised. Patients are managed according to symptoms.
- In adults, polyps are controlled by the following:
  - Upper and lower gastrointestinal endoscopy every 2–3 years.
  - Capsule endoscopy or barium follow-through every 2–3 years, followed by on-table enteroscopy, if necessary.
- An annual blood test to check the haemoglobin level is advised—if the level is low, consider the possibility of bleeding polyps or malignancy.

# Intestinal polyposis syndromes: juvenile polyposis

- Genetic testing is not routinely available.
- Juvenile polyps might develop anywhere throughout the gastrointestinal tract.
- A diagnosis can be made with fewer than three juvenile polyps, if there is a family history of the condition. The polyps might be so numerous that they require colectomy.
- Onset might be in early infancy or adulthood.
- Juvenile polyps tend to bleed and might autorotate and fall off.
- Extra-intestinal abnormalities might occur and include hydrocephalus, pulmonary arteriovenous fistulae, undescended testes, and congenital heart defects.
- In severe cases, surgery might be required, similar to FAP; otherwise, polyps can be controlled by similar means to those used in PJS.

# Intestinal polyposis syndromes:
## *MYH*-associated polyposis

MAP is commonly mistaken for attenuated FAP—the number of colorectal adenomas throughout the colon and rectum is usually <500.

• Diagnosis is made/confirmed by genetic testing.
• Recessive inheritance means that investigation of both parents and their families is required.
• Homozygotes and compound homozygotes should have colonoscopy at the time of diagnosis.
• Management of the colon is similar to FAP.
• Upper GI screening, using a side-viewing endoscope, should commence at 25 years of age—at an earlier age, if symptomatic.
• Predictive genetic testing is available for relatives—the child of an affected patient will always be a 'carrier' (heterozygote) and might be affected (homozygote) if another copy of the gene has been inherited from the other parent.
• Predictive genetic testing should be offered at the age of 18–21 years.
• Heterozygotes probably have a moderately ↑ risk of bowel cancer. Therefore colonoscopy is recommended at diagnosis, to be repeated every 5 years until the age of 80 years.

# Hereditary non-polyposis colorectal cancer

HNPCC, also known as 'Lynch syndrome', is the commonest form of hereditary colorectal cancer. The lifetime risk of bowel cancer is 50–80% and it tends to occur at an early age. Other considerations include:

• There is an excess of synchronous and metachronous colorectal cancer.
• Also ↑ risk of extracolonic cancer, including tumours in the endometrium, ovaries, stomach, small intestine, pancreas, urinary and hepatobiliary tracts, and brain.
• Diagnosis might be missed unless a thorough family history is taken.
• If HNPCC is suspected, tumour tissue should be tested for microsatellite instability (MSI) and immunohistochemical staining should be performed for mismatch repair protein.
• If the tumour proves to be MSI high, genetic testing should be performed to look for mutations in the mismatch repair genes *MLH1*, *MSH2*, and *MSH6*.
• Genetic testing can be offered to relatives if the causative mutation is identified.
• Screening should be offered to first-degree relatives.
• Colonoscopy should be performed every 1–2 years from the age of 25 years.
• Prophylactic colectomy (and total abdominal hysterectomy with bilateral salpingo-oophrectomy in ♀) is an option that can be discussed with gene carriers.

# Chemotherapy for cancer of the colon and rectum

Survival after curative surgery is directly related to the pathological stage of the disease.

Cytotoxic chemotherapy involves drugs with the potential to kill cells. Unlike surgery and radiotherapy, it has a systemic effect, treating both local and metastatic disease.

## Post-operative chemotherapy

Fluorouracil (5-FU) is used in combination with folinic acid in both early and advanced stages of cancer. Administration is mainly intravenous, either as a bolus every week for 26 weeks or as an infusion, e.g. over a 48-h period every fortnight for six cycles. The introduction of oral 5-FU prodrugs, e.g. capecitabine, enables patients to have treatment at home, ↓ hospital visits.

## Side effects

- Mucositis is a common toxicity.
- Nausea.
- Diarrhoea.
- Palmar/plantar syndrome.
- Pancytopenia.

## Combination chemotherapy

5-FU is increasingly combined with other cytotoxic drugs. For locally advanced disease, the combination regimen might be as follows:

- Oxaliplatin and 5-FU.
- Irinotecan and 5-FU.
- Mitomycin C and 5-FU.

## Nursing considerations

Information about the treatment, general emotional support, and practical help with side effects help patients cope better with their treatment.[1] Patients should be advised regarding:

- Frequent bowel actions—use loperamide or codeine phosphate as needed and advise the patient to sip fluids slowly throughout the day to maintain fluid intake.
- Encourage small meals for poor appetite, avoiding salty and spicy foods, and possibly those with a strong smell—try chewing fresh pineapple.
- Nausea—a range of anti-emetics are effective—also consider ginger, peppermint, and complementary treatments.
- Soreness of the skin on hands and feet—piridoxin cream.
- Mucositis—clean the mouth after every meal using a soft toothbrush and moisturize lips.
- Dose modification and treatment postponement might have to be considered.

1 Knowles G, Tierney A, Jodrell D and Cull A (1999). The perceived information needs of patients receiving adjuvant chemotherapy for surgically-resected colorectal cancer. *European Journal of Oncology Nursing* **3**, 208–20.

# Surgical management of colon cancer

Surgery alone cures only 50% of patients diagnosed with colon cancer. During an abdominal colonic resection, a long segment of bowel is resected to remove the primary tumour, proximal and distal margins of normal bowel, and the vascular supply to the site, including associated mesentery containing lymphatics and lymph nodes.

## Pre-operative considerations
• Bowel preparation.
• Prophylaxis of thromboembolism.
• Antibiotic prophylaxis.
• Health optimization.
• Informed consent.

Patients with a colorectal cancer who have a strong predisposition to further colonic neoplasia (i.e. long-standing ulcerative colitis or FAP patients) are advised to have their entire colon and rectum removed and offered a restorative proctocolectomy (ileo–anal pouch).

These procedures may be performed laparoscopically, depending on the available surgical expertise. If the procedure is uncomplicated, patients can recover more quickly.

## Post-operative care
• Give an IV infusion until the patient can maintain their own hydration. If surgery is fast-tracked, food can be introduced before bowel sounds are heard.
• Opiate analgesia for 2–3 days—either an epidural or PCA.
• Early mobilization—to prevent complications.
• Remove the catheter when fluid-balance issues resolve and the patient can manage without it.

## Complications
These include:
• Cardiorespiratory
• Anastomotic and/or wound dehiscence.
• Sepsis and wound infection.
• Bowel obstruction.
• Thromboembolism.
• Urinary retention and infection.
• Incidental damage to other organs, e.g. urethral injury.

There is an operative mortality rate of <5% for elective surgery, which ↑ if emergency surgery is performed.[1]

## Emergency surgery
Up to 20% of patients will present as emergency cases, the majority of which will be obstructed (exclude pseudo-obstruction). These patients should be stabilized and specialist colonic surgery should be performed during daytime hours.

---

1 Schofield G and Jones DJ (1992). Colorectal neoplasia III: treatment and prevention. *British Medical Journal* **304**, 1624–27.

## Type of surgery
- Cancer of right colon—right or extended right hemicolectomy.
- Cancer of the transverse colon—transverse hemicolectomy.
- Cancer of the left colon—left hemicolectomy.
- Cancer of the sigmoid colon—sigmoid hemicolectomy (Fig. 14.3).

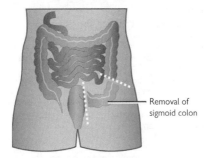

Removal of
sigmoid colon

**Fig. 14.3** A diagrammatic representation of one type of colonic resection—a sigmoid hemicolectomy. Reproduced with kind permission © Burdett Institute 2008.

# Malignant bowel obstruction

Bowel obstruction occurs with a variety of primary and metastatic malignancies; a common cause of bowel obstruction is colonic cancer. Up to 25% of patients with colonic cancer will develop intestinal obstruction. 15% of these will present with obstruction at diagnosis.

## Presentation

The patient will probably feel fatigued, dehydrated, and anorexic, and in addition may have:

- Abdominal pain—colic.
- Nausea or vomiting—can develop into a continuous and unpleasant symptom because the vomit becomes faeculent.
- Abdominal distension is variable but associated with trapped air in the bowel—occurs in 75% of patients.
- Bowel movements can vary from absolute constipation to diarrhoea.
- Sounds from the bowel might be hyperactive (borborygmi), tinkling, or absent—if ileus is present.

## Diagnosis

Abdominal X-rays or CT scans to assess dilated loops, air–fluid levels, and masses. A barium study and, occasionally, endoscopy might also be ordered.

## Management

First, resuscitate and stabilize the patient. Surgery can relieve distension and is indicated if the tumour is resectable and the patient's general condition allows it.

Malignant bowel obstruction is often caused by recurrent cancer in the advanced stages of the disease process. Considerable operative morbidity and mortality exists: risk of dying from surgery averages 15.7%. This must be weighed against the patient's life expectancy. Patients with complete obstruction survived for 29 days in one study,[1] although survival can be much longer if surgery is successful.

There are four main surgical approaches:

- Resection of a segment of bowel and re-anastomosis.
- Decompression of the bowel by stoma formation, e.g. temporary ileostomy or Hartmann's procedure.
- Bypass procedure.
- Division of adhesions.

Non-surgical options include pharmacological treatment, laser therapy, insertion of a colonic metallic stent (📖 p. 218), and conservative management. Up to one-third of patients achieve a temporary resolution of the symptoms of obstruction.

---

1 Isbister WH and Elder P (1990). Non-operative management of malignant intestinal obstruction. *Journal of the Royal College of Surgeons (Edinburgh)* **35**, 369–72.

## Nursing role

The nurse can function as the patient's advocate in steering appropriate decision-making, in addition to offering comfort and leading conservative management:

- Administration of intravenous/subcutaneous fluids to ↓ nausea and drowsiness—>500 ml/day recommended.
- A continuous subcutaneous infusion of diamorphine can help pain.
- Nasogastric suction—discontinue after 3 days if no effect is seen.
- Use antisecretory drugs (e.g. octreotide) to ↓ secretions, slow intestinal motility, and ↓ bowel distension.
- Use cyclizine, haloperidol, or levomepromazine to control any nausea.

# Partial and total colectomy

The reason for removing all or part of the colon will determine the timing of the operation; it might be the first of two operations. A total colectomy might be performed for the following two main conditions:

• Inflammatory bowel disease.
• Polyposis coli.

Patients with IBD are at ↑ risk of colorectal cancer after 8–10 years of disease. Screening colonoscopies should be instigated and mucosal histo-pathological changes reported.[1] If cancer is found, surgery to remove the whole colon, and sometimes almost the whole rectum, might be pragmatic (📖 p. 492).

Patients with polyposis coli will consider surgery a prophylactic procedure (📖 p. 484).

There are three main surgical options:

• Panproctocolectomy and the formation of an end ileostomy—rare.
• Colectomy with ileo-rectal anastomosis (IRA)—avoids a stoma.
  The colon is removed and the ileum anastomosed to the rectum.
  The mucosa of the rectal stump requires life-long surveillance.
• Restorative proctocolectomy—removes all of the large-bowel mucosa and an ileo-anal pouch is formed (📖 p. 252).

A subtotal colectomy is the partial removal of the colon, which might be performed if an individual has synchronous tumours, e.g. in the descending and sigmoid colon, or, possibly, a tumour and discrete section of colonic colitis. Individuals with HNPCC might also consider a subtotal colectomy IRA because this disease is predominantly right-sided (📖 p. 488).

## Patient information

Surgery takes up to 4 h, occasionally longer; the hospital stay could last up to 2 weeks. This is a safe and effective treatment, with only a few complications (intra-abdominal abscess or haemorrhage) reported. An ↑ in the frequency of bowel actions is to be expected (~three times/day), possibly with more urgency than previously.

Following a colectomy, attention to the diet is important because the homeostatic functions of the large bowel (storage, absorption of water, salts, and some vitamins, and consolidation of faeces) are no longer available. Menu selections should include foods high in calories and rich in protein, vitamins, and minerals, and there might be a need to limit the intake of fibre and certain spicy foods. Six to eight large glasses of liquid, such as water, juices, and milk, might be required each day. It can take up to 6 months for the body to adjust following major surgery of this kind. Some patients might find their social life and work is compromised by this surgery.

1 Tamamoto T and Keighley MRB (1999). Long term outcome of total colectomy and ileostomy for Crohn's disease. *Scandinavian Journal of Gastroenterology* **34**, 280–6.

# Megacolon and megarectum

## Dilated colon and/or rectum

### Presentation

Presents as chronic severe constipation, usually in children and young adults, usually idiopathic. Often, soiling results because a faecal bolus in the rectum inhibits anal closure and liquid stool seeps around the impaction. It can present as acute abdomen with sigmoid volvulus (twisting of sigmoid colon) which is seen on instant-contrast enema—a surgical emergency.

### Assessment

On PR examination the anal sphincter is often found to be lax; faecal impaction is evident and occasionally a palpable abdominal mass (faeces) is identified. Imaging: dilated rectum or part/whole colon. Differential diagnosis: exclude Hirschsprung's disease (📖 p. 657).

### Conservative management

- Disimpact—gentle manual evacuation might be needed (❶ care is required because the anal sphincter might already be compromised). In severe impaction, manual disimpaction should be performed under anaesthetic. Teach patients to take responsibility for their own bowel care (teenagers might be reluctant). Aim for a loose 'porridge'-like consistency of stool on permanent basis. Regular attempts to defecate after meals, even in the absence of the urge to defecate. Biofeedback can be used to teach muscular coordination (📖 p. 586). If using osmotic laxatives, titrate to response. Magnesium salts (e.g. Epsom salts) are unpalatable and the patient might have poor tolerance or compliance with them. Enemas or irrigation might be needed. Fluid intake of 2.5 L/day is necessary. Symptoms will probably last life-long.
- Surgery— only if conservative management has failed and symptoms are severe. It largely depends on where the dilated segment is (whole colon, partial, or rectum). Rectal or colonic resection is recommeded. If the whole colon is affected, ileo-anal anastomosis or ileostomy is required.

# Toxic megacolon

Toxic megacolon is a potentially fatal complication of acute, active inflammatory bowel disease or infectious colitis. It is characterized by non-obstructed segmental or total colonic dilation associated with systemic toxicity. It should not be confused with the colonic dilation that also occurs in idiopathic megacolon, in addition to pseudo-obstruction. The incidence of megacolon is low (~1–5%), but there are no precise data available. It can affect ♂ and ♀ of all ages.

## Causes
- Inflammatory bowel disease.
- Infectious colitis.
- Ischaemic colitis.
- Pseudomembranous colitis.

## Investigations
- FBC, urea and electrolytes, ESR, CRP.
- Plain abdominal X-ray.
- Stool specimens—ova, parasites, and *C.difficile*.
- Ultrasound/CT might aid management.

Colonoscopy should usually be avoided owing to the high risk of perforation.

## Diagnosis
- Radiographic evidence of colonic distension.
- At least three of the following:
  - Fever.
  - Tachycardia.
  - Anaemia.
  - Neutrophilic leucocytosis.
- In addition, at least one of the following:
  - Dehydration.
  - Altered consciousness.
  - Hypotension.
  - Electrolyte disturbance.

## Treatment
It is an acute emergency and ∴ should be managed in a high-dependency area. Pre- and post-operative considerations include:
- Frequent monitoring.
- ↓ severity of underlying inflammation.
- Nil by mouth.
- Nasogastric tube.
- Repeat abdominal X-ray every 12 h initially and daily thereafter.
- IV corticosteroids.
- IV broad-spectrum antibiotics.
- Fluid resuscitation/electrolyte depletion.
- Stop any antimotility agents.
- Blood transfusion if anaemic.

- Repositioning manoeuvres to aid decompression.
- Prevention of deep vein thrombosis.

Surgery (subtotal colectomy and end ileostomy) is indicated for:
- Progressive dilatation.
- Worsening toxicity.
- Failure of medical therapy.
- Perforation/haemorrhage.

## Further reading

Levine CD (1999). Toxic megacolon: diagnosis and treatment challenges. *Advanced Practice in Acute Critical Care* **10**, 492–9.
Sheth SG and La Mont JT (1998). Toxic megacolon. *Lancet* **351**, 509–13.

# Chronic abdominal pain

Acute abdominal pain (📖 p. 708).

Patients with chronic abdominal pain present many clinical challenges in terms of the management of their symptoms and attendant social restrictions often imposed by their condition.

▶ Once abdominal causes have been excluded (in particular, mesenteric ischaemia in predisposed patients), complete a search for organic disease, including consideration of pelvic, neurological, and musculoskeletal disorders. The wide range of disorders that can cause recurrent or chronic pain is outlined in Table 14.3.

Repeated negative findings on examination, in the context of atypical pain that does not fit the typical pattern of organic disease, should raise the possibility of a psychogenic cause of symptoms. The presence of constant unremitting pain, once malignancy has been excluded, is suggestive of the diagnosis of a functional cause of pain. The management of functional pain is based on the following three principles:

- Honest empathic explanation of the nature of the condition to the patient.
- Avoidance of potentially dangerous and addictive opiate or codeine-containing analgesia.
- Limiting the behavioural and social negative influences of the condition that exacerbate the perception of chronic pain.

Patients are best managed in specialized clinics, if available. In addition to psychological and supportive input, it is sometimes appropriate to consider the use of specialist analgesic regimens (including nerve blocks and agents for neuropathic pain). The essence of treatment in this situation is not cure but management of pain and limitation of the adverse impact on quality of life (📖 p. 700).

**Table 14.3** Disorders causing recurrent/chronic pain

| Musculoskeletal | Fibromyalgia |
| | Vertebral compression |
| Neurological | Spinal cord lesions |
| | Radiculopathy |
| Retroperitoneal | Aortic aneurysm |
| | Sarcoma or other malignancy |
| | Lymphadenopathy |
| | Abscess |
| Pelvic | Gynaecological disease |
| | Congenital or developmental cysts |
| Metabolic | Diabetes |
| | Hypercalcaemia |
| | Porphyria |
| Miscellaneous | Sickle cell disease |
| | Lead poisoning |
| Psychogenic | Somatization disorder |
| | Hypochondriasis |
| | Anxiety and depression |
| Gastrointestinal | IBD |
| | IBS |
| | Diverticulitis |
| | Idiopathic constipation |
| | Mesenteric ischaemia |
| | Malignancy |

# Irritable bowel syndrome

## Prevalence
- Peak incidence in young adults; less common with age. Many do not consult.
- More ♀ than ♂ present for health care (ratio of ♀:♂, 2:1). More likely to consult with frequent/severe symptoms.
- 850 000 GP consultations/year.
- 50% of gastroenterology out-patient department consultations.
- Affects up to 1 in 5 adults at some point in life.
- Impact on psychosocial function and work.
- Majority managed in primary care.

## Definitions
On the basis of symptoms:
- Rome II criteria—two or more of the following, for at least 25% of the time:
  - Abdominal pain, often relieved by defecation.
  - Change in stool frequency or consistency—constipation and/or diarrhoea (might alternate).
  - Bloating and/or mucus.
- Could be regular or intermittent and mild or incapacitating.
- Unusual to have symptoms at night.
- Associations:
  - Fibromyalgia and other hypersensitivities.
  - Functional dyspepsia.
  - Lethargy
  - Back pain.
  - Overactive bladder.
  - Childhood abuse (poorer outcome).
  - Depression and anxiety.

## Pathophysiology
- Unknown at present—probably multiple overlapping syndromes.
- Theories—visceral hypersensitivity, abnormal central nervous system processing of visceral pain, rectal over-sensitivity, and failure to inhibit pain pathways. Possibly a disorder of neurotransmitters in the enteric nervous system?
- Food hypersensitivity/intolerance.
- Exacerbated by emotional stress (often chronic) or adverse life events.
- Might commence after acute GI infection (gastroenteritis).
- Pain might commence with eating.
- Gut–brain axis—operates to maintain symptoms once started; a vicious circle of stress and hypersensitivity.

## Diagnosis
Diagnosis is made by exclusion: disordered colonic function in the absence of organic pathology. Consider the possibility of other bowel pathologies. Diagnosis is made using patient history and examination. Consider possibility of lactose intolerance or coeliac disease.

Patients might seek repeated reinvestigation: investigate once properly, and then reassure.

## Management
- Mild symptoms:
    - Patient education.
    - Realistic expectations.
    - Avoid caffeine and alcohol.
    - ↑ or ↓ fibre.
    - Food for ↓ gas.
    - Stress ↓.
    - Peppermint oil for bloating.
    - Probiotics?
- Moderate/severe symptoms—as above, plus the following:
    - Antispasmodics to relax gut smooth muscle (e.g. mebeverine hydrochloride).
    - Laxatives for constipation.
    - Loperamide for diarrhoea.
    - Low-dose antidepressants for pain.
    - Exclusion diet (needs dietitian supervision).
    - In the future—possibly serotonergic agents?

Complementary therapies are found helpful by some (limited evidence for hypnotherapy and acupuncture):
- Relaxation.
- Psychotherapy.
- Cognitive-behavioural therapy.

## Further reading
Camilleri M and Spiller RC (2002). *Irritable Bowel Syndrome*. WB Saunders, Edinburgh.

Patient support/IBS information/self-management programme. http://www.ibsnetwork.org.uk (accessed 14.05.07).

National Institute of Health and Clinical Excellance (2008). *Irritable Bowel Syndrome in Adults*. CG61. NICE, London.

# Rectum and anus

Structure and function  506
Stools and stool samples  508
Defecation  510
Rectal bleeding  512
Digital rectal examination  514
Proctoscopy  515
Rectal cancer  516
Tenesmus in rectal
    cancer  517
Surgery for rectal cancer  518
Radiotherapy  520
Total mesorectal
    excision  521
Management of local
    recurrence  522
Total pelvic exenteration  523
Metastastic colorectal
    cancer  524
Palliative chemotherapy and
    radiotherapy  525
Follow-up for colon and
    rectal cancer  526
Anal cancer  528
Anterior resection
    syndrome  530
Rectal prolapse  531
Haemorrhoids  532
Haemorrhoidectomy  534
Anal fissure  536
Anal fistula  538
Recto-vaginal fistula  540
Colovesical fistula  541
Anal stenosis and
    stricture  542
Pilonidal sinus  544
Perianal skin care  546
Anal warts (condylomata
    acuminata)  548

Other perianal conditions  549
Pruritus ani  550
Diarrhoea  552
Cancer-related diarrhoea  556
Faecal incontinence  558
Obstetric trauma and faecal
    incontinence  560
Anorectal testing  562
Faecal incontinence:
    conservative measures  564
Faecal incontinence: exercises
    and biofeedback  566
Anal sphincter repair
    (overlapping
    sphincteroplasty)  568
Other surgical procedures for
    faecal incontinence  570
Neosphincters for faecal
    incontinence  572
Rectocele  574
Constipation in adults:
    pathophysiology  576
Constipation in adults:
    assessment and
    investigation  578
Conservative management
    of constipation  579
Constipation: enemas and
    suppositories  580
Laxatives  582
Rectal irrigation  584
Biofeedback for
    constipation  586
Constipation: surgery  588
Constipation in cancer  590
Megarectum  592
Solitary rectal ulcer
syndrome  593

# Structure and function

Composed of the same layers as the rest of the gut: mucosa, submucosa, inner circular smooth muscle, and outer longitudinal muscle.

## Rectum

- Usually described as having three sections (Fig. 15.1).
- Compliant—accepts stools without ↑ in pressure until a level of filling is reached that stimulates conscious sensation.
- Limited range of sensations—distension (stretch receptors).
- Pain—overdistension or inflammation.

## Anus

- 3–5 cm in length.
- Proximal—columnar epithelium (similar to colon).
- Distal—squamous epithelium (similar to skin).
- Transition zone in mid-canal.
- Dentate line—rich innervation plus anal glands.
- Three anal cushions—blood-filled; enhance mucosal seal.
- Dilated = haemorrhoids (📖 p. 532).

## Anal sphincter

There are two sleeves of sphincter muscle around the anus, separated by a layer of longitudinal muscle (Fig. 15.1).

### Internal anal sphincter (IAS)

- Smooth (involuntary) muscle, which is 2–3 mm thick (thickens with age) and 2–3 cm long.
- Continuous with circular smooth muscle wall of the rectum.
- Extends along the proximal (upper) two-thirds of the anal canal.
- Responsible for passive retention of stools at rest (contributes 80% of resting anal pressure).
- Subject to idiopathic degeneration with age and disruption by anal trauma (e.g. following anal surgery or abuse).

### External anal sphincter (EAS)

- Voluntary (striated) muscle comprising three sections, which is 3–5 cm long—longer in ♂ than ♀.
- Inserts into the pelvic floor (puborectalis) proximally and extends to the subcutaneous level distally.
- ♀ have a natural 'defect' in the upper anterior EAS, above the level where the puborectalis meets the EAS.
- Responsible for resisting defecation during the recto-anal inhibitory reflex (RAIR)—functions as the 'brakes' for defecation, voluntary retention of stool.
- Subject to trauma—especially during difficult childbirth.

### Longitudinal anal sphincter muscle

The muscle is found between the IAS and EAS and is continuous with outer longitudinal muscle of the gut wall. More prominent in ♂ than ♀. Its function is unclear, but the muscle probably 'splints' the anus during defecation to enable shortening of the sphincter and facilitate stool expulsion.

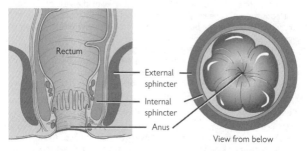

**Fig. 15.1** Rectum, anus, and anal sphincters. Reproduced with kind permission © Burdett Institute 2008.

# Stools and stool samples

▶ Use universal precautions when handling stools, particularly good hand-washing.

The normal amount of stool for a Western diet is ~150 g/day, which varies with fibre intake. Diarrhoea is defined as >200 g/24 h. Stool form is often classified on the Bristol scale (Fig. 15.2) and depends largely on water content; normal stool contains 70–80% water, with the rest of the content consisting of fibre residue and bacteria (≥400–500 species in normal gut, which is a complex but poorly understood ecosystem). The brown pigment results from bile products.

Steatorrhoea is pale, bulky, and oily stools, with an offensive odour. Stools are difficult to flush. Caused by fat malabsorption, e.g. bile duct obstruction or deficient in bile, which emulsifies fat.

Melaena is the passage of dark tarry stools—a sign of GI bleeding above the distal colon and rectum (often gastric).

## Tests

Tests are most commonly used for investigation of diarrhoea or rectal bleeding. Avoid stool collection following barium studies. Avoid taking anti-diarrhoeals or laxatives. Advise patient to eat a normal diet, if possible.

Collect a stool sample in a clean dry airtight container. Avoid contamination with urine. Keep the sample in the fridge and, ideally, deliver it to the laboratory within 30 min. Stool samples may be used:

• To observe for colour, amount, consistency, and odour.
• Faecal weight/volume—usually 2–3 day collection if true diarrhoea is in doubt (normal <200 g/day).
• Faecal fat content—normal stool <7 g of fat/day. Use a 3-day collection, with the patient taking ≥100 g of fat/day in diet. Use Sudan stain (acidify stool for uptake of stain) to detect fat malabsorption: ↑ number and size of fat droplets. Steatorrhoea is present if >7 g fat/day and can suggest small bowel disease or pancreatic insufficiency.
• Faecal osmotic gap—bacteria ferment non-absorbed carbohydrate, ↑ osmolality of stool. Use biochemistry to measure sodium and potassium levels if laxative abuse or inadvertent ingestion of osmotic agents to cause diarrhoea is suspected.
• Microscopy—detects red cells (e.g. inflammation, infection, or cancer), white cells (e.g. infection or inflammation), and ova or parasites (e.g. *Giardia*).
• Culture—for infection. Take three separate specimens, in addition to a good history, because a variety of tests/stains are used to detect unusual pathogens. Use sensitivity testing to determine appropriate treatment if infection with pathogenic bacteria is present.
• *Clostridium difficile* toxin, if suspected (e.g. diarrhoea after antibiotics).
• Pancreatic enzymes (e.g. tripsin) to determine pancreatic insufficiency.

Note: there is mandatory notification for several infectious diseases (this will be done by the laboratory).

# THE BRISTOL STOOL FORM SCALE

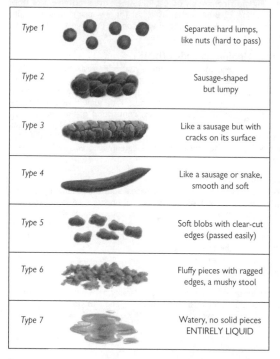

| | | |
|---|---|---|
| Type 1 | | Separate hard lumps, like nuts (hard to pass) |
| Type 2 | | Sausage-shaped but lumpy |
| Type 3 | | Like a sausage but with cracks on its surface |
| Type 4 | | Like a sausage or snake, smooth and soft |
| Type 5 | | Soft blobs with clear-cut edges (passed easily) |
| Type 6 | | Fluffy pieces with ragged edges, a mushy stool |
| Type 7 | | Watery, no solid pieces ENTIRELY LIQUID |

**Fig. 15.2** Bristol stool chart. Reproduced by kind permission of Dr. K W Heaton, Reader in Medicine at the University of Bristol. © 2000 Norgine Pharmaceuticals Ltd.

# Defecation

The gut is usually quiescent at night. Peak gut motility occurs in the morning. Awakening, mobility, eating, and drinking trigger a gastro-colic response: ↑ colonic peristalsis in response to ingesting food or drink. Rectal filling most commonly occurs following a mass movement of stool along the colon 20–30 min after breakfast (or any meal). As the rectum fills, stretch receptors in the rectal wall convey the urge to defecate to conscious perception.

## Recto-anal inhibitory reflex (RAIR)

When stools distend the rectum, there is a reflex relaxation of the IAS, enabling the stools to move into the upper anus, where they are 'sampled' by sensitive nerve endings at the dentate line (Fig. 15.3) which can distinguish solid and liquid stools and flatus. If the time is not right, there is a voluntary (but often subconscious) contraction of the EAS to stop stool expulsion and return stool to the rectum (Fig. 15.4). The RAIR lasts between 5 s and 20 s. The IAS closes again and the urge to defecate diminishes. The call to stool can be repeatedly ignored, leading to self-constipation.

## Defecation

At the correct time and place, the individual adopts a suitable posture on the toilet, with a small ↑ of intra-abdominal pressure, cessation of rectal inhibition, contraction of the rectum, and relaxation of the sphincters. Rectal contraction continues until the rectum is empty (coordinated by spinal and brainstem reflexes). Afterwards the sphincters 'snap' shut and residual stool in the anus is expelled. Note: complex social customs surround acceptable toilet behaviour. Most people consider privacy essential for defecation.

The normal frequency for defecation on a Western diet is 3 times/day to 3 times/week. Frequency varies considerably between and within individuals, depending on diet, activity, emotions, and lifestyle. ♀ defecate less frequently than ♂ on average.

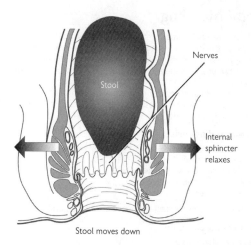

**Fig. 15.3** Stool moves down during RAIR. Reproduced with kind permission © Burdett Institute 2008.

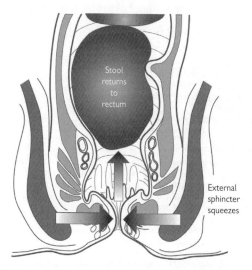

**Fig. 15.4** External sphincter squeezes to prevent stool expulsion. Reproduced with kind permission © Burdett Institute 2008.

# Rectal bleeding

This is the most common reason for referral to a colorectal clinic. Concern is because it is a symptom of colorectal cancer (which is treatable if caught early, before progression). Most rectal bleeding is not caused by cancer but usually by benign anorectal conditions. However, because of the cancer risk, all reports of rectal bleeding should be taken seriously. The patient could also be very concerned. Many patients are reluctant to present (because of embarrassment, fear of cancer, or concern about possible examination and tests).

### Differential diagnosis
- Perianal conditions (e.g. haemorrhoids or fissure).
- Inflammatory bowel disease.
- Solitary rectal ulcer syndrome.
- Diverticular disease.
- Polyps or cancer.

▶ Check that blood is actually of rectal, not vaginal, origin in ♀.

### Outlet rectal bleeding
- Bright red blood.
- Usually (not always) associated with defecation.
- Blood present on toilet paper after wiping; might drip into toilet pan.
- Possible anal pain or discomfort on defecation.
- Not usually any change in bowel habit or abdominal symptoms.
- Usually, but not always, benign anorectal conditions.
- Possibly associated mucus from haemorrhoids.

### Altered rectal bleeding
- Darker blood.
- Might be mixed with stools.
- Possible passage of mucus.
- Possible altered bowel habit or stool consistency (looser or constipated).
- Might be associated with weight loss.
- More likely to be associated with malignancy.

### Rectal bleeding clinic
Government targets now mandate a maximum of 2 weeks' wait before consultation for patients who have symptoms suggestive of colorectal cancer. Dedicated rectal-bleeding clinics are an attempt to streamline management of referrals and keep waiting times low. The patient is given rapid access after GP referral, usually with a standard referral form and a checklist for referral criteria—often nurse-led protocol-driven management. 'One-stop shop'—history, all tests, and consultation on the same day; a diagnosis is made and treatment plan formulated. Management of benign disorders is handled in the clinic, e.g. injection or banding of haemorrhoids and patient education. Ensure that the patient understands the significance of rectal bleeding and when to re-present if symptomatic (one attendance does not give lifetime protection).

## Further reading

Vance M (2004). Rectal bleeding—when to refer. In: Norton C and Chelvanayagam S (eds) *Bowel Continence Nursing*. Beaconsfield Publishers, Beaconsfield.

# Digital rectal examination

This issue has caused considerable controversy within the nursing field. Is this a legitimate nursing procedure? How is competence ensured? There have been several accusations of malpractice and even abuse. This is a legitimate nursing procedure but not an extended nursing role.[1]

**Indications**

- To determine the presence, amount, and consistency of stools in the rectum.
- To establish anal tone, the ability to contract the anal sphincter voluntarily, and sensation.
- To assess the need for, and effect of, rectal medication or manual evacuation.
- To ensure no impediment to giving rectal medication—assessment of the angle of anus and rectum.
- To perform digital rectal stimulation (📖 p. 644).
- If trained—assess the presence of a rectal mass or prostate size.
- To check for pain or stricture prior to endoscopic procedure.

Manual evacuation and digital rectal stimulation (📖 p. 644).

**Procedure**

- Ensure consent is obtained.
- Consider the need for offering a chaperone.
- Attention to privacy and dignity issues.
- Left-lateral position is customary (some patients might perform manual evacuation on the toilet).
- Use a lubricated gloved finger (note latex allergies).
- Stop if pain, bleeding, or consent is withdrawn.
- In the frail patient, consider the need for checking pulse and blood pressure before and after the procedure.
- Take extra care with fragile tissues (e.g. inflammation, radiation, or in the frail patient).
- Avoid following recent anal surgery, unless there is a medical instruction.
- Special considerations—children, history of abuse, and cultural and gender sensitivities.
- Spinal cord injury above T6 level—danger of autonomic dysreflexia (📖 p. 642).

1 Royal College of Nursing (2000). *Digital Rectal Examination and Manual Removal of Faeces*. RCN, London.

# Proctoscopy

More properly termed 'anoscopy'. Proctoscopy examines the rectum and anoscopy examines the anal canal. The rectum is better examined with a sigmoidoscope.

A plastic (disposable) or metal (sterilized and re-used) proctoscope/anoscope is 2 cm in diameter and 7 cm long (paediatric/stricture versions are smaller). Most have a light source.

The instrument is used for inspection of the anal canal and ano-rectal junction. The patient traditionally adopts a left-lateral position, with knees flexed, during the procedure. No preparation is needed, except explanation and informed consent. Digital rectal examination first to check for pain/stricture in the anal canal.

The instrument is lubricated with water-soluble gel (a local anaesthetic can be used if the patient is in discomfort). Gentle pressure is used to insert the instrument; inspect on withdrawal. The instrument will often be expelled unless the clinician keeps up gentle pressure. The following can be visualized.

• Upper anal canal—columnar epithelium (mucous membrane).
• Lower canal—squamous epithelium (skin).
• Transition zone mid-anal canal—dentate line, anal valves, and crypts are also visible.
• Haemorrhoids—usually prolapse into the lumen of the proctoscope. Can be ligated or injected.
• Fissure or fistula—inspect: might be too painful or difficult without anaesthetic.
• Biopsy—lower rectum or upper anal canal (insensitive). Biopsy of the lower anal canal is too painful except under general anaesthetic.

# Rectal cancer

Each year in the UK >10 000 people are diagnosed with rectal cancer. There is no evidence that the pathogenesis of rectal cancer is different from colonic cancer.

### Signs and symptoms

- Change in bowel habit—looser stool and/or increased frequency.
- Rectal bleeding.
- Mucus discharge.
- Tenesmus.

There could be signs of weight loss or anaemia, and more advanced cancers could cause localized pain and dysfunction.

### Screening and staging investigations

▶ Measure the distance of the tumour from the anal verge and assess its depth of penetration, the size of any lymph node enlargement, and any more distant spread. A rectal tumour up to 10 cm from the anal verge might be palpable as a hard, sometimes ulcerated, mass in the rectal wall.
  Investigations include the following.

- Endoscopy—rigid or flexible.
- Endorectal ultrasonography.
- Digital rectal examination.
- Magnetic resonance imaging (MRI) of the pelvis.

An MRI scan can accurately establish the probability of circumferential resection margin clearance around the tumour.

### Prognosis

Metastatic disease is present in ~20% of patients with newly diagnosed rectal cancer. If the disease is localized, prognosis is dependent on the following.

- The depth of invasion by the primary tumour.
- Lymph node involvement.
- Histological differentiation of the tumour.

Tumour invasion into the surrounding tissue and organs occurs more frequently in rectal cancer than colonic because its growth is not limited by a serosa. A fixed rectum is associated with a poorer prognosis. Half of recurrences are in the pelvis, rather than at distant sites.

### Further reading

Northover J, Taylor C, and Gould D (2002). Carcinoma of the rectum. In: Williams J (ed) *The Essentials of Pouch Care Nursing*. Whurr, London.

# Tenesmus in rectal cancer

'Rectal tenesmus' is characterized by a sensation of needing to pass stools, causing a painful sensation of fullness. This could cause straining and passing blood and mucus, but little stool. Tenesmus can be continuous or recurrent. It is often a presenting symptom, but can also reflect locally advanced or recurrent disease in the rectum. Tenesmus can also occur in non-cancer patients.

## Nursing assessment

Assessment includes a detailed rectal examination, abdominal examination, and ascertaining the following:
- Does the feeling come and go or is it constant?
- Is there a constant need to empty the bowels?
- Is there abdominal pain, cramping, or a persistent feeling of straining?
- Is there diarrhoea or vomiting?
- What helps/makes it worse?
- What happens on opening the bowels?

## Nursing advice

First, consider non-drug measures to ease comfort and opening of the bowels. Advise on ↑ fluid and fibre intake and improving activity levels. A combination of a softening agent and a stimulant laxative could help prevent constipation. Consider anxiolytics if there is anxiety associated with opening the bowels.

This pain tends to respond poorly to opioid analgesics,[1] so consider the following (note some are unlicensed uses)
- For muscle spasm—try benzodiazepines, nifedipine (10–20 mg oral three times daily or 20 mg twice daily, up to 60–80 mg/day), or possibly glyceryl trinitrate (GTN) ointment.
- For neuropathic pain—try a corticosteroid or anticonvulsant, e.g. sodium valproate, 200 mg oral twice daily (up to 500 mg three times daily, if necessary), plus an opioid.

## Palliation of tenesmus

Pharmacological means rarely provide good pain control and a nerve block should be considered. Radiotherapy can ameliorate the discomfort and any associated bleeding or discharge. Laser therapy can also be effective for initial palliation.

---

1 Rich A and Ellershaw J (2000). Tenesmus/rectal pain—how is it best managed. *CME Bulletin: Palliative Medicine* 2, 41–4.

# Surgery for rectal cancer

Surgery remains the cornerstone of cancer treatment, but radiotherapy and/or chemotherapy can also be used. Indicators of effective management are as follows.
- Local recurrence rates.
- Length of survival.
- Sphincter preservation.
- Degree of late morbidity—altered bowel control, urinary dysfunction, or sexual potency.

## Pre-operative nursing support
- Information-giving.
- Optimizing physical and psychological health.
- Measures to ↓ post-operative complications.

## Surgery
- Low anterior resection—indicated for proximal and mid-rectal tumours; performed in ≥80% of cases (Fig. 15.5).
- Ultra-low anterior resection—rectal dissection proceeding below the pelvic floor, or rectum completely excised.
- Abdominoperineal resection—performed if tumour is too low to staple mechanically; involves an abdominal and perineal wound and permanent colostomy (📖 p. 238).

These procedures can be performed or assisted laparoscopically depending on surgical expertise, achieving comparable oncological outcomes and shorter hospital stays.

Local resection can be either a manual transanal resection or transanal endoscopic microsurgery.

## Post-operative nursing support
Fluids can be given on the first post-operative day; food can be given on the third post-operative day because post-operative ileus usually takes 24–48 h to resolve. Enhanced recovery programmes often start fluids and food much earlier. Patients must be informed of the risks of ↑ urgency and frequency of bowel habit, which could cause minor soiling, incontinence of flatus, tenesmus, and some urinary and sexual dysfunction. After 3 months, many post-operative complications have settled, but this process can take up to 1 year.

## Role of adjuvant therapy
Surgery is curative in 60% of cases. Pre-operative and/or post-operative radiotherapy and chemotherapy can be used to enhance surgical success and improve survival, in addition to its use for palliation.[1]

---

1 Lidder PG and Hosie KB (2005). Rectal cancer: the role of radiotherapy. *Digestive Surgery* **22**, 41–8.

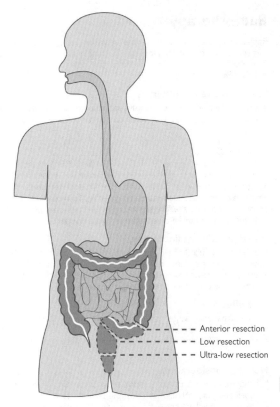

Anterior resection
Low resection
Ultra-low resection

**Fig. 15.5** Anterior resection. Reproduced with kind permission © Burdett Institute 2008.

# Radiotherapy

Radiation to the soft tissues in the pelvis can be given before or after surgery for rectal cancer alone or in combination with chemotherapy. Combination chemotherapy schedules are now being integrated with standardized radiotherapy regimens.

## Pre-operative radiotherapy

In the adjuvant setting, pre-operative radiotherapy is used more frequently than post-operative RT. This could be short course, e.g. 5 Gy × 5 days, with surgery 7–10 days later.

This is an intense treatment, with short-term and late morbidity, producing significant ↓ in local recurrence rates.[1]

A longer-course regimen is 50 Gy over a period of 5 weeks, with post-treatment assessment at 4–6 weeks. This regimen is suitable for locally advanced tumours (e.g. T2N3) which are fixed or tethered, or tumours which have been assessed radiologically (MRI) to threaten the circumferential resection margin. The downstaging effect of pre-operative chemoradiotherapy can make these tumours more operable.

## Post-operative radiotherapy

Post-operative radiotherapy does not improve survival unless combined with chemotherapy, e.g. capecitabine which is a product of oral fluorouracil. Therapy can provide symptomatic relief to patients with locally advanced tumours, which could become amenable to surgery.

## Side effects

For most patients, acute side effects resolve within 1 month. A longer-term sequence of complications can occasionally ensue, e.g. ongoing faecal continence difficulties and/or mucus discharge necessitating pad wearing (📖 p. 460).

## Nursing considerations

Patients require information about their treatment, general emotional support, and practical help with possible side effects, as follows.
• Frequent bowel actions—use loperamide or codeine phosphate as necessary.
• Urinary discomfort—encourage clear fluids.
• Dry skin—advise a shower rather than a bath and avoid rubbing and any lotions.
• Tiredness—energy returns within a few months.
• Sun sensitivity.
• Vaginal narrowing and dryness—in ♀. ♂ might have difficulty achieving an erection and ejaculation.

1 Kapiteijn E Marijnene CA and Nagtegaal ID (2001). Pre-operative radiotherapy combined with total mesorectal excision for resectable rectal cancer. *British Journal of Surgery* **81**, 1224–26.

# Total mesorectal excision

Total mesorectal excision (TME) the removal of the fatty tissue around the rectum—the mesorectum—to improve local control and survival for patients with operable rectal cancer. It relies on good pre-operative imaging to define the block of tissue for excision.

## Surgical principles

To preserve the anal sphincter and ↓ the requirement for a permanent colostomy. Tumours in the upper third of the rectum might only require a partial mesorectal excision (PME), as long as the 5 cm distal clearance is achieved. The surgical steps include the following.

- Sharp dissection.
- Recognition and preservation of the autonomic nerve plexus.
- Stapled low pelvic reconstruction.

## Outcomes

Many local recurrences in rectal cancer are regrowth of local mesorectal residues; hence this technique can achieve local recurrence rates <10%. However, such outcomes are dependent upon the meticulous dissection of the mesorectum and intact removal of the 'tumour—mesorectal package'. Formation of a short (5–7 cm) colonic pouch is advocated, anastomosed to the low rectum or anal canal for good functional outcomes.

## Complications

The most important surgical complication is symptomatic anastomotic leakage (5–15%), which is minimized by careful pre-operative assessment, use of pelvic drains, and occasionally defunctioning the bowel. Bladder and sexual function can be altered.

## Nursing care

Observe for signs of anastomotic leakage during the first 10 days: wounds draining pus, malaise, fever, generalized abdominal pain, and no stool passage. Prompt treatment is required to limit sepsis.

The autonomic pelvic nerves surround the mesorectum and, although their preservation is expected, nerve damage is possible.[1] Monitor for sexual or urinary disorders. If dysfunction persists, discuss specialist referral with the patient.

1 Maurer CA (2005). Urinary and sexual function after total mesorectal excision. *Recent Results in Cancer Research* **165**, 196–204.

# Management of local recurrence

## Predicting local recurrence of rectal cancer

Despite aggressive surgery, local recurrence is the dominant pattern of failure in managing this disease. Almost 50% of recurrences occur within 2 years of surgery. Once the cancer has spread beyond the bowel wall, the incidence of lymph node invasion rises from 14% to 43%. Local recurrence is dependent on the following.

- Surgical experience.
- Location of the tumour and its pathology.
- Circumferential margins.
- Successful TME.
- Use of chemoradiotherapy.

## Treatment

Treatment of recurrent rectal cancer depends on the treatment initially received. Surgery provides a chance of cure, which is dependent on the resectability of pelvic disease, absence of extrapelvic disease, patient preference, and fitness for surgery.

Combined chemoradiotherapy can be given to 'downstage' the disease, with assessment 4–8 weeks later and then, if appropriate, surgery tailored accordingly. Surgery achieves control in 47% of patients.[1] An *en bloc* resection is required, which could involve excision of the vagina, prostate, bladder, and part of the sacrum. Surgery can take 4–14 h.

Palliative surgery offers no benefit over non-operative management. Radiotherapy offers temporary palliation. Advances in chemoradiation can offer some patients a complete response, without surgery.

## Prognostic variables

Significant factors for survival and palliation are as follows.

- Absence of any severe symptoms—pain, obstruction, and sepsis.
- If a recurrent tumour is confined to the neorectum.
- Normal carcinoembryonic antigen (CEA) level after re-operation.

## Nursing support

Patients will face their mortality; great hope and dependence will be placed on their treatments. Establish what is important to the patient and their family now. Address supportive requirement in coping with this news, any symptoms, and potential treatment side effects.

1 Gagliardi G *et al.* (2005). Prognostic factors in surgery for local recurrence of rectal cancer. *British Journal of Surgery* **82**, 1401–5.

# Total pelvic exenteration

Radical surgery for patients with locally advanced or recurrent colorectal (pelvic) cancer. Involves the removal of one or several of the following.
- Rectum.
- Anus.
- Bladder.
- Internal genitalia.
- Bone (sacrum).

This is offered as a 'cure'. It is specialized surgery and can often require a number of investigations, such as MRI, CT, positron emission tomography, and examination under anaesthetic (EUA), before any decision on surgery is made.

An individualized plan of care is made and often requires the involvement of one or more of the following specialist surgeons, in addition to the colorectal surgeon:
- Orthapaedic surgeon.
- Plastic surgeon.
- Urologist.
- Gynaecologist.
- Vascular surgeon.
- Oncologists (if pre-operative chemoradiation is required).

## Nursing considerations
- Information-giving.
- Optimizing physical and psychological health.
- Patients will face issues regarding their mortality. They come to see the specialist with high hopes and expectations. ▶ Ensure a clear understanding is established at every meeting to enable the patient to be fully informed and thus empowered.
- Symptom control and pain could be issues that will need addressing.
- Prepare for the possibilty of a stoma (📖 p. 260).

# Metastastic colorectal cancer

Liver (hepatic) metastases develop in ~50% of patients during the course of their disease. Other less common sites for metastases are the peritoneum and lungs. Some patients have metastases at time of presentation (synchronous); others develop them metachronously.

Two main causes of disease progression are identified after apparently curative surgery:
• Occult distant metastases not found at surgery.
• Locoregional recurrence.

Although liver metastases represent the main cause of death in this disease, there now is a chance of cure for a few patients, if disease is surgically resectable.

## Surgery for liver metastases

The decision and extent of the surgical resection is based on the patient's condition and liver function. The patient will ∴ require numerous investigations and blood tests. Contraindications for surgery include the following.
• Comorbidity.
• Insufficient volume of normally functioning liver parenchyma.
• Multiple bilobar metastases.
• Poorly located lesions.

25–30% of those who have successful surgery will be alive at 5 years.

## Options for unresectable liver metastases

Palliative chemotherapy and/or locoregional treatments can be offered. Locoregional treatments include laser ablation and cryosurgery, in addition to surgical treatment, if surgery alone is not sufficiently radical. Chemotherapy can be given first to assess if the tumour can be reduced to a size which makes it amenable to surgery or another treatment.

## Patients presenting with asymptomatic primary disease and liver metastases

If feasible, surgery is the best possible option for controlling the disease. Patients expected to have a relatively long survival might opt to gain local control, before palliative chemotherapy. Less well patients might consider non-surgical management of their primary tumour only if symptomatic— either by colonic stenting or laser therapy, which are both effective treatments for symptom palliation, enabling more prompt chemotherapy.[1]

## Nursing considerations

It is imperative that patients have time to assimilate such complex information, feel able to choose between options available, and have their particular fears and hopes heard.

---

1 Biasco G, Derenzini E, Grazi G, *et al.* (2006). Treatment of hepatic metastases from colorectal cancer: many doubts, some certainties *Cancer Treatment Reviews* **32**, 214–28.

# Palliative chemotherapy and radiotherapy

## Chemotherapy

There are various treatment options for patients with advanced disease. The four main drugs used are:
- 5-Fluorouracil (5FU).
- Oxaliplatin.
- Irinotecan.
- Oral fluoropyrimidines, e.g. capecitabine/tegafur–uracil (UFT).

The trend is to use infusional 5FU in combination with oxaliplatin (FOLFOX) or irinotecan (IFL). These combinations are improving the response rate, time to progression, and overall survival. A 35% ↓ in the risk of death and an improvement in median survival of 3.7 months is reported.[1] However, there are toxicities, mainly tolerable, but occasionally severe, which might be experienced, in addition to the restrictions caused by fatigue, IV lines, and hospital-oriented treatment. The length of treatment is often 6 months or until there is tumour progression.

First-line treatment for advanced cancer is often an oral fluoro-pyrimidine, which causes less diarrhoea, stomatitis, and nausea, but hand–foot syndrome can be a problem, requiring effective skin management. These drugs could become better partners for oxaliplatin and irinotecan than 5FU.

Biological therapies have an ↑ role in conjunction with chemotherapy, e.g. epidermal growth factor receptor inhibitors (cetuximab).

## Radiotherapy

An unresectable primary tumour, e.g. a large and non-mobile tumour, might suit pre-operative chemoradiation, proceeding to radical resection in 40–80% of patients. Uncontrolled tumour growth in the pelvis can be successfully palliated with external-beam radiotherapy, with a schedule dependent on the prior radiation dose. Interstitial radiotherapy can treat pain and bleeding from locally advanced rectal tumours.

Both acute and longer-term side effects must be considered, including diarrhoea, skin reactions, fatigue, and various effects on sexual function. Side effects will ↑ if treatments are used concurrently.

## Nursing care

A person-centred approach, with emphasis on symptom control and psychological and social support is required. Achieving the patient's definition of a good quality of life should be the goal of the whole multidisciplinary team. Patients must be clear about the expectation of the treatment, the potential side effects, the time involved personally (and for the family) in receiving treatment, costs incurred, and longer-term benefits.

1 Best L, Simmonds P, Baughan C, et al. (2006). *Palliative Chemotherapy for Advanced or Metastatic Colorectal Cancer*. The Cochrane Library.

# Follow-up for colon and rectal cancer

There is a continuing debate on the subject of follow-up for patients who have had 'curative' surgery. The benefits of long-term follow-up are as follows:
• Detection of potentially curable recurrent disease.
• Detection of asymptomatic recurrence if early chemotherapy can improve quality of life and prolong survival.
• Detection of metachronous tumours.
• Provision of psychological support.
• Advice on lifestyle, diet, and optimizing health.
• Facilitation of audit, clinical governance, and continuing professional development.

There is no single strategy for follow-up. Most patients will be offered a combination of physical examination, colonoscopy, tumour markers, and radiological examinations.

The tumour marker CEA is one method of detecting recurrent disease. It requires only a blood test, but it is not always reliable.

If the colon has not already been visualized, a colonoscopy should be performed within 1 year of surgery to rule out potential synchronous or metachronous cancers or polyps. A further suggested recommendation is liver imaging 12–18 months after curative surgery.[1]

Conclusive evidence on the optimal follow-up schedule for prompt detection of recurrent disease is awaited. There are several studies examining the relative merits and appropriate frequency of employing regular CEA checks, colonoscopy, and CT by hospital surgeons, GPs, and/or specialist nurses. At present, most teams follow patients for up to 5 years before discharge from the service.

1 Association of Coloproctology of Great Britain & Ireland (2001). *Guidelines for the Management of Colorectal Cancer*. London.

# Anal cancer

Anal cancer, an uncommon cancer, arises from the cells around the anal opening (verge) or within the anal canal (3–5 cm long) up to its junction with the rectum. Symptoms include bleeding from the rectum or anus, the feeling of a lump or pain at the anal opening, and persistent or recurrent itching. Stages of anal cancer are shown in Box 15.1.

## Risk factors
- Human papillomavirus (HPV-16).
- Sexual activity.
- Smoking.
- Lowered immunity/HIV infection.

## Histological types
The position of the cancer and its histology are important considerations. Squamous cell carcinomas account for 80% of anal cancers.

## Treatment
Combination therapy, including radiation therapy and chemotherapy, is now standard treatment for most anal cancers.[1] Occasionally, very small or early tumours are removed surgically (local excision). Abdominoperineal resection might represent a rescue treatment for partial responders or in relapsing patients. Control is achieved in 80% of cases.

Chemotherapy drugs include 5FU, cisplatin, and mitomycin. They are given during week 1 and week 5 of radiation treatment, and are usually continued for several cycles. In some cases, interstitial radiation is given in addition to external beam radiation.

## Nursing care
Chemotherapy is generally well tolerated. Perianal skin care is essential during radiotherapy. Anal tissue can also be damaged, causing scar tissue to form and impairing the anal sphincter's function. Reassure the patient about the effectiveness of treatment for anal cancer, although several months are required to assess outcome.

---

1 Sato H, Koh PK and Bartolo DCC (2005). Management of anal canal cancer. *Diseases of the Colon and Rectum* **48**, 1301–15.

## Box 15.1 Stages of anal cancer

| | |
|---|---|
| Carcinoma *in situ* | Cancer in the top layer of anal tissue—a very |
| Stage 0 | early cancer |
| Stage I | Cancer beyond the top layer of anal tissue <2 cm |
| Stage II | >2 cm but no spread to nearby organs or lymph nodes |
| Stage III | Lymph node involvement around the rectum or spread to nearby organs |
| Stage IV | Cancer has spread to other parts of the body |

# Anterior resection syndrome

An altered bowel pattern following an anterior resection:
- Frequency.
- Urgency.
- Incontinence of faeces.

Any of these features might be experienced temporarily by many patients who undergo anterior resection. It could be worse for the following patients:
- Those with tumours in the lower third of the rectum.
- Those having additional treatments.
- ♀.

Improvement in reservoir capacity of the rectum seen between 3 and 6 months takes up to 1 year[1] to translate into improved quality of life.

## Nursing considerations

Patients make significant lifestyle modifications to avoid possibility of faecal incontinence. Their bowel habits might constrain physical activity and socializing. Nursing care will include:
- Address issues arising during surgical follow-up.
- Establish the degree of control possible and consider diet, fluids, exercise, and toileting.
- Recognize possible stigma, embarrassment of condition, and requirement for private, accessible, and comfortable toilet arrangements.
- Reassure that function usually improves with time.
- Management of faecal incontinence (📖 pp. 564–6).

---

1 Camilleri-Brennan J and Steele RJC (2001). Prospective analysis of quality of life and survival following mesorectal excision for rectal cancer. *British Journal of Surgery* **88**, 1617–22.

# Rectal prolapse

## Presentation

Protrusion of the rectum beyond the anal verge. Typically, prolapse occurs during straining or defecation and returns to normal position after defecation, but in severe cases may prolapse with minimal effort (e.g. walking) or even permanently, or need manual replacement. Often associated with discomfort, bleeding, copious mucus discharge, faecal incontinence (FI), and/or difficulty in evacuation. Occasionally presents as acute strangulation, which cannot be replaced manually (use ice packs and elevate the foot of the bed).

Some patients seem unaware of prolapse, even if it is major, and only complain of FI.

## Cause

There could be a history of prolonged straining, excessive exercise, or repeated heavy lifting. Or associated with neurological damage, e.g. spinal cord injury. Parity, advancing age, collagen disorders, and obesity could predispose to rectal prolapse.

## Examination

Might not be apparent during examination in the left-lateral position, even with straining. If suspected, allow the patient to strain for 1–2 min in privacy on the toilet and then observe for prolapse from behind. Is prolapse partial or circumferential? Estimate the protrusion beyond the anal verge in centimetres. Anal ultrasound might show thickened internal anal sphincter resulting from repeated trauma.

## Conservative management

Teach the patient to avoid straining, possibly with biofeedback (□ p. 586), and replace manually, as needed. Most complete rectal prolapses will require surgical repair.

## Surgery

Many different procedures/variants are available, in addition to post-operative laxatives. All patients must avoid straining and heavy lifting permanently (consider whether biofeedback is indicated). Surgery might not cure FI and there is a risk of worsened difficulty in evacuation (□ p. 576).

## Abdominal rectopexy

This procedure is used ± resection of the sigmoid colon, often with insertion of mesh or sponge. The main complication is constipation. The procedure can be performed laparoscopically. Erectile dysfunction might occur in ♂. If open surgery is performed, 4–6 weeks recovery is required; recovery is faster if surgery is laproscopic.

## Delormes procedure

A transanal procedure. Redundant mucosa is excised and the rectal wall muscle is plicated. There is ↑ recurrence rate compared with the abdominal procedure, but the hospital stay is shorter and morbidity is ↓.

# Haemorrhoids

## Presentation

Dilated anal cushions, which occur at 3, 7, and 11 o'clock positions in the anal canal, above the dentate line (Fig. 15.6). Haemorrhoids prolapse into anal lumen and might be visible externally. They are not 'varicose veins'. The probable cause is the loss of connective tissue keeping the anal cushions in place. Vessels can become dilated and often bleed with trauma (e.g. defecation), usually with bright red arterial blood. The prevalence is unknown, but the condition is common with the Western diet. It is also associated with pregnancy (impaired venous return and oestrogen levels?), advancing age (but can occur in young adults), and straining (constipation), but not always. There is a possible genetic predisposition. Equally prevalent in ♂ and ♀, but ♂ might be more likely to seek help. It occurs at all adult ages, but is rare in children. Usually classified as degree 1–4, as follows:

• First degree—internal, might prolapse into the lumen, but only seen on proctoscopy. Might look like normal cushions, but bleed.
• Second degree—prolapse out of anus on straining or defecation, return spontaneously or with minimal manual assistance to push back.
• Third degree—prolapse outside anus continuously or often, not just with straining or defecation. Often needs manual replacement and might have associated external skin tags if long-standing.
• Fourth degree—thrombosed or strangulated external haemorrhoids. Venous return impaired; haemorrhoid becomes engorged and gangrenous. May be haemorrhoidal skin tags.

## Symptoms

Depends on the degree of disease to some extent, but even large haemorrhoids could be asymptomatic. Points to consider:

• Bright red (outlet) rectal bleeding—on toilet paper after defecation or dripping into toilet.
• Pruritus.
• Possible soiling of stool or mucus, if external.
• Prolapsing or 'anal fullness' sensation.
• No change in bowel habit, but could have long-standing straining.
• Mild discomfort, rather than pain.
• Stangulated (thrombosed) haemorrhoids—acute severe pain.
• ▶ Not all perianal symptoms are caused by haemorrhoids.
• Use proctoscopy, with straining, to assess the degree of disease.
• ▶ Do not assume all rectal bleeding results from haemorrhoids—bleeding warrants further investigation, regardless of age (📖 p. 512).

## Conservative treatment

Pregnancy-related haemorrhoids usually resolve within a few months of delivery. Local over-the-counter ointments can soothe and contain local anaesthetic, mild astringent, and/or low-dose steroid (avoid prolonged use of steroids). Management depends on the severity of symptoms, as follows:

- First degree—reassure, high-fibre diet, fibre supplements, or stool softeners; adequate hydration; avoid straining by using good defecation habits (📖 p. 579); topical ointments.
- Second degree—as for first degree. If haemorrhoids remain troublesome, use injection sclerotherapy, infrared coagulation, or band ligation.
- Banding (Barron's banding or rubber-band ligation)—this is an outpatient procedure that does not require an anaesthetic. A band is inserted over the base of the haemorrhoid, which cuts off its blood supply. The haemorrhoid shrivels and drops off within 7–10 days. Probably more effective than injection.
- Injection sclerotherapy—5 ml oily phenol injected above the dentate line, which is usually painless. Injection might need to be repeated after a few months. A high-fibre diet might be as effective as sclerotherapy.
- Infrared coagulation—coagulator applied through a proctoscope for a few seconds. Necrosis and fixing of underlying tissue.
- Cryotherapy (freezing)—difficult to control the dose; often a profuse discharge afterwards. The procedure is less commonly used nowadays.
- Anal stretch—seldom used because damage to the internal anal sphincter is now recognized as a common complication.
- Third degree—surgical haemorrhoidectomy and/or skin-tag excision (📖 p. 534).
- Fourth degree—ice packs, GTN, stool softeners, and analgesia. Seldom operated on as an emergency (because of the risk of anal stenosis).

Haemorrhoids can recur, so patients need education about prevention (to avoid constipation).

### Further reading

Buchanan G and Cohen R (2004). Common anorectal conditions. In: Norton C and Chelvanayagam S (eds) *Bowel Continence Nursing*. Beaconsfield Publishers, Beaconsfield.
Hardy A (2005). Piles: separating facts from old wives' tales. *Gastrointestinal Nursing* **3**, 18–24.

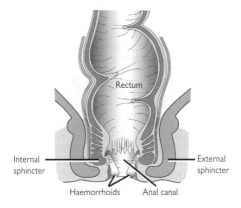

**Fig. 15.6** Haemorrhoids. Reproduced with kind permission © Burdett Institute 2008.

# Haemorrhoidectomy

Often performed on a day-case basis; can be performed under spinal or local anaesthetic.

## Open haemorrhoidectomy

- Circumferential excision—can lead to stenosis.
- Milligan Morgan technique—excise each haemorrhoid individually and remove skin bridges between them. Three separate open wounds. Diathermy can be used.
- Ferguson technique—each of three wounds closed with absorbable sutures (more common in the USA than UK).

## Stapled 'haemorrhoidectomy'

PPH—procedure for prolapse and haemorrhoids. Haemorrhoids are fixed rather than excised. An anal staple gun excises a ring of tissue above the haemorrhoids and leaves a stapled anatamosis. Might be less painful than open surgery, but is not suitable for major external haemorrhoids or skin tags.

## Post-operative care

It is usual not to use pack or wound dressings post-operatively (probably adds to pain). Discomfort can be severe and prolonged (pre-operative counselling is important to adjust the patient's expectations and ↓ anxiety about pain). Use adequate analgesia (avoid opiates because they can cause constipation; NSAIDs are more suitable). Explain that pain is normal, in addition to some bleeding, especially on defecation. Metronidazole might reduce pain (less superficial wound infection). Stool softeners are advised for as long as needed. Defecation might be very painful; again, educate patient that this is normal and strongly advise not to ignore the call to stool, avoiding constipation. Rarely, urinary retention occurs post-operatively (probably owing to pain).

Laser-doppler-guided ligation might become more widely used in future. The procedure can be performed either on a sedated out-patient basis or on a day-case basis under general anaesthetic. Sutures ligate up to six arteries that feed the haemorrhoids; there is no open wound.

There is a small risk of anal stenosis, faecal soiling, or incontinence after all procedures. The internal anal sphincter can be damaged by too deep an excision (causing passive or post-defecation soiling). Avoid haemorrhoidectomy if continence is already compromised or anus is very lax.

## Further reading

Buchanan G and Cohen R (2004). Common anorectal conditions. In: Norton C and Chelvanayagam S (eds) *Bowel Continence Nursing*. Beaconsfield Publishers, Beaconsfield.
Hardy A (2005). Piles: separating facts from old wives' tales. *Gastrointestinal Nursing* **3**, 18–24.

# Anal fissure

## Presentation

A small tear in the mucosa of the anal canal, which most commonly (≥90%) occurs in the posterior anal canal (Fig. 15.7). Can be acutely painful, especially during and after defecation. Often described by patients as 'feels like passing broken glass'. Bright red bleeding after defecation, often noticed on toilet paper. Defecation can re-open a fissure each time. Usually occurs in young adults. Pain can cause muscle spasm, which exacerbates pain and leads to chronic hypoaemia (lack of blood supply), which, in turn, inhibits healing.

A chronic fissure might have a sentinel skin tag at the lower end.

## Causes

- Anal trauma, e.g. constipation, hard stool, non-relaxing anus, or local injuries.
- Diarrhoea.
- More common after childbirth (anterior).
- Often the cause is unclear.
- Multiple fissures—consider Crohn's disease, syphilis, or anal herpes infection.

## Diagnosis

Sometimes visible on external inspection, especially with gentle traction of the anal verge. Digital anal examination might be too painful. Proctoscopy can be used to visualize higher fissures (but might be poorly tolerated). Use lidocaine gel.

## Treatment

Explanation and reassurance. Many patients heal spontaneously (can take several weeks). High-fibre diet, stool softeners, and adequate fluids to keep stool soft and easier to pass without pain. Attempt to relax during defecation (not easy). Mild oral analgesia (avoid constipating analgesics) or local anaesthetic gel. Occasionally, low-dose steroid cream for short-term relief of swelling and irritation.

### Pharmacological therapy

Up to 80% healing—GTN ointment relaxes the anal sphincter muscle spasm and promotes healing. ❶ Headache is a common side effect. Diltiazem (unlicensed use) is a newer alternative, which usually has fewer side effects. Healing takes 6–8 weeks. Botulinum toxin and nifedipine are promising new developments in management.

### Surgery

A chronic troublesome fissure might need surgery. Try pharmacological treatment first. Lateral sphincterotomy cuts the internal anal sphincter, ↓ muscle pressure and spasm, enabling healing. There is a 5–10% risk of flatus or stool incontinence. Midline sphincterotomy and anal stretch are seldom performed because they have a higher risk of incontinence. Rarely, advancement flap surgery is performed.

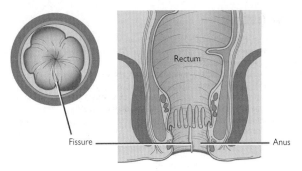

**Fig. 15.7** Anal fissure. Reproduced with kind permission © Burdett Institute 2008.

# Anal fistula

A track from the anorectum, usually with an external opening (Fig. 15.8). The prevalence is 1 in 100 000 individuals in Western Europe: 90% of cases are idiopathic and most occur in middle-aged men. Anal fistula can also be caused by Crohn's disease, previous anal surgery, or tuberculosis.

The cryptoglandular hypothesis suggests that an infected anal gland in the intersphincteric space leads to abscess formation. Glands communicate with the anal canal at the level of the dentate line. Pus tracks occur between or transect sphincters, as follows:
• Simple—one track.
• Complex—many tracks.
• Intersphincteric—between sphincters.
• Transphincteric—crosses sphincter.
• Supralevator—extends above the pelvic floor (levator ani muscles).
• Horseshoe—extends around the anus.

## Symptoms

Often acute perianal abcess—perianal pain, pus discharge, and bleeding. Pain is often relieved when the abscess discharges.

## Diagnosis

• Inspection.
• Digital examination—can feel infected tracks, but might be painful.
• Examination under anaesthetic.
• MRI to define track(s).
• Identify internal and external openings.

If tracks are more extensive it is harder to eradicate sepsis.

## Surgery

Many patients will need surgery to lay open the track, enabling it to heal by secondary intention. A chronic fistula will often need wide surgical lay-open, with curettage of granulation tissue. There is a risk of FI if sphincters are cut.

### Post-operative nursing care

Ensure the wound heals from the base out. Digitally divide any skin bridges and prevent pockets from forming on a daily basis until the wound is healed. Can be painful (use analgesia—either local gel or systemic agent). The patient or relative can be taught the procedure for management in the community. Healing can take weeks, even months.

## Alternatives

• Core out fistulectomy—but this might not clear sepsis and the fistula might recur if the track heals over at the surface.
• Advancement flap—plastic surgery.
• Seton stitch—a loose Seton stitch is semi-permanent. It is inserted to enable drainage without healing of the track. A cutting Seton stitch is gradually tightened to cut through the sphincter, while enabling the track to heal in stages (aims to prevent FI).

## New developments
Fibrin glue and biomaterials are being tried to achieve healing with or without surgery.

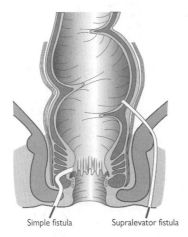

Simple fistula                Supralevator fistula

**Fig. 15.8** Anal fistula. Reproduced with kind permission © Burdett Institute 2008.

# Recto-vaginal fistula

Abnormal track or opening between the rectum and vagina.

## Symptoms
- Faecal or infected vaginal discharge.
- Occasionally passing stool per vagina (PV) spontaneously or when defaecating.
- Flatus passed PV.
- Pain, burning, or itching.
- Odour.
- Possible secondary dysuria and urinary tract infection.

## Diagnosis
- Inspection.
- CT scan.
- EUA.
- Might need to image track—ultrasound or MRI.
- Methylene blue in rectum might leak onto a vaginal tampon if the track is uncertain.

## Causes
- Extended fourth-degree obstetric tear (might have been missed at original obstetric repair or failure to heal).
- Pelvic irradiation.
- Crohn's fistula.
- Malignancy.
- Occasionally idiopathic.
- Perforated diverticular disease.
- Can also be congenital.

## Treatment
- Treat any infection—small opening could close spontaneously (but usually not if Crohn's disease or radiation is the cause).
- Most patients will need surgery.
- Control Crohn's disease optimally and ensure good nutrition for healing.
- Perineal or transabdominal approach—depends on position.
- Tracks might cross anal sphincters—danger of FI if laid open.
- Often poor healing if prior radiotherapy.
- Seton stitch is possible (📖 p. 538).

## Management
Very difficult and distressing for patient. Incontinence pads do little to disguise odour. Irritation might benefit from skin care products or local anaesthetic gel. Live natural yoghurt is reported to be soothing.

# Colovesical fistula

Abnormal track or opening between the colon or rectum and bladder. Often secondary to diverticular disease (50–70% of diverticular fistulae). More common in ♂ and in ♀ after hysterectomy (uterus protects).

## Symptoms

- Air or stool in urine.
- Urinary tract infection.
- Pyelonephritis possible.

## Management

Will usually need surgery to close. Surgery usually one stage with bowel resection and bladder closure. A catheter is required post-operatively to enable bladder to heal.

# Anal stenosis and stricture

No clear distinction between stenosis and stricture.

### Stenosis
Permanent narrowing of a tube or passageway. Can be congenital or acquired. Acquired causes include scarring, growths, radiation, inflammation (e.g. inflammatory bowel disease or tuberculosis), or extra-gut compression.

### Stricture
Acquired by scarring, often post-operatively (e.g. extensive haemorrhoidectomy, fistula surgery, or sphincterotomy).

### Symptoms
- Evacuation difficulty.
- Constipation.
- Incomplete evacuation.
- Thin 'ribbon' or 'pencil' stools.
- Might be pain or bleeding on defecation.

### Diagnosis
- Inspection.
- Digital rectal examination.
- Anoscopy (might need a paediatric proctoscope).
- Examination under anaesthetic.
- Might bleed easily.

### Conservative management
- Patient education and reassurance.
- Soften stool—diet or softening laxatives.
- Evacuation techniques—↓ straining (📖 p. 579).
- Anal dilators—progressively larger sizes are available. Can be used to prevent further stenosis or gradually dilate anus. Use 1–2 lubricated dilators per day and/or before defecation. Briefly insert the dilator into the anal canal; the left-lateral position is probably best, but use sitting on the toilet can also be helpful.

### Surgery
- Superficial—might just incise.
- Deeper—risk of FI if sphincter is divided. Might need rotation flap repair or extensive reconstruction.

# Pilonidal sinus

Pilonidal sinus ('nest of hairs') is also known as sacral fistula, hair cyst, sacral dermoid, and jeep driver's disease (it is common in the armed forces) (Fig. 15.9).

Infection of a hair follicle in the natal cleft between the buttocks. It has a cystic structure and is often several centimetres in diameter. Leads to abscess formation and extends to subcutaneous fat. Other hairs become incorporated and promote a foreign-body reaction. Not all sinuses contain hairs. Subcutaneous sinuses are lined with granulation tissue and filled with debris (e.g. skin, scales, hair, and keratinocytes). The sinus usually discharges in the midline, often at the top end of the natal cleft. Occasionally there can be multiple fistulae, with many openings.

## Cause

Unknown. Most commonly occurs in hirsute men <40 years (?because they are hairier). There might be a congenital predisposition (a family history is common). Obesity, inactivity, and local irritation/friction can predispose to the condition. Often there is a history of local micro-pressure or prolonged sitting. It is rare in children and in adults >40 years.

## Presentation

If not infected, might be an asymptomatic lump or a soft lump with fistula tract; hairs might protrude. If infected, it is a red, swollen, and acutely painful abscess, discharging pus (possibly blood-stained). Many fistulae become chronic. After many years, squamous cell carcinoma might develop.

## Treatment

• Asymptomatic/mild symptoms—shaving and good hygiene.
• Acute symptoms—painkillers and surgical drainage, often under local anaesthetic. Post-operative shaving and hygiene needed to promote healing.
• Can be excised and sutured, but could recur if infection and granulation tissue is not excised adequately.
• Tendency to recur, especially if the tract is not drained adequately.
• Might need wide surgical excision and healing by secondary intention if it becomes chronic.
• Occasional need for plastic surgery.
• Antibiotics usually unhelpful.

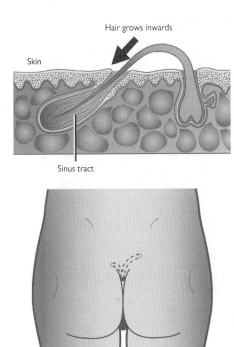

**Fig. 15.9** Pilonidal sinus. Reproduced with kind permission © Burdett Institute 2008.

# Perianal skin care

See also pruritus ani (🕮 p. 550). Three factors enable the skin to protect the body: integrity, lipid content (barrier to fluid absorption or loss), and pH (slightly acidic, pH 5.5; 'acid mantle'). Risk factors for perianal skin problems are shown in Table 15.1.

Soreness often results from a complex interaction of several factors. Perianal dermatitis is inflammation of the perianal skin, which often results from an excess of moisture (incontinence or sweating), mechanical irritation (e.g. friction), chemical (e.g. alkaline pH, enzymes contained in stool, and activity of bacteria) irritation, or a combination of factors. Untreated, the skin can become ulcerated and prone to secondary infection. Frail older people, immobile people, the immunocompromised, and those with urinary and faecal incontinence are at ↑ risk.

The most common cause of anal soreness is FI. Stools are more likely to contain traces of digestive enzymes if diarrhoea occurs or the colon has been removed and stools contain the small bowel contents, e.g. ileo-anal pouch or ileo-anal anastomosis.

## Assessment

Find the cause using the following.
- Detailed history.
- Symptoms—soreness, pain, burning, stabbing, 'passing glass' (e.g. anal fissure), itching, pruritus (e.g. pain, burning, and itching), discomfort, bulging/dragging (e.g. prolapse).
- When—all the time, or during or after defecation?
- Where—perianal (outside), proctalgia (inside), or pelvic pain?
- Associated events—related to activity or diet?
- Observation of the perianal area for conditions listed in Table 15.1.
- Proctoscopy might be indicated.
- Swabs can be taken if infection is suspected.

## Treatment of soreness

Treat the underlying cause if possible, especially FI (🕮 p. 558). Treatment can be prolonged and frustrating. Detailed advice on hygiene and skin care should be given. Products: there is little research on effectiveness. Advise the patient to use a good pad for urinary incontinence. Use a faecal collecter for severe diarrhoea in bedbound patients. Soap and water has been superseded by a combined cleaner and moisturizer, with pH balance. Barrier cream or film might protect.

Refer patients with persistent non-healing dermatitis to a dermatologist.

## Further reading

Norton C (2006). Perianal skin care. *Gastrointestinal Nursing* **4**, 18–25.

**Table 15.1** Causes of and risk factors for perianal soreness

| Problem | Examples |
| --- | --- |
| Alkalinity | Stool (FI/soiling) |
| | Urinary incontinence |
| | Sweat |
| | Skin products (cleaners or moisturizers) |
| Anorectal conditions | Pruritus ani |
| | Haemorrhoids |
| | Anal fissure |
| | Anal fistula |
| | Rectal prolapse |
| | Proctitis |
| | Neoplasia: |
| |   Anal cancer |
| |   Bowen's disease |
| |   Rectal cancer (especially villous adenoma with copious mucus production) |
| Friction | Diarrhoea (frequency of defecation/wiping) |
| | Mucus leakage |
| | Pads/underwear |
| | Pressure sores |
| | Abrasions from digitation or sexual activity |
| Dermatological conditions | Psoriasis |
| | Contact dermatitis/allergy |
| | Eczema |
| | Lichen sclerosus |
| | Oestrogen deficiency (atrophic changes) |
| Infection | Condylomata acuminate (anal warts) |
| | Bacterial infection |
| | *Candida albicans* |
| | Herpes simplex |
| | Shingles (zosteriform herpes) |
| | Infestation |
| Advanced age or compromised health | Malnutrition |
| | Ageing skin |
| | Immobility |

# Anal warts (condylomata acuminata)

Perianal manifestation of genital warts ('venereal' warts). They are caused by a virus, the human papilloma virus (HPV), of which over 90 types have been identified, many sexually transmitted. HPV types 6 and 11 are the commonest. Warts can be found on or around the penis, anus, or vagina, and are the most common viral sexually transmitted infection (STI) in the UK. The highest rate of new cases is in 20–24-year-old ♂ and 16–19-year-old ♀. Warts are usually benign; very rarely, oncogenic viruses infect, with malignant potential. In 1999, 72 000 new cases were reported in the UK.[1] Up to 1 in 100 sexually active people have warts.

## Risk factors

Transmitted by skin-to-skin contact. The main risk is unprotected sex with an infected partner. Anal sex can predispose to anal, rather than genital, warts. Immunocompromised patients are at risk. Warts can be associated with HIV infection. Condoms do not offer full protection if the infected area is not covered.

## Appearance

Skin-coloured/whitish soft lumps on warm or moist hairless skin; harder lumps on dry hairy skin. Single or multiple warts are common, and they can occur in various sizes. In severe cases, warts can form a perianal 'carpet'. They can take weeks or months to appear after infection.

## Symptoms

Patients could be asymptomatic carriers (common—no visible warts but can still infect other people). Warts might not cause any problems or they could be sore and itchy.

## Investigations

None needed (but test for other STIs).

## Treatment

Usually takes place at genitourinary medicine clinics. Warts can take several months of repeated treatments to clear. One option is to leave warts untreated, but they often take months to clear spontaneously (and are infectious until cleared). Warts can spontaneously recur without reinfection. Treatments include:

- Chemical/topical—podophyllin, trichloroacetic acid, and podophyllotoxin. ❶ Avoid in pregnancy.
- Laser or electrocautery—to 'burn' the warts.
- Cryotherapy (freezing) with liquid nitrogen (spray or application)—might need several treatments.
- Surgery—small warts can be removed by local scissor excision under local anaesthetic. Extensive warts might need formal surgical excision. Often done piecemeal to avoid extensive scarring.

## Prevention

Avoid unprotected sex and sex with multiple partners.

1 Gilson R and Mindel A (2001). Recent advances: sexually transmitted infections. *British Medical Journal* **322**, 1160–4.

# Other perianal conditions

## Hidradenitis suppurativa

Occulsion of appocrine glands, which become infected. Occurs perianally, mostly in young adult ♂ (but can also occur in the axilla, groin, and perineum, more commonly in ♀). Associated with obesity, sweating, poor hygiene, and endocrine disorders. Bacterial proliferation causes spread to adjacent glands and secondary infection. Rupture of glands causes scarring and fibrosis.

### Presentation

Multiple tender red lumps. In chronic disease, there can be multiple interconnecting sinuses and scarring.

### Treatment

- Antibiotics—if mild.
- Drain acute abscesses.
- Chronic severe disease—might need to be widely laid open. Skin grafts or a temporary stoma might also be required.
- Meticulous wound care post-operatively.
- Patient instruction on hygiene to avoid recurrence.

## Perianal haematoma

Presents as a tender 2–4 cm olive-shaped lump at the anal verge. It is bluish in appearance, with a clotted venous saccule. The cause is unknown.

### Diagnosis

Distinguish from external haemorrhoids. Haematoma does not prolapse from higher in the anal canal; it only occurs on the skin surface. Diagnose by inspection, digital examination, or proctoscopy if in doubt.

### Conservative management

- Ice packs and analgesia.
- Reassurance.
- Many cases subside spontaneously.

### Surgical management

If very troublesome, the haematoma can be incised under local anaesthetic: blood is released and the pain relieved. This is more difficult if the haematoma has been present for >24 h because a thrombus will have formed. Conservative management is usual. A residual skin tag might remain once the haematoma is resolved.

# Pruritus ani

## Symptoms
Perianal itching, burning, irritation, and pain.

## Causes
The most common cause is ineffective anal cleaning after defecation, FI, or minor faecal soiling. Faecal residue on the skin sets up a chemical reaction. Other causes are listed in Table 15.2. Once established, a vicious circle of irritation, scratching, and further skin damage results.

Dry anal wiping with paper does not always completely remove faecal residue from the perianal area. Small amounts of stool can also inadvertently be passed with flatus and any stool remaining can very soon make the skin sore. Patients who are not aware of soiling are very offended by the suggestion that they might need to improve their perianal hygiene. When examining the patient, soiling might be evident. Wiping the anus with wet cotton wool and demonstrating the soiling to the patient can help to confirm the situation.

## Treatment
Treat FI (📖 pp. 564–6). Detailed advice on post-defecation cleaning (e.g. wet wiping/washing). Barrier cream or film can help, but can exacerbate the problem. Avoid soaps, bubble baths, and strong chemicals for washing and laundry. Allow air to the area. Desist from scratching (gloves should be used at night in extreme cases). Avoiding some foods might help (e.g. citrus, caffeine, alcohol, and chocolate).

**Table 15.2** Causes of pruritus ani

| Anorectal conditions | Haemorrhoids |
| --- | --- |
| | Fissure |
| | Fistula |
| | Prolapse |
| | Proctitis |
| Dermatological | Psoriasis |
| | Eczema |
| | Contact dermatitis (e.g. faeces) |
| Infection | Anal warts |
| | *Candida albicans* |
| Malignant | Rectal cancer |
| | Villous adenoma |
| | Bowen's disease (perianal carcinoma *in situ*) |

# Diarrhoea

## Definition

There is no consensus on a definition. Patients could report ↑ frequency of normal stool or faecal incontinence as 'diarrhoea'. Types of diarrhoea:

- Acute—sudden onset, often food-related infective gastroenteritis (e.g. *Escherichia coli*, *Shigella* spp, or *Salmonella* spp), and usually self-limiting. Might be related to exotic travel (some evidence for prophylactic probiotics taken before and during travel); observe sensible precautions in at-risk zones.
- Chronic—>4 weeks of defecation >3 times/day. Loose stools, 200 g of stool weight per 24 h, and usually non-infective.
- Stool water content ≥70–90%.
- Frail older people or patients with neurological disease—might present with 'spurious diarrhoea', which is thick offensive brown liquid overflow from rectal impaction that usually leaks passively.

## Pathophysiology

- Common— gastroenteritis; irritable bowel syndrome (IBS) (might alternate with constipation), in younger patients, pain and bloating, or could coexist with psychological disturbance; diet (Table 15.3), e.g. alcohol, caffeine, or artificial sweeteners such as sorbitol; lactose-intolerance (especially in non-Caucasians); medication (e.g. antibiotics, antacids, or laxative abuse).
- Less common—IBD, colorectal cancer, coeliac disease, microscopic colitis, bacterial overgrowth, radiotherapy, chronic pancreatitis, or after gut surgery (e.g. gastrectomy, resection of terminal ileum and ileocaecal valve, or colectomy).
- Rare—villous gut tumour (secreting), tumour that stimulates gut secretion (e.g. VIPoma, gastrinoma, or carcinoid), infection (e.g. HIV patients), or thyrotoxicosis.

Large volume of watery stools if the cause is in the small bowel, frequent small volumes in the large bowel, or pancreatic/biliary pale bulky oily stools that are difficult to flush (steatorrhoea). Pain after eating with nausea/vomiting indicates possible obstruction. There are four main types of diarrhoea:

- ↓ absorption—maldigestion (enzyme deficiency) or malabsorption (inflammation or infection).
- Osmotic diarrhoea—large amounts of osmotic material in gut lumen (drugs, lactase deficient, or enteral feeds), which stops on fasting.
- Secretory diarrhoea—even on fasting. Excess GI secretion versus reabsorption.
- Abnormal motility—rapid transit or motility disorders (e.g. IBS).

Nocturnal diarrhoea is usually organic (not IBS).

See Table 15.4 for differential diagnosis.

**Table 15.3** Dietary causes of diarrhoea

| Condition | Food |
|---|---|
| Excess ingestion of non-absorbable/ poorly absorbable carbohydrate | Sorbitol in elixirs, sugar-free foods and gum, and mints; pears, prunes, peaches, and orange juice |
| | Fructose from soft drinks, apples, honey, pears, cherries, dried dates, dried figs, grapes, pears, and prunes |
| | Mannitol in sugar-free products and mints |
| | Bran and other fibre supplements |
| Magnesium-induced diarrhoea | Antacids |
| | Laxatives |
| | Food supplements |
| Stimulation of GI motility | Caffeine—coffee, tea, and cola |
| Lactose intolerance | Milk |

**Table 15.4** Differential diagnosis of chronic diarrhoea by probable site of disease

| Site | Relatively common | Uncommon |
|---|---|---|
| Large bowel | IBS | Microscopic colitis |
| | IBD | |
| | Colon cancer | |
| | Villous adenoma | |
| Small bowel | Coeliac disease | AIDS |
| | Bacterial overgrowth | Whipple's disease |
| | Crohn's disease | Tropical sprue |
| | Lactase deficiency | Lymphoma |
| | Parasitic infection | Small bowel ischaemia |
| | Terminal ileal resection | Amyloidosis |
| | | Ulcerative jejunitis |
| | | Radiation enteritis |
| | | Zollinger–Ellison syndrome |
| Hepatobiliary/ pancreatic | Chronic pancreatitis | Pancreatic cancer |
| | Post cholecystectomy | Cystic fibrosis |
| | | Extrahepatic biliary obstruction |
| | | Chronic cholestatic liver disease |

### History and investigation

Assess history (e.g. onset, recent travel, symptoms, pain, and bleeding), comorbidities, medical history and medications, family history, psychological factors, and diet. Examination for:
- Weight loss.
- Skin (dehydration).
- Abdominal mass.
- PR examination (e.g. impaction or fistula).
- Rash (e.g. coeliac disease or IBD).
- Fever (e.g. IBD or HIV).
- Anaemia (e.g. IBD, coeliac disease, or cancer).
- Neuropathy (e.g. vitamin $B_{12}$ deficiency or diabetes).
- Enlarged liver (secondary tumour?).
- Abdominal mass (e.g. IBD or cancer).

If indicated by the history and examination, perform the following investigations:
- FBC.
- Biochemistry.
- Stool sample.
- Sigmoidoscopy.
- Biopsy.

Consider colonoscopy, gastroscopy, and small bowel biopsy, a small bowel follow-through study, and pancreatic function tests. A hydrogen breath test (for bacterial overgrowth) might also be helpful. Collect stools over a period of 3 days, perform a laxative screen, check faecal fat levels, and measure fasting stool volumes.

### Management

- Address dehydration, electrolyte balance, and malnutrition, if necessary.
- Treat the underlying cause.
- Trial of antibiotics for bacterial overgrowth.
- Anti-diarrhoeal medication—loperamide, 2–16 mg/24 h (avoid in acute infective and fulminant ulcerative colitis), codeine phosphate (more side effects and can be habit-forming), or co-phenotrope.
- Severe—octreotide (subcutaneous).
- Colestyramine for bile salt malabsorption.
- Diet—exclude alcohol, sorbitol, caffeine, and foods with known sensitivities (e.g. milk). There is some evidence of a benefit from using a BRATT diet in cancer patients (i.e. bananas, rice, cooked apples, white toast, and decaffeinated tea). Pectin can bind stools. Fibre can help (e.g. adds bulk and binds stools) or worsen symptoms (i.e. ↑ peristalsis; avoid large volumes of cereal fibre because it can cause an obstruction). Avoid spices. Use a lower-osmolality tube feed or add a bulking agent for tube-fed patients.
- Chronic diarrhoea can be exhausting and demoralizing. Patients need emotional support and practical advice on skin care (📖 p. 546).

# Cancer-related diarrhoea

More common presenting symptom of colorectal cancer than constipation. Less common than constipation in advanced cancer, but can be severe. Occurs in 10% of patients with advanced cancer. There is a threat of dehydration, malnutrition, weight loss, and exhaustion, and an impact on social function and sense of control. Patients might be reluctant to complain or fear withdrawal of treatment, and so might tolerate even severe symptoms.

Symptoms can include frequency, urgency, incontinence, blood in stools, abdominal pain, and perianal soreness. Often associated with vomiting, which carries a risk of acute dehydration and electrolyte imbalance.

❶ Distinguish from impaction and associated overflow 'spurious diarrhoea'.

## Risk factors

↑ risk if chemotherapy and radiotherapy are combined.

### Radiotherapy

Although 5–15% of cases are immediate, the condition can persist. Characterized by mucosal damage (especially in the small bowel because of a rapid turnover of epithelial cells), inflammation, atrophy, and malabsorption of bile salts. Aim to ↓ radiation enteritis by focusing radiation as much as feasible. Avoid irradiating the small bowel, if possible.

### Chemotherapy

Occurs in 50–80% of cases during therapy. Many drugs cause diarrhoea as a side effect (e.g. 5FU, methotrexate, and irinotecan). If associated with vomiting, it can limit the tolerance to chemotherapy.

### Surgery

Gut resection (e.g. colectomy, gastrectomy with dumping syndrome, ileo-caecal valve resection, low anterior rectal resection, or short bowel syndrome, if the small bowel is resected).

### Secretory tumours

- Pancreatic, VIPoma, or endocrine tumours (can be ≥3 L in 24 h). Villous adenoma is associated with copious mucus secretion.
- Secondary gut infection in immunosuppressed patients (gastroenteritis, C. difficile—possible pseudomembranous colitis—or Candida spp).
- Tube feeding (bulking additives can help).
- Bile salt malabsorption (terminal ileum resected, radiotherapy).

## Management

- Assessment of cause(s).
- Constipating agents (e.g. loperamide, codeine phosphate, or octreotide).
- Bulking agents can absorb some fluid (but can worsen symptoms).
- Colestyramine for bile salt malabsorption.
- Pancreatic enzymes for pancreatic insufficiency.
- Steroid retention enema for proctitis.
- Adjust diet (📖 p. 554).
- Support and reassurance.

## Further reading

Andrewes TY and Norton C (2006). Constipation and diarrhoea In: Kearney N and Richardson A (eds) *Nursing Patients with Cancer*. Churchill Livingstone, Edinburgh.

# Faecal incontinence

FI can be defined as involuntary loss of stool, which is a social or hygienic problem. 'Anal incontinence' denotes involuntary loss of stool or flatus.

The prevalence of FI is ~5% in community-dwelling adults, with 1% of the population having a regular and life-limiting problem. In community surveys, the prevalence is equal in ♂ and ♀. Prevalence rises to >25% of people in nursing home care. FI is a very embarrassing condition and many people are reluctant to report symptoms, making active case-finding in patients with GI disorders very important.

## Pathophysiology

FI is a symptom not a diagnosis. It can result from any combination of the following mechanisms.

- Anal sphincter disruption or weakness, e.g. as a result of obstetric trauma, iatrogenic injury during anal surgery, impalement injuries, or idiopathic anal sphincter degeneration. Typical symptoms are as follows:
  - Urgency and urge faecal incontinence (usually external sphincter disruption).
  - Passive faecal soiling (usually internal sphincter disruption).
- Diarrhoea, loose stools, or intestinal hurry for any reason (e.g. inflammation, diet, anxiety, or IBS).
- Local anal pathology (e.g. haemorrhoids, rectal prolapse, or skin tags).
- Neurological disorders affecting sensory or motor function (e.g. spinal cord injury, multiple sclerosis, spina bifida, or any neuropathy).
- Severe constipation with faecal impaction and 'overflow spurious diarrhoea' (e.g. in frail and dependent people).
- Difficulty with toilet access or drug side effects.

## Assessment

Nursing assessment takes time and needs adequate privacy for the patient to relax and tell their story. A bowel diary and symptom questionnaire might give added information. Assessment will include the following.

- History of the problem and former bowel habit.
- Current symptoms—severity and frequency (Box 15.2).
- Diet (especially fibre) and fluid (especially caffeine) intake.
- Medication and other medical conditions.
- Effects of symptoms and limitations on lifestyle.
- Coexistence of urinary incontinence (~50%).
- Ability to use the toilet independently.
- Availability and involvement of carers.
- Multiple causes often coexist.

▶ Consider the possibility of serious bowel pathology (e.g. rectal bleeding, unexplained change in bowel habit, anaemia, or weight loss) and whether further investigations are indicated.

**Examination**
- General observation will give an idea of the patient's mobility and ability to self-toilet.
- Perianal inspection for anal conditions (📖 p. 547), scars, and skin excoriation.
- Digital rectal examination for anal resting and squeeze tone, and the presence and consistency of stools.
- Abdominal examination for masses, distension, or scars.
- Neurological examination if neuropathy is suspected.

The condition of many patients can be improved by conservative measures (📖 pp. 564–6) without recourse to further investigations.

Those who do not respond to conservative measures, or if surgery is contemplated, should have anorectal physiology studies (📖 p. 562) and anal ultrasound.

**Further reading**

National Institute for Clinical Excellence (2007). *Faecal Incontinence: The Management of Faecal Incontinence in Adults: Guideline CG 49*. NICE, London.

Norton C and Chelvanayagam S (2004). *Bowel Continence Nursing*. Beaconsfield Publishers, Beaconsfield.

Patient Information. http://www.bowelcontrol.org.uk (accessed 14.05.07).

---

**Box 15.2 Checklist for FI symptom assessment**

- Onset of symptoms.
- Usual bowel habit.
- Changes in bowel habit.
- Stool consistency (Bristol stool form scale 📖 p. 509).
- Amount and frequency of FI.
- Urgency or urge FI.
- Passive soiling.
- Difficulty wiping clean after toilet.
- Nocturnal bowel symptoms.
- Abdominal pain and bloating.
- Evacuation difficulty:
  - Straining.
  - Incomplete evacuation.
  - Pain.
  - Digitation.
- Control of flatus.
- Rectal bleeding or mucus.
- Products used to manage FI.

# Obstetric trauma and faecal incontinence

Up to 30% of women have some anal sphincter damage during a vaginal delivery. There might also be damage to the pudendal nerve. These conditions are not always symptomatic.

## Classification of obstetric tears
- First degree—superficial vaginal mucosa or perineal skin laceration.
- Second degree—extending into the perineum and vaginal submucosa.
- Third degree:
  - 3a—partial disruption of external anal sphincter (<50%).
  - 3b—complete disruption of external anal sphincter (>50%).
  - 3c—disruption extending into internal anal sphincter.
- Fourth degree—extending to anal or rectal mucosa (might extend along posterior vaginal wall into the rectum (cloacal deformity, rectum opening into vagina).
- Rectovaginal fistula—abnormal opening between rectum and vagina (rare without fourth-degree tear, but can persist after repair of fourth-degree tear).

## Risk factors
- First baby.
- Forceps delivery (greater risk than with ventouse delivery).
- Large baby (>4 kg).
- Abnormal presentation.
- Prolonged (or very precipitant) second stage of labour.
- Midline episiotomy.
- Mediolateral episiotomy if used too liberally.
- ↑ maternal age.
- Caesarean section (CS) is protective, but not completely.
- FI is more likely to develop if the patient already has altered continence (e.g. urgency, IBS, or flatus incontinence).

## Management
Careful inspection is used to detect trauma, which should be repaired by a trained surgeon who has experience in repair; surgery should be performed in an operating theatre, usually under epidural anaesthetic. Overlap repair can give better results than end-to-end repair. Surgery involves careful closure of tear in layers. Post-operatively use antibiotics and stool softeners; pelvic muscle exercises might also help. Check for symptoms at the post-natal check. It is not known if these women are more likely to develop faecal incontinence in later life. Discuss future deliveries (elective CS versus careful trial of vaginal birth—no evidence which is better). If the patient is symptomatic, she might opt for CS.

## Further reading
Norton C (2002). Faecal incontinence following pregnancy. In: Maclean AB and Cardozo L (eds) *Incontinence in Women*. RCOG Press, London.

# Anorectal testing

Anorectal testing comprises a series of tests of anorectal muscle and nerve function. They are usually performed in combination, depending on symptoms.

## Indications

Testing is indicated if the cause of FI is in doubt, conservative measures have failed to restore continence, or surgery is contemplated. Testing is also useful in neurological bowel management and suspected Hirschsprung's disease.

## Patient preparation

No bowel preparation is usually given, although tests might be difficult to perform or interpret if the rectum is loaded (consider use of suppositories or an enema if this is found). ▶ Many patients will find these tests very embarrassing and every effort should be made to explain the procedures, maintain dignity, and gain fully informed consent. Testing is contraindicated after very recent anorectal surgery and might be traumatic for patients with a history of anal abuse.

## Sphincter function

This is most usually assessed using pressure (i.e. manometry using air-filled, water-perfused, or solid-state anal catheters; (Fig. 15.10)). Electromyography (EMG) activity of the sphincters can also be measured. This test should not be performed within 20–30 min of anal examination because this will affect the results obtained. The following parameters are recorded.

- Functional anal canal length—distance from the rectal verge to the anal verge.
- Resting anal pressure—a marker for function of the internal anal sphincter.
- Squeeze increment over resting pressure—an indication of external anal sphincter function.
- Squeeze endurance or fatigue rate—external sphincter function.
- Cough reflex.
- Some equipment is computerized and multi-channel recordings can enable sophisticated three-dimensional mapping of the sphincter—vector manometry.

## Sensation

A balloon is slowly distended into the rectum to assess the sensation of rectal filling. The patient reports the first sensation, an urge to defecate, and maximum tolerated volume. Some equipment will measure rectal compliance and pressure (e.g. Barostat).

Anal and rectal sensation can also be measured using a low-amplitude electrical current. A catheter with an electrode is introduced into the anus and the current is slowly ↑ until the patient can feel it. Recordings continue until a consistent threshold is established. This is then repeated in the rectum. Impaired sensation might indicate neuropathy. Hypersensitivity might indicate inflammation or IBS.

## Recto-anal inhibitory reflex (RAIR)

A balloon is rapidly inflated in the rectum and the anal pressure is observed for the expected temporary fall in resting pressure and its gradual recovery to baseline. Absence of RAIR might indicate Hirschsprung's disease.

## Pudendal terminal motor latency (PTML)

This test is of doubtful reliability and limited clinical relevance. A special finger-mounted electrode is used to stimulate the pudendal nerve during rectal examination and record the time taken for anal contraction in response.

## Further reading

National Institute for Clinical Excellence (2007). *Faecal Incontinence: The Management of Faecal Incontinence in Adults: Guideline CG 49.* NICE, London.

Nicholls T (2004). Anorectal testing. In: Norton C and Chelvanayagam S (eds) *Bowel Continence Nursing.* Beaconsfield Publishers, Beaconsfield.

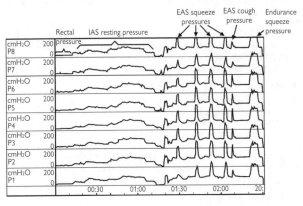

**Fig. 15.10** Manometry trace produced using a station pull-through technique (MMS software). Reproduced with kind permission © Burdett Institute 2008.

# Faecal incontinence: conservative measures

The choice of options will depend on the patient's symptoms and wishes. The following interventions are often used in combination.

### Patient education

Enables the patient to understand their normal bowel function and likely causes of current symptoms; empowers self-management. Simple diagrams help.

### Diet and fluid modification

Hard stool benefits from ↑ fibre intake. Loose/soft stool might benefit from ↓ fibre intake or soluble fibre to bind stools. Lactose intolerance is ↑ common. ↓ caffeine and sorbitol intake might help loose stools.

### Toilet habit

Aim for a predictable stable bowel habit with formed stools. Patient teaching can assist.

### Toilet access

People with physical disabilities might access the toilet more quickly/easily if adaptations are made to the toilet or their clothing. Mobility or transfer aids might be indicated.

### Medication

- Hard stool—stool softeners or bulking agents.
- Loose/soft stool with frequency—anti-diarrhoeal medication, e.g. loperamide 2–16 mg/day. Take medication 30 min before eating to dampen the gastrocolic response. Loperamide syrup can be taken if capsules constipate too much. Codeine phosphate or co-phenotrope can be taken if loperamide is not tolerated/fully effective.
- If FI seems to be worsened because of side effects of other medication (e.g. loose stools), consider whether alternatives are possible.

### Bowel retraining

Patients with urgency can build up confidence again by behavioural retraining. When the urge is felt, hold on for as long as possible. Gradually ↑ time deferment is possible and ↓ anxiety.

### Effective rectal emptying

Patients with FI associated with incomplete rectal evacuation might benefit from constipation measures (including suppositories, enemas, and evacuation techniques; 📖 p. 579).

### Rectal irrigation

📖 p. 584.

## Other measures

Nicotine is a colonic stimulant, so smoking cessation might help. FI is associated with obesity, so weight ↓ and general fitness measures might be helpful. Counselling or psychotherapy might be beneficial if FI is associated with excessive anxiety or depression.

## Products for FI

An anal plug is a foam plug that actually sits at the rectal outlet, not in the anus. It is designed to prevent FI. Many patients find it too uncomfortable to tolerate, but this is unpredictable so it is worth a try. An anal plug is best tolerated by patients with impaired rectal sensation (e.g. spina bifida).

A faecal collection bag is a modified ileoestomy bag. It is only suitable for completely immobile patients, usually with profuse diarrhoea (e.g. intensive care units). Great care is needed to apply the bag correctly. More recently, intra-rectal tubes with collection bags have become available for use in intensive care settings.

Pads do little to absorb faeces, protect skin, or disguise odour.

See also skin care (📖 p. 546).

## Further reading

National Institute for Clinical Excellence (2007). *Faecal Incontinence: The Management of Faecal Incontinence in Adults: Guideline CG 49*. NICE, London.

Norton C and Chelvanayagam S (2004). *Bowel Continence Nursing*. Beaconsfield Publishers, Beaconsfield.

Patient Information. http://www.bowelcontrol.org.uk (accessed 14.05.07).

# Faecal incontinence: exercises and biofeedback

Anal sphincter exercises teach the patient to strengthen the striated (voluntary) EAS through an intensive exercise programme (similar to pelvic floor exercises for urinary incontinence). Can also speed reaction and improve coordination of the EAS. Assessment will determine current strength of voluntary squeeze, how long this can be held for, and how many repetitions the patient can do before fatigue. A challenging target should be set to improve function: maximal squeeze, gentler submaximal squeeze to build endurance, and fast-twitch contractions to speed reaction time. A typical patient might start with 50 repetitions of each exercise per day. It takes 4–6 weeks to see any benefit and up to 6 months for maximal benefit. The patient must be motivated.

▶ Check the patient is performing the correct action (not abdominal or buttock squeezes).

## Biofeedback

Use of manometry or EMG to show the patient whether exercises are being performed correctly and monitor progress. The measurement device is often connected to a computer in the clinic, but small hand-held units are also available (for possible home use).

Feedback techniques can also be used with a rectal balloon to teach the patient to feel rectal contents sooner (for an insensitive rectum) or to tolerate larger volumes in the rectum (for an oversensitive rectum). The patient can learn to coordinate rectal distension with anal contraction.

## Electrical stimulation

Skin surface or anal probe electrodes are used to assist with exercises if the patient has limited function or sensation. Stimulation of striated muscle at 35–50 Hz produces an involuntary contraction which should, with repetition, eventually strengthen the muscle. It might also sensitize the area and enable the patient to locate the correct muscle for exercises.

## Further reading

National Institute for Clinical Excellence (2007). *Faecal Incontinence: The Management of Faecal Incontinence in Adults: Guideline CG 49*. NICE, London.
Norton C and Chelvanayagam S (2004). *Bowel Continence Nursing*. Beaconsfield Publishers, Beaconsfield.
Patient Information. http://www.bowelcontrol.org.uk (accessed 14.05.07).

# Anal sphincter repair (overlapping sphincteroplasty)

### Indications

- Persisting anal sphincter defect after obstetric trauma.
- Acute anal sphincter trauma (e.g. impalement injury).
- Post-fistula repair (beware further sepsis).

Only usually considered for major symptoms of FI that are unresponsive to conservative management.

### Investigations

- Anal ultrasound or MRI to confirm sphincter defect.
- Usually manometry to confirm impaired sphincter function.

### External anal sphincter repair

The transperineal approach involves upward dissection to identify the two ends (Fig 15.11). Overlap repair is more usual than end-to-end repair. Fibrous/scar tissue can help the security of the suture line. Covering colostomy has no benefit. The wound can be left open to heal by secondary intention if closing the wound would produce tension on sutures. Combination with plication of puborectalis lengthens the anal canal and/or reconstruction of the perineal body (which has cosmetic and hygiene functions, but has an unproven benefit for continence).

### Internal anal sphincter repair

Very difficult to identify and repair (1–2 mm). Repair is usually unsuccessful and seldom attempted in isolation.

### Pre-operative management

Not usual to prepare bowel.

### Post-operative management

- Early eating and drinking.
- Analgesia and mobilization.
- Meticulous wound care—secondary infection can lead to wound breakdown and operative failure.
- Avoid constipation—stool softeners to take home for 1–2 weeks.
- No proven benefit of anal sphincter exercises or biofeedback, although biofeedback might help if symptoms remain.
- Repeat repair is possible if the first repair is inadequate (equally good results). Re-operation often has reasonable short-term results.

### Long-term prognosis (5 years)

Few patients have perfect continence: flatus incontinence, urgency, and some soiling is common. Up to one-third of patients report a new evacuation difficulty. No evidence on >10 years results . The likely success rate is difficult to predict for an individual patient, but realistic expectations are important for the patient.

## Further reading

Madoff RD, Pemberton JH, Mimura T, *et al.* (2005). Surgery for fecal incontinence. In: Abrams P, Cardozo L, Khoury S, and Wein A (eds) *Incontinence*. Health Publications, Plymouth.

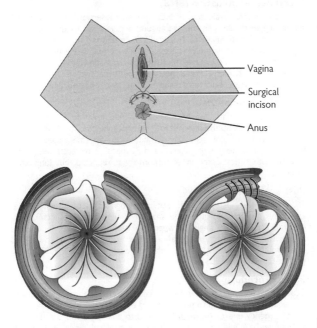

Vagina

Surgical incison

Anus

**Fig. 15.11** Anal sphincter repair. Reproduced with kind permission © Burdett Institute 2008.

# Other surgical procedures for faecal incontinence

## Sacral nerve simulation (SNS)

Peripheral nerve evaluation (PNE) involves insertion of temporary stimulating leads through the sacral foramen, with an external battery box (Fig. 15.12). Stimulate for 2–3 weeks and monitor symptoms.

If temporary stimulation is successful, a neuromodulating electrode is implanted in a sacral spinal nerve (usually S3) and a stimulator is implanted in one of the buttocks. This is a specialized and expensive new procedure, but it has promising short-term results; its long-term effects are unknown.

## Injectable biomaterials

A variety of materials have been tried experimentally on a small scale. The aim is to bulk up the deficient internal anal sphincter and ↑ anal pressure. Bioplastique® collagen, Teflon®, autologous fat (the patient's own body fat transplanted), Durasphere®, and Permacol® have each been tried in very small series. Some initial response was reported, but long-term results are unknown.

## Post-anal repair

Plication of the posterior puborectalis through an incision behind the anus. The aim is to lengthen the anal canal, tighten the sphincter, and obtain a more acute angle between the rectum and anus (anorectal angle). This was a common operation before anal ultrasound. Nowadays, direct sphincter repair is used for sphincter disruption (📖 p. 568). Long-term results are generally poor.

## Secca procedure

Radiofrequency ablation. Few data on safety or effectiveness. The original technique was developed to prevent gastro-oesophageal reflux. High-energy radiofrequency energy (heating) is applied to anal canal mucosa through needles and an endoscope to 'tighten' the anal sphincter by collagen contraction. It is an out-patient procedure with local anaesthetic.

## Antegrade continence enema (ACE)

📖 p. 588.

## Colostomy

If all else fails to restore acceptable continence for social functioning, the patient might experience improved quality of life with a colostomy. Troublesome mucus discharge might occur (an incontinent anus might eventually need proctectomy if troublesome) and the patient could be prone to hernias (collagen deficiency). Informed choice is essential.

## Further reading

Madoff RD, Pemberton JH, Mimura T, et al. (2005). Surgery for fecal incontinence. In: Abrams P, Cardozo L, Khoury S and Wein A (eds) *Incontinence*. Health Publications, Plymouth.

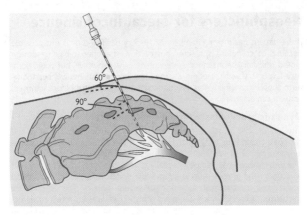

**Fig. 15.12** Sacral nerve stimulation. Reproduced with kind permission © Burdett Institute 2008.

# Neosphincters for faecal incontinence

If the patient has major FI and other surgery has failed or is not possible because of complete sphincter destruction, the only remaining option would normally be a stoma. A neosphincter is expensive, but could compare favourably with a lifetime of stoma equipment. Patients will need long-term support and follow-up. Full understanding is essential before informed consent can be given.

## Dynamic graciloplasty (gracilis neosphincter)

The long gracilis muscle is mobilized from its insertion into the knee and wrapped around the anal canal, to preserve the blood and nerve supplies in groin (Fig. 15.13). An electrical stimulator is implanted in the abdomen. Once the wound has healed, gradually change the stimulation parameters to convert the gracilis muscle from a fast-twitch to a slow-twitch (good endurance) muscle over a period of several weeks. This is complex specialized surgery, which can have a high complication rate (e.g. infection, pain over the implant site or in leg wound, and new difficulty in evacuation). It is expensive. The battery in the neosphincter will need replacing after 5–7 years.

## Artificial anal sphincter

Implantation of an inflatable cuff around the anus, which is connected to a deflation pump (within the labia in ♀ and scrotum in ♂) and fluid reservoir within the abdomen (Fig. 15.14). The pump is deflated to enable defecation. This is complex specialized surgery, which can have a high complication rate (e.g. infection, rejection of implant, pain over the implant site or around the pump or reservoir, or new difficulty in evacuation). There is a high risk of rejection and need for revision surgery; only 50% of procedures are successful overall, but these patients can have very good continence. Long-term results are unknown. The procedure has a high cost. Meticulous asepsis is essential to avoid infection/rejection.

## Gluteus maximus transposition

The gluteus maximus muscle is mobilized and wrapped around the anus; a double wrap (both gluteus muscles) is possible. There are usually poor functional results, and the technique is seldom used. The unstimulated gracilis muscle (inner thigh) is also used sometimes, but poor results are common.

## Further reading

Madoff RD, Pemberton JH, Mimura T, *et al.* Surgery for fecal incontinence. In: Abrams P, Cardozo L, Khoury S and Wein A (eds) *Incontinence*. Health Publications, Plymouth.

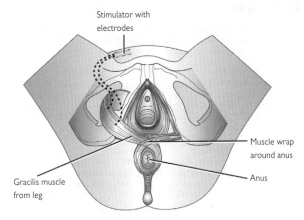

**Fig. 15.13** Gracilis neosphincter (dynamic graciloplasty). Reproduced with kind permission © Burdett Institute 2008.

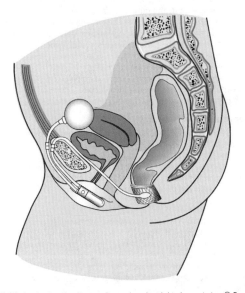

**Fig. 15 14** Artificial anal sphincter. Reproduced with kind permission © Burdett Institute 2008.

# Rectocele

A rectocele is a herniation of the rectovaginal septum, resulting in a bulging of the rectum forwards into the vaginal lumen (Fig. 15.15).

## Symptoms

Sensation of a bulge or dragging. Incomplete evacuation, straining to evacuate, needing to digitate vaginally or perineally to complete evacuation, and sexual discomfort. Major symptoms include backache and discomfort on standing for long periods. Rectocele can be associated with soiling in some ♀. Stools often become 'trapped' in rectocele during attempted defecation. However, many patients are asymptomatic.

## Causes

Childbirth, straining, and possibly congenital collagen weakness. It is exacerbated by obesity (possibly) and ageing. Some degree of rectocele is probably normal in older parous ♀. It is associated with anterior vaginal wall and vaginal vault prolapse and enterocele (small bowel herniation into the vaginal vault) in some ♀.

## Diagnosis

- Vaginal examination—supine, at rest, and during straining.
- Sims speculum enables the best visualization of the posterior vaginal wall—standing, at rest, and during straining.
- Proctogram—barium paste can be seen in bulge, at rest, or during defecation. Might see trapping of barium after defecation of paste is thought complete by the patient. Surgery could be indicated for a 2–3 cm non-emptying rectocele.
- First degree—small rectocele on straining.
- Second degree—moderate rectocele on straining.
- Third degree—rectocele reaches into introitus on straining.
- Fourth degree—rectocele reaches beyond the introitus.

## Conservative management

Patient teaching and reassurance. Some patients are happy to digitate to support the posterior vaginal wall during defecation. Modify stool consistency (firmer or looser, as indicated) to ease evacuation. Teach good defecation dynamics and avoid excessive straining (📖 p. 579). Vaginal pessary helps some patients. Manage associated constipation. Suppositories, enemas, or irrigation help some patients.

## Surgical management

For cosmetic/comfort reasons or trapping rectocele. A gynaecologist will perform posterior vaginal repair or sacrocolpopexy (if associated with vaginal vault prolapse). A colorectal surgeon will perform transrectal repair (usually with resection of excess tissue), with insertion of mesh to reinforce if necessary. The patient must avoid straining after repair because it can cause recurrence. Complications include new sexual dysfunction or faecal incontinence.

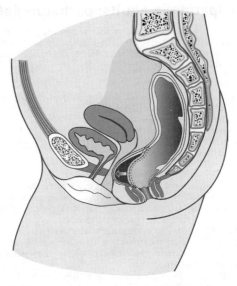

**Fig. 15.15** Rectocele. Reproduced with kind permission © Burdett Institute 2008.

# Constipation in adults: pathophysiology

There are 3 million GP consultations for constipation per year; 10% of district nurses' time is spent remedying constipation. In the UK, £50+ million is spent on laxatives per year. Myths abound. (For childhood constipation 📖 pp. 660–4.)

## Definition

Fewer than 3 stools/week and/or straining, hard stools, or a sense of incomplete evacuation ≥25% of the time.

Associated symptoms include the following.

• Abdominal discomfort, pain, and bloating.
• Lethargy and malaise.
• 'Spurious diarrhoea' in frail impacted patients.

## Prevalence

Constipation is prevalent in 5–10% of the general population and in ≥50% of individuals in nursing homes and neurological patients. However, more people believe that they are constipated than fit the definition. There are two main types of constipation (which can coexist).

• Slow colonic transit—faeces are not propelled along the colon adequately. The longer the transit time, the more water is reabsorbed from the stools, resulting in hard, often pellet-like, stools that are difficult and often painful to pass.
• Evacuation difficulty—stools arrive in the rectum but cannot be expelled easily. Ineffective pushing and/or failure to relax the anus and pelvic floor ('anismus' or pelvic floor dyssynergia).

Underlying causes of constipation include the following (often a combination).

• Poor diet (e.g. amount, frequency, and fibre), dehydration, and immobility.
• Local anal pathology (e.g. haemorrhoids)—patient avoids defecation.
• Neurological disorders affecting sensory or motor function (e.g. spinal cord injury, multiple sclerosis, spina bifida, or any neuropathy).
• Pregnancy.
• Depression and apathy (e.g. nursing-home population).
• Endocrine disorders (e.g. hypothyroidism, diabetes mellitus, hypercalcaemia, and hypokalaemia).
• Difficulty with toilet access (e.g. disability and hospitalization) or lifestyle (ignore call to stool).
• Drug side effects (e.g. analgesics, especially opioids such as those prescribed post-operatively or for palliative care).
• Bowel disorders—IBS (often alternates with bouts of diarrhoea) and diverticular disease.
• Idiopathic (might be associated with laxative abuse or anorexia nervosa).
• Rarely—severe motility disorder, e.g. pseudo-obstruction.

## Further reading

Emmanuel AV (2004). Constipation. In: Norton C and Chelvanayagam S (eds) *Bowel Continence Nursing*. Beaconsfield Publishers, Beaconsfield.

# Constipation in adults: assessment and investigation

Takes time and requires adequate privacy for the patient to relax and tell their story. A bowel diary and symptom questionnaire give added information. Assessment will include the following.
- History of the problem and former bowel habit.
- Current frequency and form of stools.
- Current symptoms (e.g. straining, sense of incomplete evacuation, need to assist digitally, pain, bloating, and bleeding) and their severity and frequency.
- Diet (especially fibre), eating pattern, and fluid intake.
- Medication (include laxative history) and other medical conditions.
- Effects of symptoms and limitations on lifestyle.
- Coexistence of FI.
- Ability to use the toilet independently.
- Availability and involvement of carers.

## Examination
- General observation—patient's mobility and ability to self-toilet.
- Perianal inspection—anal conditions (e.g. haemorrhoids), scars, and skin excoriation.
- Digital rectal examination for presence and consistency of stool and ability to relax the anus on bearing down.
- Abdominal examination for masses, distension, or scars.
- Neurological examination if neuropathy is suspected.

▶ Consider the possibility of serious bowel pathology (e.g. rectal bleeding, unexplained change in bowel habit, anaemia, or weight loss) and whether further investigations (e.g. colonoscopy) are indicated. Consider also if a blood screen (e.g. thyroid function tests) is indicated. Usually no further tests are indicated.

Severely long-standing constipation that fails to respond to simple measures might require a colonic transit study or proctogram (📖 p. 46).

## Further reading
Muller-Lissner SA, Kamm MA, Scarpignato C, et al. (2005). Myths and misconceptions about chronic constipation. *American Journal of Gastroenterology* **100**, 232–42.

# Conservative management of constipation

- Reassurance and patient education.
- Make sure toilet is accessible.
- Address diet, fluids, and mobility, if possible.
- Eat regularly and do not skip meals (stimulates peristalsis).
- ↑ fibre slowly and mix types.
- Unrefined bran can cause bloating, mineral malabsorption, and even impaction.
- 1.5 L fluids (but excessive fluids will not help).
- Immobile—passive exercise or abdominal massage can help.
- Treat comorbidities (e.g. hypothyroidism or depression).
- Change constipating medications, if feasible (e.g. alternative analgesia or iron supplementation in pregnancy).

## Attempt to establish toilet routine

- Establish regular toileting pattern ~30 min after breakfast or evening meal (capitalize on the gastrocolic response).
- Sit comfortably and well-supported on the toilet.
- Ideally, attempt a semi-squat position if feasible (e.g. support feet on a footstool).
- Relax and breathe normally (do not hold breath and valsalva/strain).
- Use abdominal muscles to push.
- Relax anus.
- Attempt for maximum of 10 min.
- Practice on a daily basis.
- If an urge to defecate occurs at another time, do not ignore it.
- Consider short-term laxatives or evacuants (📖 p. 582) to establish a pattern.
- Severe constipation—fibre can worsen symptoms if transit is slow. A ↓ fibre diet might be beneficial.
- Refer for specialist investigations if initial management fails.

## Further reading

Muller-Lissner SA, Kamm MA, Scarpignato C, *et al.* (2005). Myths and misconceptions about chronic constipation. *American Journal of Gastroenterology* **100**, 232–42.

Patient Information. http://www.bowelcontrol.org.uk (accessed 14.05.07).

Patient Information. http://www.digestivedisorders.org.uk (accessed 14.05.07).

# Constipation: enemas and suppositories

Enemas and suppositories might be more predictable in effect and timing than oral laxatives. Not all patients have sufficient dexterity or find suppositories acceptable. They are especially useful for evacuation difficulties in neurogenic constipation. A carer or community nurse might need to aid administration (if acceptable to patient and available).

The aim of treatment is to stimulate a complete rectal evacuation. Try to achieve the desired result with the least intervention in the following hierarchy.

## Suppositories

Moisten or lubricate suppositories before insertion. Position the suppository against the rectal mucosa as high as possible (the agent will not work if it is embedded in stool). There is controversy regarding whether the blunt or pointed end should be inserted first—no good evidence exists for either method. Usual hierarchy:

- Glycerin—one suppository as required . If no effect, use two suppositories. A paediatric size is available. Lubricates stool and has a slight stimulant effect on the rectal mucosa.
- Bisacodyl—one suppository in the morning. Has a rectal stimulant effect.
- Carbalax (phosphate). Has a stimulant effect.

## Enemas

If suppositories are ineffective, try:

- Microenemas (5 ml)—sodium citrate.
- Tap water enemas—use 50–200 ml of warm tap water.
- Arachis oil (peanut oil) enema—as a softener for hard stool. ❶ Do not use in nut allergic patients.
- Phosphate enemas (large volume or 100–130 ml)—acts osmotically. Can also be used as preparation before flexible sigmoidoscopy. Use with care if the tissue is fragile (e.g. after pelvic irradiation) or if electrolyte disturbance is probable (e.g. hyperphosphataemia and perforation are rare, but have been reported).

It is customary to administer rectal preparations with the patient in the left-lateral position, but sitting on the toilet might be more practical for some patients. Consider if self-administration is feasible.

See also rectal irrigation (📖 p. 584) and digital stimulation/manual evacuation (📖 p. 644), which some constipated patients find helpful, especially those with neurological disorders and associated faecal incontinence (e.g. spina bifida).

# Laxatives

Almost all laxatives seem to become less effective with prolonged use, so keep use to the minimum effective dose and for the minimum time period. However, some patients do need to use laxatives for the long term if all other measures for constipation have failed, in particular neurological patients and those on opiate analgesia. It might be wise to try to find several effective agents and rotate their regimens to avoid a lessening effect with time.

Laxatives are greatly overused and there is little evidence for choice. Abdominal discomfort and bloating could be a result of laxatives rather than constipation. Expensive preparations cost 20 times more than cheap forms. Re-evaluate the patient regularly. Figure 15.16 gives a suggested flowchart for use.[1]

## Categories

- Bulking agents (artificial fibre), e.g. ispaghula husk, methylcellulose, and sterculia (if diet is inadequate and stool is hard); might cause bloating.
- Stool softeners, e.g. docusate sodium.
- Colonic stimulants, e.g. bisacodyl, senna, docusate sodium, and sodium picosulfate. These agents stimulate peristalsis. There is no evidence of colonic damage with long-term use.
- Osmotic agents, e.g. lactulose, and macrogols (which are also licensed for disimpaction). Possibility of dehydration in vulnerable patients.
- Prokinetic agents, e.g. tegaserod (which is in development and has a direct effect on the enteric nervous system).

## General principles

- Try non-drug options (📖 p. 579) first.
- Start with a low dose of a cheap preparation and discontinue as soon as possible.
- Difficulty in evacuation/hard stool—use softener or rectal preparation.
- Slow transit—use a stimulant.
- If long-term use is probable, find several agents and rotate their regimens.

1 Emmanuel AV (2002). The use and abuse of laxatives. In: Potter J, Norton C and Cottenden A (eds) *Bowel Care in Older People*. Royal College of Physicians, London.
Patient Information. http://www.bowelcontrol.org.uk (accessed 14.05.07).
Patient Information. http://www.digestivedisorders.org.uk (accessed 14.05.07).

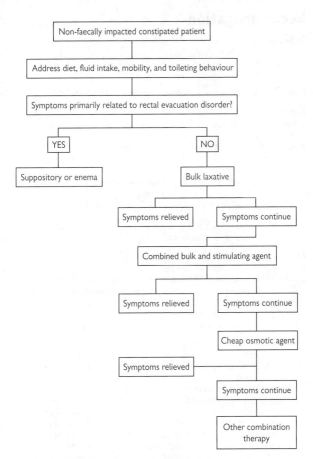

**Fig. 15.16** Flowchart for managing constipation.

# Rectal irrigation

## Indications
- FI and/or difficulty in evacuation.
- Most used in neurologically impaired patients (e.g. spina bifida).
- Incomplete evacuation and rectocele.

Rectal irrigation does not work for all patients (reasons unclear).

## Equipment
- Nelaton urethral catheter—might not retain fluid if anal sphincter is incompetent.
- Foley urethral catheter with balloon inflated.
- Stoma irrigation cone and water bag—need dexterity and hand strength to hold in place.
- Shandling rectal catheter and reservoir—inflatable balloon to keep catheter in place and prevent fluid leakage.
- Transanal irrigation kit (Coloplast Ltd, Peterborough): floor standing with hand pump.[1]
- Electrical pump—↑ infusion speed, but cumbersome (difficult to disguise and travel) and expensive.

## Fluids
- Tap water—body temperature.
- Saline—for children and if there is a risk of electrolyte disturbance.
- Can add aperients, e.g. phosphate enema or senna liquid (unlicensed use).
- No evidence regarding optimal volumes. Children: 20 ml/kg body weight is often recommended. Adults: start with 300–500 ml, ↑ if needed, up to 2 L reported.

## Technique
Use after meals to capitalize on gastrocolic response. Daily or alternate day use is usual. Evening administration might fit better with work or school schedules.
- Ensure privacy and adequate time is available.
- Assemble the equipment, fill the water bag, and sit on the toilet.
- Insert the catheter/cone (using lubricant gel if necessary) and then gradually infuse the fluid. It might take 10–20 min with a gravity fill (might be difficult to sit if the patient has disabilities). ❶ Pressure necrosis might occur if the patient has sensory impairment.
- When the fill is complete, remove the catheter or cone (can leave *in situ* for 5–10 min) and possibly massage abdomen.
- Attempt to evacuate.

Some authors suggest repeated smaller fills, but this can be time-consuming. After irrigation, the patient could experience anal leakage of fluid (use a pad as a precaution). Abdominal cramps can occur because of stimulation of peristalsis (usually tolerated and lessens with practice).

---

1 Christensen P, Bazzocchi G, Coggrave M, et al. (2006). A randomised, controlled trial of transanal irrigation versus conservative bowel management in spinal cord injury patients. *Gastroenterology* **131**, 738–47.

# Further reading

Crawshaw A (2004). How to establish a rectal irrigation service. *Gastrointestinal Nursing* **2**, 29–31.

Gardiner A, Marshall J, and Duthie GS (2004). Rectal irrigation for relief of functional bowel disorders. *Nursing Standard* **19**, 39–42.

# Biofeedback for constipation

The aim is to re-establish normal 'defecation dynamics' and spontaneous (laxative-free) evacuation; the patient relearns the voluntary (but usually subconscious) components of bowel evacuation. Biofeedback is used if other conservative measures have failed (e.g. diet, exercises, and establishing a bowel routine). Use of equipment to give the patient 'feedback' about function. Several modalities are possible.

- Insertion of a rectal balloon filled with 50 ml of air or water gives a sensation of rectal fullness. The patient attempts to expel the balloon (lying or sitting position). Observe and teach the patient, as appropriate:
  - Paradoxical anal sphincter contraction: teach relaxation.
  - Appropriate anal relaxation.
  - Use of abdominal muscles to 'brace and bulge', creating downward propulsive effort.
  - Avoid straining (holding breath and valsalva).
- Use of surface or intra-anal EMG to show the patient muscle activity, e.g. anal sphincter squeeze and relaxation, and activity of abdominal muscles.
- Use of manometry equipment to demonstrate anal and rectal pressures at rest and during attempted stool expulsion.

Biofeedback sessions might take place weekly or monthly over a 4–6 month period. The patient must practice the 'exercises' daily (Box 15.3). It is best to stop all laxatives (except in neurological patients). Use glycerin suppositories as a rescue if no stool is passed for 3–5 days. The patient might feel worse at first. About two-thirds of patients with chronic idiopathic constipation respond, and this response is usually sustained at least in the medium term. Results might not be as good in patients with neurological or anorectal (e.g. megarectum, solitary rectal ulcer syndrome, or rectocele) disorders.

## Box 15.3 Patient instructions for biofeedback

### Sitting properly

The way you sit on the toilet can make a big difference to the ease of opening your bowels. The 'natural' position (before toilets were invented) is squatting. Although actually squatting is not very practical, many people find that adopting a 'semi-squat' position helps a lot. One of the footstools that toddlers use to reach a sink is ideal, 8–12 in (20–30 cm) high. Position this just in front of your toilet and rest your feet flat on the stool, keeping your feet and knees about 1 ft (30 cm) apart. Lean forwards, resting your elbows on your thighs. Try to relax.

### Breathing

It is important not to hold your breath when trying to open your bowels. Relax your shoulders and breathe normally.

### Pushing without straining

The best way to open your bowels is by using your abdominal (stomach) muscles to push. Leaning forwards, supporting your elbows on your thighs, and breathing gently, relax your shoulders. Make your abdominal muscles bulge outwards to 'make your waist wide'. Now use these abdominal muscles as a pump to push backwards and downwards into you bottom. Keep up the gentle but firm pressure.

### Relaxing the back passage

The final part of the jigsaw is to relax the back passage. To locate the muscles around the back passage, first squeeze as if you are trying to control wind. Now imagine that the muscle around the anus is a lift. Squeeze to take your lift up to the first floor. Now relax, down to the ground floor, down to the basement, and down to the cellar.

### Putting it all together

The above instructions tell you WHAT to do, but do not tell you HOW to do it. It sounds simple, but coordinating everything takes practice.
• Sit properly.
• Breathe normally.
• Push from your waist downwards.
• Relax the back passage.

Keep this up for about 5 min, unless you have a bowel action sooner. If nothing happens, don't give up. Try again tomorrow. It often takes several weeks of practice until this really starts to work.

## Further reading

Horton N (2004). Behavioural and biofeedback therapy for evacuation disorders. In: Norton C and Chelvanayagam S (eds). *Bowel Continence Nursing*. Beaconsfield Publishers, Beaconsfield.

# Constipation: surgery

Surgery is very rarely indicated, even for severe constipation. Patients will need extensive counselling and realistic expectations. A few patients seem keen to pursue surgical options and can be very disappointed if symptoms of abdominal pain and bloating persist after an operation.

## Subtotal colectomy and ileo-rectal anastomosis (IRA)

Usually results in permanent diarrhoea, although a few patients report persisting constipation.

## Colonic resection

Removal of a segment of the colon (typically descending and sigmoid). Performed less frequently than IRA. Results are often poor or short-lived; the remaining colon might still be constipated.

## Rectocele repair

📖 p. 574.

## Antegrade continence enema (ACE)

The appendix is brought onto the abdominal surface in the right iliac fossa, as a small catheterizable stoma, for antegrade irrigation of the colon. The procedure is most commonly performed in children with spina bifida; results seem less predictable in adults. Irrigate with water and/or a stimulant laxative or enema, with the patient sitting on the toilet.

## Percutaneous endoscopic colostomy (PEC)

Insertion of an irrigation port into the left colon during endoscopic examination. PEG or gastrostomy tubes can be used; dedicated PEC tubes are becoming available. There is a risk of infection because bacteria can colonize the track. Irrigate with water and/or a stimulant laxative or enema, with the patient sitting on the toilet (📖 p. 584).

## Sacral nerve stimulation

A neuromodulating 'pacemaker' wire is implanted into the nerves at the sacrum (usually at S3; 📖 p. 570), with a battery stimulator in the buttock. The procedure is experimental for constipation at present, but early results are promising. The mechanism of action is unclear.

## Stoma formation

If a partial colectomy with end colostomy is formed, some patients (especially those with slow gut transit) will develop a constipated stoma. For this reason, an end ileostomy is often preferred as a definitive procedure. This is obviously a major undertaking for a 'benign' condition.

# Constipation in cancer

Patients with cancer often have ↑ risk factors for constipation (Box 15.4), especially in advanced disease. Constipation often causes great distress to the patient and can worry carers. It is, perhaps, symbolic to patients of ↓ control of bodily functions.

Use proactive management to prevent problems, if possible. Palliative care is a particular problem and 50% of patients are constipated on admission to a hospice.

Constipation can present as impaction with overflow 'spurious diarrhoea' (especially opiate-induced constipation, which is present in 10–15% of hospice patients).

Opiates slow peristalsis, ↑ fluid reabsorption, possibly ↑ sphincter tone, ↓ rectal sensation, and generally ↓ arousal levels.

The underlying cause(s) must be identified by detailed assessment (&#x1F4D6; p. 578) and may be factors specific to the cancer.

## Management

Maintain hydration, nutrition, and mobility, if possible. Ensure oral care to enable chewing; the patients should have frequent small meals, with as much fibre as they can tolerate (often limited by bloating and discomfort).

Good bowel habits and posture (&#x1F4D6; p. 579) should be encouraged. Ensure the patient has as much privacy as possible. Address the patient's posture and comfort on the toilet with relevant aids (e.g. grab rails or padded seat).

Many patients will need preventive laxatives, especially if they are taking opiates. However, these agents can cause fear of FI if the patient is dependent on others for toileting.

Oral preparations should be taken as for other types of constipation; use a trial-and-error approach to find the best treatment for each individual.

Rectal preparations might be more predictable in terms of results, but they might not be tolerated by the patient. Note that administration by a relative might not be acceptable.

Manage constipation due to spinal cord compression as for spinal injury (&#x1F4D6; p. 644).

In patients with a terminal illness, sitting might be impossible. The patient could require manual evacuation if all other methods of management fail.

**Box 15.4 Risk factors for constipation in cancer patients**

- Opioid analgesia (high risk).
- Oral problems (e.g. *Candida* spp infection during chemotherapy)—low food intake.
- Anorexia/poor diet.
- Immobility or general muscle weakness.
- Difficulty with sitting on the toilet and the risk of pressure sores.
- Lack of privacy (if carers are needed for toileting).
- Depression/confusion.
- Dehydration (vomiting or poor intake).
- Tumour (bowel or spinal).
- Comorbidities of advancing age (e.g. metabolic disorders).
- Drug side effects (e.g. diuretics, iron supplements, antidepressants, antacids, or vincristine chemotherapy).

# Megarectum

Dilated colon and/or rectum.

## Presentation

- Chronic severe constipation.
- May present in children and young adults. ?Idiopathic, or result of long-standing constipation.
- Often, soiling by a faecal bolus in the rectum inhibits anal closure and liquid stool seeps around the impaction.
- Abdominal pain.
- Megarectum can present as acute abdominal pain with sigmoid volvulus (twisting of sigmoid colon, which is seen on instant contrast enema).
  ► This is a surgical emergency.

## Assessment

- Often, a lax anal sphincter or faecal impaction is found on digital rectal assessment.
- An abdominal mass (faeces) might be palpated.
- Imaging might detect a dilated rectum or partial/whole colon.
- ❶ Exclude Hirschsprung's disease (📖 p. 657).

## Conservative management

Disimpact; gentle manual evacuation might be needed (► take care because the anal sphincter might already be compromised). If constipation is severe, manually disimpact under anaesthetic. Use patient teaching to encourage the patient to take responsibility for their own bowel care (teenagers might be reluctant). Aim for a loose 'porridge'-like consistency of stools on a permanent basis. Make regular attempts to defecate after meals, even in the absence of the urge to defecate. Use biofeedback to teach muscular coordination (📖 p. 586). If using osmotic laxatives, titrate to response. Magnesium salts (e.g. Epsom salts) are unpalatable and the patient might have poor tolerance of or compliance with the regimen. Enemas or irrigation might be needed. The patient should drink 2.5 L of fluids per day. Symptoms will probably be lifelong.

## Surgery

If conservative management fails and symptoms are severe, surgery should be considered. The surgical approach depends on where the dilated segment is (i.e. whole colon, partial colon, or rectum). Aim for a 'porridge'-like stool consistency. Rectal or colonic resection may be used. If the whole colon is affected, ileo-anal anastomosis or ileostomy is used.

# Solitary rectal ulcer syndrome

A rare syndrome in which the patient develops one large rectal ulcer, usually on the anterior rectal wall.

## Symptoms

- Rectal bleeding and mucus, especially on defecation (can be profuse).
- Rectal pain.
- Frequent desire to defecate, often with multiple attempts throughout the day (can be 20–30 attempts/day).
- Tenesmus.
- Excessive straining, often unproductive of stool.
- Seldom symptomatic at night.
- Patients might have history of repeated anorectal digitations to remove stool.

## Cause

Thought to be the result of long-standing straining to defecate. Digitation can damage the rectal mucosa. Associated with internal rectal intussusception (telescoping of the mucosa) and sometimes rectal prolapse. Thought to be the result of chronic trauma to the mucosa from straining, although some patients report no previous history of defecation difficulties and solitary rectal ulcer syndrome seems to be idiopathic.

## Diagnosis

Seen on rectal endoscopy, with diagnosis confirmed by biopsy.

## Conservative management

Educate patient about the genesis of symptoms. Aim to stop straining behaviour and allow the ulcer to heal (can take many months if the ulcer is large and deep). Limit attempts to defecate (maximum of three attempts in 24 h). This is very hard for most patients, but it is essential if the ulcer is to resolve. Avoid all straining (📖 p. 587). Caffeine, certain foods (individual), and alcohol are found by some patients to exacerbate symptoms; it is worth experimenting with diet. Rectal steroids (e.g. Proctofoam®) help some patients.

## Surgery

Occasionally, the ulcer is resected; this procedure is often unsuccessful and the ulcer returns if the patient does not stop their straining behaviour.

# Inflammatory bowel disease

Introduction 596
Pathogenesis of Crohn's disease: epidemiology
   and environmental factors 597
Pathogenesis of Crohn's disease: genetics 598
Presentation of Crohn's disease 600
Initial investigation of Crohn's disease 602
Extra-intestinal manifestations of Crohn's disease 604
Further investigation of Crohn's disease 606
Nutritional treatment for Crohn's disease 608
Medical management of Crohn's disease 610
Surgical management of Crohn's disease 612
Pathogenesis of ulcerative colitis 614
Presentation of ulcerative colitis 616
Investigations for ulcerative colitis 618
Medical management of ulcerative colitis 620
Surgical management of ulcerative colitis 622
Extra-intestinal manifestations of inflammatory
   bowel disease 624
Chronic disease management: general 626
Chronic disease management: ulcerative colitis 628
Chronic disease management: Crohn's disease 629
Procedure protocols: infliximab infusions 630
Procedure protocols—methotrexate 632
Procedure protocols: other immunosuppressants 634
Osteoporosis management 636

# Introduction

Inflammatory bowel disease (IBD) affects about 1 in 400 in the UK.

! Do not confuse with irritable bowel syndrome (IBS) (📖 p. 502).

Two main forms are recognized: ulcerative colitis (UC) and Crohn's disease (CD). A lack of a firm histopathological distinction between these two main forms is known as indeterminate colitis. There are other less common types such as microscopic colitis (including collagenous colitis and lymphocytic colitis), which share much of the same management. Bowel inflammation can also be caused by radiotherapy or diversion colitis.

Although UC and CD share many features, there are also important differences in management, which will be highlighted in this chapter.

IBD has a profound impact on the individual, both physically and often psychologically. Needs are complex and unpredictable. Often an IBD nurse specialist is seen as the lynchpin for coordinating care, providing a range of services from direct clinical care, to education and telephone helplines.[1]

The principal aim of treatment in both UC and CD is to induce and maintain clinical remission, with a ↓ in symptoms and a satisfactory quality of life for the individual with the disease.

When selecting therapies for treatment of active disease, consider the following to help make a decision in collaboration with the patient regarding appropriate therapies.

- Activity/severity.
- Site of disease.
- Lifestyle and behaviours.
- Previous response to medications.
- Side effects.
- Patient preference.

Medication choice will need to be tailored to the individual to ensure compliance and the best chance of response. It is also essential to have an understanding of the different preparations and qualities of available therapies, to be able to tailor drug therapy to the individual optimally.

1 Younge L and Norton C (2007). Contribution of specialist nurses in managing patients with IBD. *British Journal of Nursing* **16**, 208–12.

# Pathogenesis of Crohn's disease: epidemiology and environmental factors

CD is characterized by transmural inflammation affecting any part of the GIT (mouth to anus). The condition has a tendency to develop fistulae or strictures within the bowel. The cause of CD is unknown, although a number of theories exist.

## Epidemiology

- The prevalence of CD is 50–100 cases/100 000 population.
- Between 4 and 11 new cases/100 000 population are identified in the UK each year.
- Most patients present between 20 and 60 years of age.
- The condition is more common in ♀ than ♂.
- 15% of patients diagnosed have a family member with UC or CD.
- Identical twins are often diagnosed together.

## Environmental factors

- Cigarette smoking is probably the strongest environmental risk factor for the development of CD and predicts a worse course of disease.[1] The reason for this is unclear.
- Infectious agents, such as *Mycobacterium paratuberculosis* and the measles virus/MMR vaccine have been proposed as causal factors, but evidence to support this remains unconvincing.

### Other factors

- Intestinal permeability has been suggested as a possible causal factor in the development of CD. It is suggested that a leaky intestinal barrier intensifies antigen absorption which, in turn, heightens the inflammatory response.

1 Birrenbach T and Bocker U (2004). Inflammatory bowel disease and smoking: a review of epidemiology, pathophysiology, and therapeutic implications. *Inflammatory Bowel Diseases* **10**, 848–59.

# Pathogenesis of Crohn's disease: genetics

During the past decade, rapid advances have been made in defining the genetic origins of IBD. New studies continue to illuminate the relationship between the genotype and the phenotype: in other words, between the genetic make-up and disease characteristics. Particular emphasis has been placed on the genes NOD2 (CARD15), OCTN1, and OCTN2 (IBD5).

NOD2 (CARD15), discovered in 2001, is considered to be important in the inflammatory response. Expression of these proteins is thought to be associated with small bowel disease and the presence of fibrostenosing disease. The precise action has yet to be confirmed, but four main theories have been proposed:

- NOD2 maintains the gut mucosa at a certain level of inflammation. In healthy gut mucosa, this produces a localized inflammatory response that suppresses any possible infection. In CD, this process is not as well regulated and the localized inflammation becomes more severe and widespread.
- NOD2 functions as an antibacterial factor, controlling the expression of Paneth cells in the inflammatory response. Paneth cells are found at the base of crypt formation in the gut mucosa of the small bowel. In CD, this response is greater; the Paneth cells trigger a heightened inflammatory response.
- NOD2 might have a role in apoptosis (cell death). This theory emerges from the belief that the pathogenesis of CD might involve dysregulation of apoptosis by mutated forms of NOD2.
- NOD2 negatively influences the activation of other inflammatory signals preventing the activation of defence responses.

There is a possible relationship between OCTN1 and OCTN2 genes on chromosome 5 and perianal disease. Research on the mutations in the OCTN1, OCTN2, and DLG5 genes has suggested an up to 10-fold ↑ in susceptibility to CD if these mutations are present.

Understanding of the genetics of CD is still in its infancy. This area does however raise the possibility of screening, prevention, and early intervention in the future.

## Further reading

Gaya D, Russell R, Nimmo E, et al. (2006). New genes in inflammatory bowel disease: lessons for complex disease? Lancet **367**, 1271–84.

# Presentation of Crohn's disease

It is considered useful to classify CD in terms of the site, extent, and pattern of disease, because this affects medical management, surgical options, and prognosis. The site of disease also affects the presentation; exacerbations tend to produce similar features.

## Clinical features

### All sites of disease
- Altered bowel habits.
- Abdominal pain.
- Pyrexia.
- Lethargy.
- ↓ appetite and weight loss.

### Small bowel disease
- Nausea and vomiting.
- Bloatedness/abdominal distension.
- Apthous ulceration.
- Duodenal ulcers—post-bulbar, difficult to heal, or associated with elevated ESR.
- Abdominal pain—epigastrium and right iliac fossa are common sites.
- An abdominal mass is sometimes palpated, particularly in the right iliac fossa.

### Colonic Crohn's disease
- Severe diarrhoea.
- The rectum is often spared.
- Patchy inflammation of the colon.
- Rectal bleeding.
- Passing mucus rectally.
- Toxic dilatation of the colon.

### Perianal Crohn's disease
- Usually associated with ileocolonic disease.
- Recurrent fistulae, abscesses, and skin tags.
- Severe rectal pain.
- Varying bowel habits from constipation to diarrhoea.

## Pattern of disease

CD can be either fibrostenotic or fistulating in presentation.
- Fibrostenotic disease occurs because inflammation of the bowel causes narrowing of the bowel lumen. Initially, strictures will respond to steroids, but over a period of time, the tissue develops into scar tissue and becomes fibrotic. This could lead to intestinal obstruction.
- Fistulating disease occurs because inflammation penetrates the bowel mucosa. This can result in connections developing with adjoining structures, such as the bladder, vagina, and small bowel. Sometimes, the connection is with the skin (Plate 17).

# Initial investigation of Crohn's disease

## Assessment of activity/severity of disease

The severity of CD can be more difficult to assess objectively than that of UC. Presenting symptoms, indicating an ↑ in disease activity, commonly include the following:
- Diarrhoea.
- Abdominal pain.
- Anorexia.
- Weight loss.

Rectal bleeding is not always present and is dependent on the localization of disease. Other signs to look for can include:
- Abdominal tenderness/mass on palpation.
- Oral ulceration.
- Anal skin tags/fistulae.
- Postprandial pain (after eating)—indicative of obstruction.
- Anaemia.

A number of pathological, endoscopic, radiological, and histological investigations are used to confirm the diagnosis of CD. Scoring systems are available to assess disease activity; the most commonly used scale is the Crohn's Disease Activity index[1]. Their use regarding objectivity of symptom reporting/assessment can be controversial.[2]

## History and examination

When assessing the patient with suspected CD, a number of factors should be taken into consideration, including:
- Recent travel.
- Medication.
- Smoking.
- Family history.

A full bowel assessment should be undertaken, examining the following:
- Stool frequency and consistency.
- Urgency.
- Rectal bleeding ± mucus.
- Abdominal pain.
- Malaise.
- Fever.
- Weight loss.
- Abdominal and anorectal examination.
- Extra-intestinal manifestations of CD (Table 16.1).

Additionally, pulse, blood pressure, temperature, and weight should be documented.

---

1 Best W, Becktel J, Singleton J, et al (1976) Development of a Crohn's disease activity index. National Coperative Crohn's Disease Study. *Gastroenterology* **70**, 439–44

2 Forbes A (1998). *Inflammatory Bowel Disease: A Clinician's Guide* (2 edn) Arnold, London.

## Initial investigations
### Pathology
- Full blood count.
- Urea and electrolytes.
- Liver function tests.
- Serum $B_{12}$, iron, and folate.
- ↑ CRP and ESR.

### Stool samples
- For culture and sensitivity, and ova and parasites.
- To exclude infection.

### Abdominal X-ray
In an acute presentation of CD, an abdominal X-ray might also be appropriate to assess for toxic dilation, perforation, or obstruction of the bowel.
Other possible complications:
- The presence of joint pains (arthralgia) or frank arthritis.
- Inflammation of the iris or uveitis.
- Presence of erythema nodosum, pyoderma gangrenosum, or aphthous ulcers.
- Anal fissures, fistulae, or abscesses.
- Other fistulae.
- Fever during the previous week.

# Extra-intestinal manifestations of Crohn's disease

Numerous non-gut manifestations of Crohn's disease may arise (Table 16.1). See also 📖 p. 624.

**Table 16.1** Extra-intestinal manifestations of CD

|  | Common (5–20%) | Uncommon (<5%) |
|---|---|---|
| Related to disease activity | Aphthous ulcers<br>Erythema nodosum<br>Finger clubbing<br>Ocular<br>Conjunctivitis<br>Episcleritis<br>Iritis<br>Arthritis<br>Osteoporosis | Pyoderma gangrenosum |
| Unrelated to disease activity | Gallstones<br>Sacroilitis<br>Arthralgia (small joint)<br>Nutritional deficiency | Liver disease<br>Fatty liver<br>Primary sclerosing cholangitis<br>Ankylosing spondylitis<br>Renal stones<br>Osteomalacia<br>Sweet's syndrome<br>Systemic amyloidosis |

# Further investigation of Crohn's disease

## Sigmoidoscopy and colonoscopy

Colonoscopy is more appropriate for CD because it enables the clinician to visualize the terminal ileum and to take a biopsy. CD on endoscopy could demonstrate the following.
- Patchy inflammation throughout the colon.
- Inflammation at the terminal ileum.
- Rectal sparing.

Sigmoidoscopy might be considered to enable visualization of the left side of the colon and mucosal biopsy.

## Gastroscopy

In patients with small bowel disease, a gastroscopy might be considered to assess for oesophageal and gastric CD.

## Histology

Biopsies taken during endoscopy might reveal:
- Transmural infiltration (inflammation penetrating the bowel mucosa).
- Lymphocytic infiltration (evidence of inflammatory response).
- Presence of granuloma.

## Small bowel radiology

A barium meal and follow-through study is the best means of assessing the small bowel, it enables the following to be assessed.
- Distribution of the disease.
- Depth of the inflammation.
- Presence of strictures.
- Presence of fistulae.

## Capsule endoscopy (📖 p. 222)

A non-invasive, pain-free, fully ambulatory diagnostic procedure specifically for investigating the small intestine. Can enable direct visualization of mucosal abnormalities for assisting:
- New diagnosis of CD.
- Diagnosis of suspected active episode in a patient with known CD.

## Ultrasound

Ultrasound scans may be used to assess for the following:
- Thickened bowel loops.
- Inflammatory masses.
- Collections of fluid associated with abscess cavities.

## White cell scanning

Radio-labelled white cell scanning identifies areas of inflammation and ∴ active segments of CD.

## CT scanning

A CT scan enables the assessment of complications of CD. Thickening of bowel loops and their location are easily ascertained, in addition to information regarding the length of strictures and fistulae.

## MRI

MRI enables non-invasive 3-dimensional images to be collected. MRI is considered to be better than CT scanning in obtaining clear information regarding fistulae tracts, particularly in perianal disease.

## Further reading

Carter M, Lobo A, and Travis S (2004). Guidelines for the management of IBD in adults. *Gut* **53**, V1–16.

Cohen RD (ed) (2003). *Inflammatory Bowel Disease: Diagnosis and Therapeutics (Clinical Gastroenterology)*. Humana, Press Totowa, NJ.

Kamm MA (1999). *Inflammatory Bowel Disease. Medical Pocketbooks.* Taylor & Francis, London.

Rampton DS and Shanahan F (2005). *Inflammatory Bowel Disease (Fast Facts Series)*. Health Press, Oxford.

# Nutritional treatment for Crohn's disease

## Aims
• Maintain or improve current nutritional state.
• Induce remission.
• Maintain remission.

Dietary therapy is used in CD not only in a supportive role for medical and surgical management, but also as the primary treatment.

## Supportive dietary therapy
The nutritional status of patients with CD should be assessed regularly, especially during a flare-up. Patients might be unable to maintain adequate intake because of:
• Poor appetite.
• Nausea.
• Food intolerances.
• Partial or complete bowel obstruction.

The addition of vitamin and mineral supplements, high-calorie drinks, or supplemental feeding with liquid diets might be needed, and, very occasionally, parenteral nutrition (PN) is used if oral diet is not possible or there is very extensive small-bowel disease or resection (📖 p. 380).

Many patients with CD are unable to tolerate high-fat or high-fibre diets (which lead to ↑ diarrhoea and pain) and some benefit from dairy-free diets. Patients should be referred to specialist dietitians and discouraged from avoiding foods in a haphazard and unnecessary manner. If there is subacute obstruction, a low-residue or liquid diet is needed until the obstruction is resolved through medical/surgical management.

## Diet as the primary therapy
It is also possible to use diet as a primary therapy for CD by means of liquid diets.[1, 2] These have been shown in some studies to be as effective as steroids in inducing remission, with none of the side effects. However, this is controversial. This is of particular benefit for the undernourished and children who are still growing. The usual method is 2–3 weeks of liquid feeding (elemental, e.g. EO28, semi-elemental, e.g. Pepdite®, or polymeric, e.g. Modulin®), followed by a gradual and planned reintroduction of normal foods with supplemental liquid feeding.

It is unclear exactly how liquid diets achieve healing and remission, but it is probably due in part to:
• ↓ of dietary/bacterial antigens and proinflammatory eicosanoids (fatty acids).
• Restoration of optimum nutrition.
• ↓ of intestinal permeability.

1 O'Sullivan M and O'Morain C (2001). Liquid diets for Crohn's disease. *Gut* **48**, 757.

2 Woolner JT, Parker TJ, Kirby GA, *et al.* (1998). The development and evaluation of a diet for maintaining remission in Crohn's disease. *Journal of Human Nutrition and Dietetics* **11**, 1–11.

All the above lead to healing of the gut mucosa.

Despite the obvious benefits of providing nutrition and avoiding steroid use, there are problems associated with liquid diets:

• Supportive and specialized input from the medical/nursing staff and dietary team is essential, with rapid access to help and advice during treatment.
• Patients must be well motivated—it can be very difficult socially and psychologically to give up normal meals for several weeks.
• Some patients are unable to take the feeds orally because of unpalatability—nasogastric feeding might be an option for those who are willing. Occasionally, longer-term feeding through a PEG tube can help in more severe cases or if there is oesophageal CD (rare).
• The use of liquid diets might cause osmotic diarrhoea, which can respond to taking the drinks more slowly or diluting them.

If remission is achieved through liquid diet, resuming a normal diet immediately will usually cause a relapse. Gradual and phased reintroduction by means of an exclusion diet such as the low-fibre fat-limited exclusion (LOFFLEX) diet is used, subject to local practice. In this way, problem foods can be identified and then avoided, to help maintain remission. With continued support through this phase, many patients can eventually identify an appropriate individual diet, avoiding some foods but maintaining a healthy nutritional status through alternatives. Patients report that the most common symptom-provoking foods include dairy products, wheat, and caffeine.

# Medical management of Crohn's disease

In established CD, knowledge regarding the site of disease can help with treatment choices.

There is little evidence to support the use of maintenance 5-aminosalicylic acid (5-ASA) therapies in CD, although some clinicians and patients choose to use maintenance regimens and there may be a role in reducing post-operative recurrence of disease after ileal resection.

## Ileocaecal Crohn's disease

The use of oral budesonide is recommended for mild to moderate exacerbations. In studies, the drug has proved most effective in right-sided disease and has a better side-effect profile than prednisolone.[1] If remission is not achieved, treatment with a standard tapering dose of prednisolone is recommended.

The use of antibiotics (e.g. ciprofloxacin and metronidazole) should be reserved for moderate localized disease for which there is a suspicion of septic complications. However, side effects and limited tolerability by patients restrict antibiotic use.

In severe disease, there is a better evidence base for initial treatment with oral prednisolone, with early introduction of immunosuppressant therapy for those patients who relapse on dose ↓ or withdrawal. Infliximab is indicated for those patients who prove immunosuppressant intolerant or unresponsive, although surgery should also be discussed at this time.

## Colonic Crohn's disease

Colonic CD can be managed in a similar fashion to UC, with the use of targeted steroid and 5-ASA therapy, depending on distribution of disease, including topical treatments. If systemic corticosteroid therapy is indicated, there is little evidence to favour the use of budesonide over prednisolone. Immunosuppressant therapy should be considered early in patients with relapsing disease, although the slow action of this group of drugs does not promote their use as first-line therapy in active disease. Infliximab can be used, as appropriate, in patients who prove refractory to other treatments or situations in which surgery is contraindicated.

## Extensive small bowel disease

Active disease can require a tapering dose of oral steroid therapy and, again, early consideration of the introduction of immunomodulatory therapy. The use of polymeric or elemental diets can provide an alternative for patients who are not keen on steroid therapy, although the evidence for its effectiveness as a sole therapy is really only clear in children and adults with mild disease.

1 Rutgeerts P, Lofeburg R, Malchow H, *et al.* (1994). A comparison of budesonide with prednisalone for active Crohn's disease. *New England Journal of Medicine* **331**, 842–5.

Infliximab should be considered in refractory patients who do not respond to first-line therapy and, whilst exercising caution, its use can also be considered in patients with known stricturing disease.

## Fistulating/perianal disease

The management of perianal and fistulating CD is recognized as one of the most challenging problems in IBD. The use of antibiotics (e.g. ciprofloxacin and metronidazole) can be beneficial in the presence of sepsis or abscesses, and treatment is usually for an extended period. Unfortunately, many patients relapse when the drugs are withdrawn, and there are side effects associated with long-term use, particularly paraesthesia (tingling and sensory loss) with metronidazole.

Immunosuppressants (e.g. azathioprine and mercaptopurine) seem to have efficacy in perianal disease, although the response can be very slow.

An induction regimen of infliximab (given intravenously at 0, 2, and 6 weeks, dose based on body weight; (🕮 p. 630) can produce dramatic closure of fistulae, but the presence of sepsis or an abscess must be excluded with confidence before initiating treatment.

The use of topical and oral tacrolimus has been studied with some success in perianal disease, although numbers remain small.

In many cases, the underlying intestinal disease could be a significant contributory factor to the perianal symptomology and should be addressed as part of the management strategy.

## Oesophageal/gastric/duodenal Crohn's disease

Although uncommon, CD affecting these areas is an indicator of a poor disease prognosis. Acute exacerbations might respond to a proton-pump inhibitor, in addition to any other therapies the patient might already be taking.

### Other medication considerations

If oral corticosteroids are used, it is considered good practice to prescribe concomitant calcium as a bone protector (🕮 p. 636).

If required, oral steroid courses should be kept as short as possible, with alternatives used wherever feasible. Give the patient a steroid card.

Patients requiring more than two courses of oral steroids should be counselled and commenced on steroid-sparing therapy wherever possible (e.g. azathioprine, mercaptopurine, or methotrexate).

If the patient has small bowel disease or an ileostomy avoid enteric-coated medication as it may be poorly absorbed.

Extreme caution in relation to pregnancy (both genders).

# Surgical management of Crohn's disease

Patients require surgery for CD if medical treatment has failed or to manage sepsis or complications. Because the effects of medical options for Crohn's disease are often not sustained, ~80% of patients will need surgery at some point. 50% of these patients will go on to require further surgery, with recurrence of inflammation at the surgery site and/or elsewhere. Surgery is ∴ not a cure for CD, as it is for UC.

Because of the likelihood of repeated surgery, resection is always conservative. If <1 m of small bowel is left after multiple resections, 'short bowel syndrome' could result, leading to severe diarrhoea and inadequate absorption of nutrients. In such cases, PN will be necessary (🕮 p. 148).

## Indications
- Emergency—perforation of bowel or severe haemorrhage.
- Acute—small bowel inflammatory obstruction or small bowel and/or colonic inflammation that is unresponsive to medical management.
- Chronic—small bowel obstruction due to fibrostenotic stricture.
- Repair of fistula or abscess (perianal or internal).
- Severe dysplasia or malignancy (rare).

The common surgical procedures are:
- Stricturoplasty or resection for ileal strictures (Fig. 16.1).
- Ileocolic resection for terminal ileal/colonic inflammation (Fig. 16.2).

Other procedures include the following:
- Colonic resection.
- Ileorectal anastamosis.
- Panproctocolectomy with ileostomy.
- Laying open of perianal fistula.
- Insertion of seton suture (keeps fistula open and prevents abscess).
- Drainage of perianal or abdominal abscess.
- Dilation of stricture.
- Ileo-anal pouch often quoted as contraindicated (controversial).

The preparation for surgery will depend on the operation performed. If surgery is elective rather than emergency management, patients are reviewed in joint medical/surgical clinics if possible. They should have the opportunity to discuss the implications of surgery for physical function and body image. In all cases, it is important to maintain and, if necessary, improve nutritional status beforehand, using supplemental feeding or PN as required. If the patient requires a temporary or permanent stoma, counselling and siting will be indicated (🕮 p. 262).

## After surgery
Following simple resections, diet will be gradually reintroduced and, in most cases, function will return to normal. Terminal ileal resection might lead to bile-salt malabsorption, with consequent diarrhoea requiring the use of a bile salt sequestrant such as colestyramine. Regular vitamin $B_{12}$

injections might also be required because vitamin $B_{12}$ is primarily absorbed in the terminal ileum.

Following significant colonic resection, stools might remain loose and the use of an anti-diarrhoeal agent, such as loperamide, might be necessary. Patients requiring a stoma will require much support and information, both before and after surgery, from the medical, surgical, and stoma care teams.

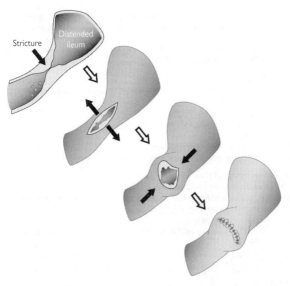

**Fig. 16.1** Surgical stricturoplasty of ileum. Reproduced with kind permission © Burdett Institute 2008.

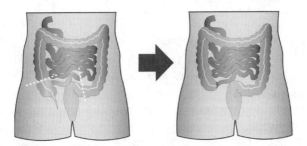

**Fig. 16.2** Ileocolic resection. Reproduced with kind permission © Burdett Institute 2008.

# Pathogenesis of ulcerative colitis

The prevalence of UC is ~100–200 cases/100 000 population. The cause is unknown, but a number of genetic, physiological, immunological, and environmental theories have developed. Unlike CD, UC affects only the large bowel and rectum.

## Genetics

No clear genetic predisposition to ulcerative colitis has been identified, although predisposition in some groups suggests a genetic contribution. However, there are a number of emerging theories suggesting how the condition develops and manifests. The strongest evidence explores familial traits and antigens (HLA and pANCA markers).

### Familial traits

- 15% of patients who are diagnosed with UC have a family member with UC or CD.
- UC is more likely to occur at a younger age in familial cases (28 years compared with 35 years for familial and non-familial traits, respectively).
- Concordance is higher among identical twins than non-identical twins.
- UC is more common in Jewish than non-Jewish communities.

### HLA (human lymphocyte antigen) links

- HLA links have been considered in UC for many years. A study found that the presence of HLA–B27 in conjunction with exposure to bacteria ↑ the risk of development of UC. In the general population, ~4% of individuals carry this gene.
- A variety of HLA-A and HLA-B have been associated with pancolitis.
- HLA–DRB1*0103 has been associated with severe disease presentations and extra-intestinal manifestations. This group of patients are between 5 and 11 times more likely to require surgery.

### pANCA4

- The identity of and the function of pANCA4 antigen is unclear. There is a strong association between the presence of the antigen and the development of primary sclerosing cholangitis.
- It does not indicate an ↑ in genetic risk.

## Physiological

- A number of mucosal abnormalities are noted in UC.
- In UC, the colonic mucosal barrier is impaired, which leads to ↑ intestinal permeability and an ↑ inflammatory response because the gut mucosa allows antigens into the submucosa (Fig. 16.3).

## Immunological

A number of complex theories have been proposed regarding the immune response and UC. When the disease is active, the lamina propria of the mucosa becomes heavily infiltrated with a mixture of acute and chronic inflammatory cells. There is a predominant ↑ in IgG within the mucosa, resulting in the release of numerous cytokines and amplification of the inflammatory process.

## Environmental

- Smoking—ex-smokers are three times more likely to have UC than smokers. This is attributed to the effect of nicotine in suppressing the inflammatory response.
- Appendectomy—the removal of the appendix at an early age has been associated with a preventative effect on the development of UC.
- Anti-inflammatory drugs—this group of drugs can trigger exacerbations of UC. This is thought to be because of an effect of altering the mucosal barrier.

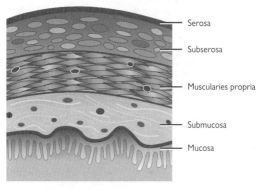

Serosa

Subserosa

Muscularies propria

Submucosa

Mucosa

**Fig. 16.3** Diagram of bowel wall. Reproduced with kind permission © Burdett Institute 2008.

# Presentation of ulcerative colitis

UC is characterized by inflammation of the mucosa and submucosa of the colon; it always affects the rectum and can progress to involve all or varying extents of the colon. The site and extent of UC will usually determine medical and surgical management. Four headings are used to describe UC.

- Pancolitis—affects the whole of the colon and rectum (19% of patients).
- Left-sided colitis—affects the descending colon and rectum (left-sided and distal colitis affects 33% of patients).
- Distal colitis—affects the rectum and sigmoid colon.
- Proctitis—affects the rectum only (48% of patients).

It is estimated that 50% of patients with UC will relapse in any given year and it is likely that a significant number of patients will have frequently relapsing or continuous disease. It is estimated that 20–30% of patients will need colectomy at some point. The majority of patients remain fully capable of work.

## Clinical features

- Change in bowel habits—usually ↑ bowel frequency and urgency and occasionally constipation.
- Rectal bleeding.
- Passing mucus rectally.
- Abdominal pain.
- Loss of appetite.
- Lethargy.

## Extra-intestinal manifestations

(📖 p. 624)
- Primary sclerosing cholangitis.
- Arthralgia.
- Colorectal cancer.
- Uveitis/iritis.
- Erythema nodosum.
- Pyoderma gangrenosum.

## Colorectal cancer surveillance

UC patients are at higher risk of developing colorectal cancer (CRC) than the general population: 2% at 10 years, 8% at 20 years, and 18% at 30 years since onset of UC.[1] Highest risk: extensive disease, family history CRC, and primary sclerosing cholangitis. Colonoscopic surveillance is recommended, but early dysplasia may be difficult to spot (newer chromoendoscopy techniques may improve detection). Random biopsies risk missing any lesion present. 5-ASA or sulfasalazine treatment may be protective and should probably be taken long term in those who tolerate it.[2]

1 Chambers W, Warren B, Jewel D, *et al.* (2005). Cancer surveillance in ulcerative colitis. *British Journal of Surgery* **92**, 928–36.

2 Moum B and Ekbom A (2005). Ulcerative colitis, colorectal cancer and colonoscopic surveillance. *Scandinavian Journal of Gastroenterology* **40**, 881–5.

## Defining the severity of UC

A number of endoscopic tools are used to assess disease severity. The tool in use for the longest time is the Truelove and Witts[3] framework for assessing severity at initial presentation (Table 16.2).

**Table 16.2** Defining the severity of UC[3]

| Feature | Mild | Moderate | Severe |
|---|---|---|---|
| Motions/day | <4 | 4–6 | >6 |
| Rectal bleeding | Small | Moderate | Large amounts |
| Temperature | Apyrexial | Intermediate | 37.8°C on >2 out of 4 days |
| Pulse rate | Normal | Intermediate | >90 bpm |
| Haemoglobin | >11 g/dl | Intermediate | <10.5 g/dl |
| ESR | <20 mm/h | Intermediate | >30 mm/h |

3 Truelove SC and Witts LJ (1955). Cortisone in ulcerative colitis: final report on a therapeutic trial. *British Medical Journal* **2**, 1041–8.

# Investigations for ulcerative colitis

The aim of any investigation in UC is to confirm the diagnosis, assess severity and extent of disease, and detect complications.

## History and examination

As for CD (📖 p. 602).

## Pathology

A full blood count, a urea and electrolyte count, liver function tests, determination of ESR, and measurement of level are usually performed. This enables identification of anaemia, abnormal renal or hepatic function, and the level of inflammation within the individual. Remember that ↑ ESR and CRP level are indicative of active IBD; however, they are not bowel specific and levels may be normal (especially in distal UC).

## Abdominal X-ray

In an acute presentation of IBD, an abdominal X-ray might also be appropriate to assess for toxic dilation of the colon (📖 p. 498). It can also assess the disease extent of UC or presence of proximal constipation.

## Stool cultures

It is always necessary to exclude infective causes of diarrhoea, e.g. *Escherichia coli*, *Salmonella* spp, *Shigella* spp, *Campylobacter* spp, and *Clostridium* spp.

## Sigmoidoscopy and colonoscopy

A sigmoidoscopy is usually performed in all patients presenting with bloody diarrhoea to assess the severity and disease extent (Table 16.3). Colonoscopy might be preferred to sigmoidoscopy in mild to moderate disease because it gives a more thorough assessment of the disease extent. In more severe cases, endoscopic investigations might be deferred until the clinical condition improves to ↓ the risk of perforation.

Colonoscopy surveillance for CRC is suggested for patients with pancolitis after 8–10 years and left-sided disease after 15–20 years.

## Histology

In UC, the histology changes are predominately confined to the mucosa and submucosa. In active disease, there will typically be an acute inflammatory reaction with neutrophil infiltration, crypt abscesses, and goblet cells depleted of mucus. None of these features are unique to UC, but they are highly suggestive of it.

## Further reading

Carter M, Lobo A and Travis S (2004). Guidelines for the management of IBD in adults. *Gut* **53**, V1–16.

Forbes A (1998). *Inflammatory Bowel Disease: A Clinician's Guide* (2nd edn) Arnold, London.

Travis S (1998). Ulcerative colitis. In: *Medicine*. Medicine Publishing Group, London, pp.15–20.

**Table 16.3** Endoscopic appearance of colitis

| Mild | Moderate | Severe |
| --- | --- | --- |
| Diffuse erythema | Granular mucosa | Intense inflammation |
| Loss of vascular pattern | Petechial haemmorrhage | Purulent exudate |
| Contact bleeding | Spontaneous bleeding | Discrete ulcers |

# Medical management of ulcerative colitis

In patients with an established diagnosis of UC, the extent of disease should be known and will help guide the medical treatment, once other causes for the symptomology have been excluded.

## Proctitis

The use of prednisolone or mesalazine suppositories is usually effective in managing inflammation.

## Left-sided disease

Foam or retention enemas, used nightly ± suppositories, can effectively bring a flare into remission. For more extensive left-sided disease, water-based retention enemas, containing steroids or mesalazine, might be required, although these can be messy and difficult for patients to retain.

If the patient is currently taking an oral maintenance 5-ASA preparation, such as mesalazine, the dose can be ↑ in conjunction with topical treatment for mild to moderate flare-ups.

Severe proctitis or left-sided disease, or a flare-up that has not responded to the above measures, will usually require treatment with a tapering dose of oral prednisolone, typically starting with a dose of 40 mg for 1–2 weeks, ↓ by 5 mg/week until the drug is discontinued.

## Extensive or total colitis

A mild flare might respond to an ↑ in oral 5-ASA ± topical treatment, but typically will require treatment with oral steroids (as above).

Severe or fulminant disease, defined by a high bowel frequency in association with fever, tachycardia, ↑ inflammatory markers (e.g. ESR), anaemia, low serum albumin level, or systemic symptoms such as malaise, will require hospital admission and treatment with IV steroid therapy, plus resuscitation, as required, with fluids and/or a transfusion. If symptoms do not settle, treatment with intravenous ciclosporin or infliximab should be considered. There is, however, a significant risk that surgical intervention will be required and this must be discussed with the patient; support should be given to prepare for this outcome (e.g. involve the stoma care nurse).

## Assessing response to therapy

This is an essential part of the management of an acute episode to determine success of treatment intervention and guide management. Improvement and response can result in the following:
- ↓ in bowel frequency.
- ↓ in the presence of blood and mucus.
- An improved sense of well-being.
- ↓ in urgency.
- Improvement in endoscopic appearance.

A majority of episodes will respond to therapy within 2 weeks, at which time treatment can be tapered and maintenance regimens can be commenced or recommenced. Common maintenance therapies for ulcerative colitis include the following:

- Mesalazine.
- Balsalazide.
- Olsalazine.
- Sulfasalazine.

Maintenance therapy will be discussed further on 📖 p. 628.

## Immunosuppressant therapy

Patients who present with severe or fulminating disease, or who have steroid-refractory or steroid-dependent disease despite maintenance therapy with oral 5-ASA, should be counselled and started on immunosuppressant therapy to achieve improved remission. Standard immunosuppressant therapies include azathioprine and mercaptopurine, and these should be first-line choices.

Any patient commencing immunosuppressant therapy must be counselled regarding the side effects of this group of drugs, including the risk of neutropenia (about 1/300 risk). Measurement of thiopurine methyl transferase (TPMT) prior to commencing therapy can identify patients at higher risk of this effect. An agreement to undertake regular monitoring of blood counts must be undertaken by the patient and healthcare provider, with implementation of robust systems for checking the results (📖 p. 634).

# Surgical management of ulcerative colitis

## Indications

Surgery is needed for UC if medical treatment fails. If patients have severe or fulminant colitis, surgery is indicated if there are signs of toxic megacolon ( P. 498) developing despite intensive treatment with IV steroids and ciclosporin. Rarely, surgery is needed as emergency management for perforation of the colon or severe haemorrhage. Surgery is also recommended for chronic symptoms with steroid dependence and/or lack of efficacy of immunomodulatory drugs, or intolerance of the latter. Chronic UC can lead to poor overall health and a much reduced quality of life. About 25–30% of patients with extensive colitis will require surgery .

Occasionally, surgery is performed for severe dysplasia or high risk presence of CRC ( p. 492).

In nearly all cases, the entire colon and rectum are removed. Even if the extent of disease is subtotal, removing only the affected section could result in the remaining colon becoming affected and there will still be a risk of colon cancer developing.

Initially, most patients will have a subtotal colectomy and temporary ileostomy, leaving a rectal stump in place. After a period of recovery, there are three options:

• Formation of an ileo-anal pouch or an ileo-anal anastamosis ( p. 252).
• Removal of the rectal stump (proctectomy), leaving a permanent ileostomy.
• Leave rectal stump *in situ* and keep under surveillance for cancer.

The pouch functions as an artificial rectum, but because of a lack of a colon, the stools are liquid and frequent (typically four to seven stools during the daytime) and there might be nocturnal waking or incontinence in ~20% of cases. Inflammation of the pouch (pouchitis) can develop, requiring medical treatment similar to that for proctitis; if inflammation is severe, removal of the pouch might be necessary. Despite the issues outlined above, this option is favoured by younger patients who wish to avoid a stoma.

The final decision regarding which option is most suitable does not have to be made initially, allowing plenty of time to consider the implications of each option. For detailed nursing care and considerations, refer to stoma care ( Chapter 8).

In all cases, much support is needed for the both the patient and his/her family from the combined medical/surgical team, with input from stoma care nurses at an early stage if possible. There are many issues of concern to patients regarding body image, stoma or pouch function, sexuality, fertility, pregnancy, work, and social life after surgery. Much time might be required for discussing questions, with a partner or family member present, if appropriate. Some patients can benefit from meeting with another who has had surgery, and most will need to approach the idea gradually if time allows.

# Extra-intestinal manifestations of inflammatory bowel disease

Not only do patients with IBD suffer with symptoms relating directly to the bowel and the effect inflammation has on its function, but they may also suffer from what are termed 'extra-intestinal manifestations'. Their clinical course can vary with the course of IBD, but extra-intestinal manifestations could precede, or dominate, any gastrointestinal symptoms (📖 p. 604).

Up to 25% of patients with IBD suffer from extra-intestinal manifestations. It is not fully known why these extra-intestinal symptoms occur. It is a possibility that the inflammation in the colon is only another manifestation of what is a systemic disease.

## Musculoskeletal manifestations

- Arthritis occurs in up to 20% of patients—the main types seen in UC are peripheral arthritis, ankylosing spondylitis, and sacroileitis.
- For those with peripheral arthropathies, a wide range of joints could be involved, from large joints (e.g. knees) to smaller joints (e.g. fingers). A relapse in bowel symptoms is associated with symptoms of arthritis in 29% of patients. The majority of these symptoms of arthritis are seronegative arthropathies, such as ankylosing spondylitis and reactive arthritis.
- The incidence of finger clubbing is ↑ in CD.
- ↓ bone mass density, resulting in osteoporosis or osteopenia, has been reported in 3–77% of patients with IBD (may be steroid related).

## Skin

- Oral lesions (CD).
- Erythema nodosum can be seen in UC or CD, but occurs most often in CD. It shows itself as raised inflamed bumps or nodules, most commonly on the legs. These bumps look red and angry and are very painful to touch. Its appearance generally parallels IBD disease activity and usually responds well to steroid therapy.
- Pyoderma gangrenosum occurs in 5% of patients with UC and 2% of patients with CD. It can manifest itself in wound sites post-operatively and looks like large areas of ulceration, with a necrotic and infected centre and a dusky purple outline. These ulcers can be very large, painful, and distressing for the patient, who might find the link between bowel and skin diseases confusing. Skin biopsy is used to rule out any other causes for ulceration, making pyoderma gangrenosum essentially a diagnosis of exclusion (📖 p. 292).

## Ocular manifestations

- Episcleritis occurs in 3–4% of IBD patients and causes local, tender inflammation. It can be treated with topical steroids.
- Uveitis is a more serious condition. It can mirror the activity of the colonic inflammation and presents with pain, blurred vision, and photophobia. There is a risk of scarring and possible blindness if it is not treated promptly, so patients complaining of these symptoms need a quick and early diagnosis.

## Primary sclerosing cholangitis

(🕮 p. 446)

- Primary sclerosing cholangitis is an injury that occurs to the bile duct that comprises inflammation, thickening, and stricture formation. Its link to UC is very well accepted and it is the most serious of the common extra-intestinal manifestations. Long-term complications include cholestasis which leads to liver cirrhosis and portal hypertension.
- Studies have shown a prevalence of between 3% and 10% in patients with UC. It is more common among ♂, and 95% of patients will have substantial colitis, leading to an ↑ risk of colorectal carcinoma (patients need regular screening colonoscopy).
- Patients often present with abnormal liver function tests, particularly high serum alkaline phosphatase levels, and diagnosis is most specifically made using endoscopic retrograde cholangiography. Treatment is limited and tends to aim for the prevention of scarring of the biliary tree. Although treatment options are available, none are curative, and patients might eventually need liver transplantation (🕮 p. 420).

## Renal stones

- There is an ↑ incidence of renal stones in CD, particularly in patients with ileal disease post-resection.

## Other rarer extra-intestinal manifestations

- Amyloidosis—occurs in <1% of patients; can be fatal.
- Pancreatitis—often related to medication, e.g. azathioprine.
- Bronchopulmonary inflammation.
- Pleuropericarditis.

## Further reading

Kelly P, Patchett S, McCloskey D, et al. (1997). Sclerosing cholangitis, race and sex. *Gut* **41**, 688–9.

Lamers CBHW (1997). Treatment of extra-intestinal complications of ulcerative colitis. *European Journal of Gastroenterology and Hepatology* **9**, 850–3.

Orchard TR, Wordswoth BP, and Jewell DP (1998). Peripheral arthropathies in inflammatory bowel disease: their articular distribution and natural history. *Gut* **42**, 387–91.

Rankin GB (1990). Extra-intestinal and systemic manifestations of inflammatory bowel disease. *Medical Clinics of North America* **74**, 39–50.

Tavarela Veloso F (2004). Skin conditions in inflammatory bowel disease. *Alimentary Pharmacology and Therapeutics*, **20**, 50–3.

Weiss A and Mayer L (1997). Extra-intestinal manifestations In: Allan RN, Rhodes JM, Hanauer SB, et al. (eds) *Inflammatory Bowel Diseases*. Churchill Livingstone, Edinburgh.

# Chronic disease management: general

### Lifestyle issues

Although most patients will be completely well between relapses, active UC or CD can cause many problems and be very disruptive. Bouts of frequent urgent bloody diarrhoea ± cramping abdominal pain, fatigue, and loss of appetite can leave a patient housebound or severely restricted. Activities that are taken for granted, such as shopping, (even short) journeys, or going somewhere new can become fraught with difficulties. The impact of CD on each individual will depend on the extent and severity of the disease, frequency of relapse, need for hospitalization, personality type, and social circumstances. In some cases, the effects can be devastating. Many patients feel unable to plan ahead because of the uncertainty of a relapsing/remitting condition.

Common concerns or difficulties include the following.

- Body image—effects of symptoms, medication (e.g. steroids), and surgery might lead to feelings of self-disgust and poor self-esteem.
- Relationships—when unwell, there might be an inability to participate in usual activities. Low self-esteem and embarrassment could make it difficult to form new relationships.
- School/college/career—UC most commonly first presents in young adulthood when the individual is often trying to finish education or start a career. There might be problems with repeated absences, especially if diagnosis has not been disclosed. There could be discrimination or lack of support.
- Sexuality and fertility—illness and poor body image can cause a loss of libido. Those wishing to become pregnant or who are pregnant might be very concerned about the possible adverse effects of their medication. Fertility is ↓ in ♂ taking sulfasalazine. Pregnancy must be avoided by those on methotrexate because of its teratogenicity (possible damage to developing fetus). As yet, there is limited evidence for the safety of newer agents such as infliximab and ∴ patients are advised to avoid them during pregnancy. Most other medications should be continued, but advice should be sought from the specialist team. Contraception advice is crucial. Discussion of sperm/egg banking and possible later IVF in patients with incomplete families.
- Financial issues—some patients are unable to work periodically or permanently. Those with severe disease may be eligible for Disability Living Allowance and should be referred for appropriate advice. Travel or health/life insurance may be an issue. The National Association for Colitis and Crohn's Disease (NACC) offers useful addresses.

Although most patients have the support of close family and friends, the fact remains that UC and CD affect body parts and cause symptoms that are considered by many to be deeply embarrassing. Patients can suffer a great deal of distress and feel that there are few, if any, to whom they can disclose the worst aspects of their disease. Members of the health-care team caring for them must be aware of this and allow time for unburdening, if possible. Membership of a support organization, such as NACC might help.

Factors that can affect the course of UC or Crohn's include:
- Smoking—has a protective role against developing UC. It is not uncommon for colitis to flare up on stopping smoking. The best advice for a smoker with UC who wishes to quit would be to wait until they were in good remission first.
- Diet—finding and adhering to a 'safe' diet can be very beneficial (📖 p. 110).
- Stress—the role of stress in contributing to disease activity is, as yet, poorly understood. In addition to the stress caused by UC itself, many patients can attribute the onset of a flare-up to a particularly stressful event, such as separation or moving house. It is important to recognize this stress and find ways to ↓ it.
- Holidays—particular care must be taken to guard against gastro-intestinal infection, which could trigger a relapse. In some cases, it is advisable to carry prophylactic antibiotics and steroids to treat 'travellers' diarrhoea' that does not settle within 1–2 days. It is vital that travel insurance covers IBD.

The best possible outcome for any patient with UC or CD will ensue if they can accept and become knowledgeable about their condition without becoming overly self-absorbed, make positive lifestyle choices, develop coping strategies, and receive support and care from their families, colleagues, and healthcare team, as needed.

# Chronic disease management: ulcerative colitis

## Maintenance treatment

The aim of maintenance treatment is to prolong remission for as long as possible. Usual maintenance treatment:

- For UC extending beyond the rectum, a maintenance dose of 5-ASA is recommended both to prolong remission and as a protective measure against the development of CRC. This is in addition to any immuno-modulatory medication used.
- For proctitis, 5-ASAs can be discontinued when the patient is well.

Patients might be tempted to stop medication or ↓ it to a subtherapeutic dose when they are well. The possible risks involved should be explained, particularly if immunomodulation is used. Adherence to treatment will be enhanced if patients are given an explanation of their disease process, the medication they are using, and any monitoring necessary. Leaflets and self-help books can help with this. If symptoms start to recur, rapid treatment can ↓ the severity of the episode. It might be difficult to obtain a speedy assessment in the hospital out-patient clinic but, increasingly, IBD nurse specialists are setting up telephone helplines that enable a prompt response. If possible, patients should be encouraged to develop a self-management plan with their specialist doctor/nurse, whereby they can initiate treatment for a new flare (e.g. ↑ oral 5-ASA or adding a topical preparation to the regimen); patients should make contact with their healthcare team if symptoms do not improve.

# Chronic disease management: Crohn's disease

## Maintenance treatment

The aim of maintenance treatment is to prolong remission once it has been achieved, either by medical or surgical means. Chronic management of CD includes:

- Unlike use in UC, 5-ASA preparations do not seem to prolong remission, except after small bowel surgery.
- Patients might be tempted to stop all medications when they are well, particularly those with a greater risk of side effects. ∴ if immunomodulation is used, the importance of continuing this, in addition to regular blood monitoring, must be stressed.
- Adjunctive treatments, such as vitamin $B_{12}$, colestyramine, and anti-diarrhoeal agents, should be continued.

Adherence to treatment can be enhanced if patients have a basic knowledge of their disease process and a clear understanding of the purpose of their medication. Leaflets and self-help books can help with this. If symptoms start to recur, rapid treatment can ↓ the severity of the episode. It might be difficult to obtain a speedy assessment in the hospital outpatient clinic but, increasingly, IBD nurse specialists are setting up telephone helplines that enable a prompt response. If possible, patients should be encouraged to develop a self-management plan with their specialist doctor/nurse, whereby they can initiate treatment for a new flare (e.g. restarting 5-ASA or elemental diet); patients should make contact with their healthcare team if symptoms do not improve.

# Procedure protocols: infliximab infusions

Infliximab is a chimeric anti-TNF-$\alpha$ monoclonal antibody, which binds to tumour necrosis factor $\alpha$ (TNF-$\alpha$) and inhibits its biological activity. TNF-$\alpha$ is a pro-inflammatory cytokine.

## Indications for treatment

Infliximab is recommended in patients who fulfil the following criteria[1]:
- Patients who have severe active IBD.
- Patients whose disease is refractory to treatment with standard therapy or who have been intolerant of, or experienced toxicity from, these treatments.

## Exclusion criteria for infliximab

- Current sepsis/infection.
- Abscess—if unsure, perform an abdominal CT scan or ultrasound to exclude presence of an abscess.
- Pregnancy/breastfeeding.
- Previous sensitivity to infliximab.
- Moderate/severe heart failure.
- Tuberculosis—chest X-ray before the first infusion to exclude TB.

## Dosage

- Severe active IBD and fistulizing CD—5 mg/kg body weight at 0, 2, and 6 weeks.
- Maintenance treatment—5 mg/kg body weight every 8 weeks.

## Patient preparation

Before treatment with infliximab, patients must be screened for any contraindications to treatment with a full past medical history. Patients must also be counselled on the potential side effects of treatment, which can include infusion reactions, ↑ risk of infection. A baseline set of vital observations should include blood pressure, pulse, temperature, $O_2$ saturation, respiratory rate, and weight. IV access must be obtained. Premedication with an antihistamine or corticosteroid is useful in ↓ the incidence of infusion reactions, particularly in patients not on corticosteroid or immunosuppressant therapy, and a slower infusion rate is also useful if there were previous infusion reactions.

1 National Institute for Health and Clinical Excellence (NICE) (2002). *The Effectiveness and Cost Effectiveness of Infliximab for Crohn's Disease. Technology Assessment.* http://guidance.nice.org.uk/TA40 (accessed 15.05.07).

## Procedure

Follow the manufacturer's guidelines for reconstitution. Infliximab should only be administered by physicians with appropriate knowledge of, and training with, the drug and treatment of IBD.

The drug must be infused intravenously through an infusion pump over a period of 2 h, with close observation and monitoring of vital signs every ~15–30 min. This must be done in a safe environment, with access to emergency equipment and oxygen. The patient should also be monitored for ~1–2 h post-infusion for infusion reactions. On discharge, the patient should be educated about the possibility of a delayed infusion reaction and given tips on dealing with this and also an alert card (which is included with each vial of infliximab). Re-treatment with infliximab is a decision made by the gastroenterologist following a full assessment of response.

# Procedure protocols: methotrexate

Methotrexate is a folic acid antagonist and is classified as an anti-metabolic cytotoxic immunosuppressant agent. It is not licensed for IBD, but its use in this area is underpinned by studies in Canada[1], which have found that it can induce and maintain remission in CD.

### Indications for use

Methotrexate is used in patients with resistant CD who have failed or are intolerant of treatment with immunosuppressants or corticosteroids. In some cases, it can be used for treatment of resistant UC (generally after azathioprine therapy), but there is less evidence for this.

### Dose

Patients are prescribed 25 mg of methotrexate, to be given orally or by intramuscular (IM) injection once weekly. It is usual to administer 12 once-weekly doses of methotrexate (25 mg), followed by maintenance on a ↓ dose of 15 mg orally once weekly. Response to treatment is usually seen within 4 weeks. The length of treatment is based on the patient's response to treatment and compliance as well as tolerance of any side effects.

### Contraindications

- Known sensitivity.
- Renal impairment.
- Liver impairment.
- Pleural effusion/fibrosis.
- Haematological impairment.
- Pregnancy—both ♂ and ♀ considering pregnancy are excluded because of the teratogenic effects of methotrexate. Patients should also be advised against pregnancy for at least 3 months after discontinuation of treatment. Adequate contraception for both ♂ and ♀ before the commencement of treatment must be agreed.
- Breastfeeding.

### Precautions

- Alcohol intake >7 units/week or not willing to abstain.
- Underlying infection.
- Chickenpox or shingles.
- Kidney stones.
- Obese patients might have a prolonged excretion of methotrexate.
- Concurrent administration of any drugs with nephrotoxic or hepatotoxic potential, but specifically aspirin, NSAIDs, diuretics, and ciclosporin.

1 Feagan B, Rochon J, Fedorak R, *et al.* (1995). Methotrexate for the treatment of Crohn's disease. *New England Journal of Medicine* **332**, 292–7.

## Administration considerations

Patients should be counselled on the effects and side effects of treatment, and written informed consent should be obtained, especially because to date the drug lacks a licence for IBD. A full assessment of the patient's past medical history and the contraindications to treatment is essential before commencement.

Local policy should be adhered to regarding the administration of IM methotrexate because the drug should always only be administered by adequately trained staff. Strict cytotoxic guidelines should be followed, including handling and administration of the drug (syringes should be pre-filled by the pharmacy), use of protective clothing, and disposal of equipment. The administration of methotrexate should take place in a designated cytotoxic area, with appropriate facilities for dealing with drug spillages.

## Monitoring

Measurement of the full blood count and a liver function test are advisable before, and within 4 weeks of, starting therapy and then monthly for the duration of treatment.

## Further reading

Buckton S (2003). Using immunosuppression therapy: implications and consequences. *Gastrointestinal Nursing* **1**, 32–5.

Forbes A (1998). *Inflammatory Bowel Disease. A Clinician's Guide* (2nd edn) Arnold, London.

# Procedure protocols: other immunosuppressants

The immunosuppressants azathioprine and 6-mercaptopurine (unlicensed indications) are effective therapies for IBD. They are indicated in both active disease and maintenance and remission of CD and UC in those patients who have steroid-dependent or resistant disease (unlicensed use).

## Monitoring azathioprine and 6-mercaptopurine

Many patients respond well to immunosuppressive therapy, although some go on to develop various side effects, including gastro-intestinal intolerance or severe myalgia and bone-marrow suppression. ∴ regular monitoring of blood counts, liver function tests, and urea and electrolytes are essential in the management of the patient taking immunosuppressive agents. The frequency of monitoring is dependent on local guidelines, but the BSG guidelines should be followed.[1]

## Abnormal blood parameters

- White cell count <4 × 109 cells/L or a fall of 50% from the previous count.
- Platelets <150 000/µl or a fall of 50% from the previous count.
- Haemoglobin below the normal range.
- Low neutrophil count.
- Low leucocyte count.
- Abnormal liver function tests.
- Abnormal urea and electrolyte count.

If an abnormal blood test is noted, the patient's care should be discussed with the consultant gastroenterologist. It might be appropriate to ↓ the dose or even stop the medication.

Weekly blood monitoring should continue until blood parameters have returned to normal. The patient should then be contacted and the management plan discussed.

If azathioprine monitoring is undertaken by the secondary care team, all results should be communicated to the GP.

## Non-compliance with monitoring

Considering the potential side effects of azathioprine, if patients are not compliant with blood monitoring, every effort should be made to contact them.

It might be appropriate to suggest to the GP that further prescriptions of azathioprine should not be issued until a blood test has been completed.

## Further reading

Buckton S (2003). Using immunosuppression therapy: implications and consequences. *Gastrointestinal Nursing* **1**(6), 32–5.
Forbes A (1998). *Inflammatory Bowel Disease. A Clinician's Guide* (2nd edn) Arnold, London.

---

1 Carter M, Lobo AJ, Travis SP (2004). Guidelines for the management of inflammatory bowel disease in adults. *Gut* **53**(Suppl 5), V1–16.

# Osteoporosis management

Osteoporosis is characterized by low bone mass or bone mineral density (BMD) deterioration that leads to fragile bones and risk of fracture. Nationally, it affects one out of three ♀ and one out of 12 ♂, with one out of four ♀ >60 years of age suffering an osteoporosis-related fracture.

## General risk factors for osteoporosis
• Premature menopause/amenorrhoea.
• Family history.
• Previous unintentional fractures.
• Poor calcium intake.
• Malabsorption.
• Anorexia.
• Smoking.
• High alcohol intake.
• Other conditions, including steroid treatment, thyroid abnormalities, long-term immobility, and other bone diseases.

## Osteoporosis and inflammatory bowel disease
↓ BMD has been reported in 3–77% of patients with IBD. Studies are inconsistent because the subjects included had a great variation in disease.

Osteoporosis has been found to be:
• More common in CD than UC.
• ↑ in patients with low weight or body mass index.
• ↑ in patients who have undergone steroid therapy.

Steroid therapy ↓ BMD by suppressing oestrogen and testosterone, which stimulate bone growth.

## Diagnosis and investigation
Dual energy X-ray absorptiometry (DEXA) is a low-dose radiation scan that can detect osteopenia or osteoporosis. Ultrasound has also been used.

BMD measurements are expressed using standard deviation from the mean. A T-score shows comparison with the young adult average, and a Z-score compares values with the average for their age.

## Screening
It is recommended that all patients undergo DEXA when they are diagnosed with IBD. Current guidelines recommend repeat DEXA every year if steroid treatment is given, and every other year if osteoporosis is established. It should also be repeated if a fragility fracture occurs.

X-ray can be used to identify fracture. Biochemical measurement of blood and urine can establish bone renewal.

## Treatments for osteoporosis
- Hormone replacement therapy in post-menopausal women (with caution/counselling on risks vs benefits).
- Bisphosphonates.
- Calcitonin.
- Seek and treat vitamin D deficiency.

## General lifestyle advice for osteoporosis prevention
- Good calcium intake—1500 mg/day (1 pint of skimmed milk contains 700 mg of calcium).
- Stop smoking.
- Take weight-bearing exercise.
- Enjoy sunshine.
- Menopausal women should discuss hormone replacement therapy with their GP.
- Drink sensible amounts of alcohol.

## Further reading
Scott EM, Gaywood I, and Scott BB (2000). Guidelines for osteoporosis in coeliac disease and inflammatory bowel disease. *Gut* **46**(Suppl 1), i1–8.

# Neurological bowel care

Bowel care in neurological patients  640
Autonomic dysreflexia  642
Digital rectal stimulation and
    manual removal of faeces  644

# Bowel care in neurological patients

## Common problems in neurological patients
- Independent toileting (mobility, dexterity, clothing, toilet facilities, grab rails, and hygiene).
- Privacy and dignity issues if dependent on carers.
- Often prone to both constipation and faecal incontinence (FI)—difficult to balance these two conditions.

## Multiple sclerosis (MS)
Constipation affects 30–40% of patients with MS, whereas at least 50% of patients with MS have FI. These two conditions often coexist and can be more severe in advanced MS. They are major limiting factors on quality of life.

### Disrupted sensation and motor function of the anorectum
- Constipation—poor rectal sensation, slowed motility, loss of the ability to relax the anus voluntarily, immobility, and polypharmacy.
- FI—poor rectal sensation and lax anal muscles. Difficulties with toilet access, transfer, and dependence on carers.

There is very limited evidence for the following interventions:
- Bowel habit and routine.
- Diet and fluids.
- Caution should be used with laxatives because they could cause FI.
- Biofeedback mild help in early/mild disease.
- Digital stimulation or manual evacuation might be needed.

## Spinal cord injury
All patients will need active bowel management after spinal cord injury. If the patient cannot manage independently, they might need community services.

Constipation results from slowed peristalsis (nerve damage and immobility). FI often results if the patient does not have a bowel routine (no sensory or motor function). Need to balance avoiding both constipation and FI.

### Injury above the 12th thoracic vertebra (T12)
Upper motor neurone or reflex bowel. Bowel management may use diet, establishing a routine, often nocturnal laxatives and/or suppositories/micro-enema, and/or digital stimulation (📖 p. 644). May need manual evacuation to complete evacuation. The anus is normally closed and FI is unusual unless the reflex is stimulated. Beware autonomic dysreflexia in injuries to T6 and above (📖 p. 642).

### Injury below T12
Lower motor neuron or flaccid bowel (sacral reflex arcs are disrupted). With a flaccid rectum and anus there is a risk of FI if the rectum is full. Management is similar to that for upper motor neuron, but digital stimulation is ineffective; often requires routine manual evacuation (📖 p. 644).

## Stroke

FI is common (30%) immediately after stroke, and is related to severity. At 6 months, 10% of stroke patients still have FI. There is a loss of cortical awareness and inhibition. Constipation (may be neurogenic, or due to immobility, loss of sensation, dependence, and medications).

## Cauda equina syndrome

Low spinal cord damage (e.g. injury, post-surgical (laminectomy), cord compression, or tumour). Sensory and motor functions of the bladder, lower bowel, and genitalia are partially or completely disrupted. Bowel symptoms are usually constipation and lax anus; FI occurs if stools are loose because there is no anorectal sensation or control. Difficult to balance constipation and FI. Routine and predictability is the aim of management. Laxatives tend to produce FI. Many patients need to use manual evacuation.

## Spina bifida

Congenital anomaly of the sacral spinal cord. Many children use irrigation (☐ p. 584). Management is similar to that for cauda equina syndrome above.

## Parkinson's disease

The predominant symptom is constipation, which can result from the disease process (↓ peristalsis), anti-Parkinson medication, poor mobility, and poor coordination between abdominal muscles pushing and anal sphincter/pelvic floor muscle relaxation. FI is unusual, unless stools are loose (because of limited voluntary control).

## Learning disability (LD)

Developmental intellectual impairment. FI is related to LD severity: 3% of patients have mild LD and at least 80% of patients have profound LD. Often related to constipation and 'overflow' soiling. Start to train children at the normal chronological age. It can take time and persistence. Reward positive actions (e.g. defecation in the toilet/potty). See vulnerable groups (☐ p. 675).

## Further reading

Coggrave M (2004). Effective bowel management for patients after spinal cord injury. *Nursing Times* **100**, 48–51.

Norton C (2004). Bowel management in multiple sclerosis. *Gastrointestinal Nursing* **2**, 31–5.

Smith L and Smith P (2004). Bowel control and intellectual disability. In: Norton C and Chelvanayagam S (eds). *Bowel Continence Nursing*. Beaconsfield Publishers, Beaconsfield.

Wiesel P and Bell S (2004). Bowel dysfunction: assessment and management in the neurological patient. In: Norton C and Chelvanayagam S (eds). *Bowel Continence Nursing*. Beaconsfield Publishers, Beaconsfield.

White H (2004). Making toilets more accessible for individuals with a disability. In: Norton C and Chelvanayagam S (eds). *Bowel Continence Nursing*. Beaconsfield Publishers, Beaconsfield.

# Autonomic dysreflexia

Potentially life-threatening condition that only affects people with complete spinal cord injury (SCI) above T6 (and occasionally above T10). Most patients will have been through a spinal cord injury centre and know the symptoms and management well.

## Symptoms

Pounding headache, restlessness, dizziness, shortness of breath, blurred vision, and nasal congestion. Symptoms above the level of injury include:
- Flushing (redness).
- Profuse sweating.
- Goose pimples.
- ↑ blood pressure.
- ↓ pulse (bradycardia).

If not treated promptly, collapse, seizures, stroke, and even death can result.

## Cause

Any noxious stimulus below the level of injury that would cause pain, discomfort, or irritation in a person without SCI (e.g. kinked catheter, urinary infection, anal fissure, faecal impaction, endoscopy, or rectal examination or other procedure). It can be triggered by routine bowel care in prone individuals.

## Mechanism

A noxious stimulus causes sympathetic nerve reaction, ↑ blood pressure due to vasoconstriction. Parasympathetic outflow through the vagus nerve slows the heart to compensate for hypertension. Cord transection prevents the usual regulation of the parasympathetic system: the parasympathetic system ↓ the heart rate (above the level of injury) to attempt to ↓ blood pressure.

## Prevention

Monitor the condition of susceptible patient with SCI during bowel care (observe for signs or symptoms, ask patient to report any changes, consider need to monitor pulse and blood pressure (BP) in patients known to experience autonomic dysreflexia). Ask the patient to report any dysreflexic symptoms. Avoid a loaded bowel (with regular bowel care). In patients prone to dysreflexia, local anaesthetic (e.g. lidocaine gel) can be used for bowel care/rectal examination. Consider local anaesthetic for any rectal/colic examination, despite the patient lacking sensation.

## Treatment

Stop any procedure and remove anything that might cause pain if possible (this is usually sufficient). Elevate the head immediately (❶ do not lie the patient down) and treat hypertension if trigger cannot be found (e.g. nifedipine or glyceryl trinitrate). Monitor BP regularly for at least 2 h if the reaction is unexpected/unusual. Consider the need for hospitalization in a community patient if BP is uncontrolled (it is an emergency situation if BP is severely elevated).

# Digital rectal stimulation and manual removal of faeces

☞ This issue has caused a lot of controversy in nursing.
- Is this a legitimate nursing procedure?
- How is competence ensured?
- Some accusations of malpractice and even abuse.

This is a legitimate nursing procedure and not an extended nursing role.[1] The National Patient Safety Agency states that some patients must have manual evacuation and the nurse should provide this.[2]

## Digital rectal examination
(☐ p. 514.)

## Manual evacuation: indications
- Faecal impaction/rectal loading that has not responded to other measures (e.g. laxatives and enemas). Note the use of macrogols for disimpaction.
- Inability to defecate (e.g. terminally ill or unconscious patient).
- Neurogenic bowel dysfunction if unresponsive to other means (especially lower motor neuron damage, e.g. low spinal cord injury): manual evacuation will be a routine part of regular bowel care.
- Some patients can manage their own procedure.
- Carers—consider acceptability to both parties.

## Manual evacuation: procedure
- Ensure consent is obtained.
- Consider the need to offer a chaperone.
- Pay attention to privacy and dignity issues.
- A left-lateral position is customary (some patients perform manual evacuation on the toilet).
- Use a lubricated gloved finger (note latex allergies).
- Remove stool with finger.
- Stop if pain, major bleeding, or consent is withdrawn (note: minor bleeding is common, especially as many neurological patients have haemorrhoids).
- Frail patient—consider the need for checking pulse and BP before and after the procedure.
- Take extra care with fragile tissues (e.g. inflammation, radiation, or frail patient).
- Avoid if recent anal surgery, unless there is a medical instruction.
- Special considerations:
  - Children.
  - History of abuse.

---

1 Royal College of Nursing (2000). *Digital Rectal Examination and Manual Removal of Faeces.* RCN, London.
2 National Patient Safety Agency (2004). *Ensuring the Appropriate Provision of Manual Bowel Evacuation for Patients with an Established Spinal Cord Lesion.* NPSA, London.

- Cultural and gender sensitivities.
- Spinal cord injury above T6—danger of autonomic dysreflexia (📖 p. 642).

## Digital rectal stimulation

A single gloved lubricated finger is inserted into the rectum and a circular motion used to stimulate the rectal mucosa, which in a reflex bowel should elicit a rectal contraction and anal relaxation. Stimulate for up to 30 s, then remove finger and observe for stool passage (may take several minutes to start). May be repeated at approximately 5 min intervals until no further stool obtained.[3]

3 Coggrave M (2004). Effective bowel management for patients after spinal cord injury. *Nursing Times* **100**, 48–51.

# Paediatric bowel care

Congenital anomalies 648
Imperforate anus 650
Paediatric stoma care 652
Problem-solving in paediatric stoma care 654
Antegrade continence enema 656
Hirschsprung's disease 657
Spina bifida 658
Constipation in children: causes 660
Constipation in children: assessment and management 662
Constipation in children: other issues 664
Toilet training 665
Toddler diarrhoea 666
Inflammatory bowel disease in children 668

# Congenital anomalies

Bowel dysfunction in children can manifest from the following congenital abnormalities:
- Embryological development, e.g. anorectal malformation.
- Instrinsic autonomic nerves of the gut.
- Sensory and motor nerves of the spine, e.g. neural tube disorders.

## Tracheoesophageal fistula and oesophageal atresia

Tracheo-oesophageal fistula is an abnormal opening between the trachea and the oesophagus, with obvious implications. Oesophageal atresia can also occur in conjunction with tracheo-oesophageal fistula or alone. It is often associated with imperforate anus. Oesophageal atresia results in the oesophagus ending in a closed blind pouch before it reaches the stomach. These abnormalities require early surgical intervention. If primary repair is not possible because of the severity of the abnormality, the baby will require a gastrostomy tube inserted into the stomach for feeding. Severe cases involving the trachea will often necessitate the baby also requiring a tracheostomy to aid breathing and prevent food bolus or mucus from entering the lungs.

## Necrotizing enterocolitis

The specific cause is unknown, but the condition arises because of mesenteric vasoconstriction, leading to intestinal ischaemia and infective gangrene. Initial treatment is conservative, by resting the bowel. Parental feeding and IV antibiotic therapy are needed. Should stricture or perforation occur, the diseased bowel must be resected and a temporary ileostomy must be formed. Closure of the stoma too early can result in diarrhoea, creating perianal skin problems.

*Signs and symptoms*
- Rectal bleeding.
- Abdominal distention.
- Bilious vomiting.
- Abdominal erythema.
- Lethargy.

*Investigations*
- Abdominal X-ray.

*Treatment*
- Antibiotic therapy.
- Laparotomy, ischaemic bowel resection, ileostomy.
- Once thriving, closure of ileostomy.

## Meconium ileus

Cystic fibrosis is a genetically determined disease that affects the intestinal, bronchial, salivary, and sweat glands, in addition to the pancreas. Of infants born with cystic fibrosis, ~10% are born with meconium ileus. This occurs because of the deficiency of pancreatic enzymes that are released into the intestinal tract. The meconium thickens and adheres to the intestinal mucosa, resulting in an obstruction. Perforation and peritonitis can occur if the obstruction is not relieved.

*Signs and symptoms*
- Failure or delay in passing meconium.
- Abdominal distension.
- Thick meconium, which is palpable on examination.

*Treatment*
- Gastrograffin enema.
- Surgery—a temporary loop ileostomy.

## Anorectal atresia

Atresia is defined as the absence of a normal opening or failure of a structure to be tubular. Anal atresia is the congenital absence of a normal anal opening, which presents in varying degrees of abnormality, from anal stenosis and imperforate anus to anorectal agenesis. Anorectal atresia results from the abnormal division of the cloaca during fetal development.

## Anorectal agenesis

Agenesis, or failure of the terminal bowel to develop, accounts for 75% of all anorectal atresias. It can be complicated by vaginal, vesical, or urethral fistulae. The prognosis depends on the site of the abnormality, i.e. whether it is high atresia (supralevator) or low atresia (translevator). Surgical outcomes are good, particularly in low atresias.

*Investigations*
- Perineal examination.
- Invertogram.
- MRI.
- Water-soluble contrast studies.

*Possible long-term outcomes of anorectal atresia*
- Faecal incontinence (FI).
- Constipation.
- Flatus incontinence.
- Sexual dysfunction.

*Treatment*
- High anal atresia: surgical reconstruction, colostomy, anal dilatation.
- Low anal atresia: simple surgical incision, surgical reconstruction, anal dilatation.

## Anal stenosis

Anal stenosis normally manifests at birth. The affected infant will have a small anal aperture, perhaps containing only a dot of meconium. If defecation is possible, a ribbon-like stool is likely to be passed. The abdomen might be distended. Faecal impaction and secondary megacolon can occur.

# Imperforate anus

Also known as 'anorectal malformation', imperforate anus is the absence of an anus or the presence of an incomplete anus. Imperforate anus occurs in 1 out of 3000 live births. Imperforate anus is evident from a failure to pass meconium. There are several variations of the deformity, which depend on the site at which the large bowel ends within the body.

## Low imperforate anus

The bowel stops slightly short of the site at which the anus should be, or the anus is present but is small or in the wrong place, so ectopic anus, anal stenosis, or anorectal stricture may occur. Treatment involves opening or moving the anus to connect it to the bowel. The operation is known as an 'anoplasty' and can be performed at birth.

## High imperforate anus

This is more complex. The patient commonly presents with either a bowel that ends in a blind pouch or a fistula between the bowel and the vagina (♀) or urethra (♂).

## Signs and symptoms

- In babies, the back passage is absent, tiny, or in the wrong place.
- Distended abdomen.
- Unable to pass meconium.
- Vomiting.
- Sacral abnormalities.
- If a fistula is present, meconium is present in the vagina or urethra.
- Two-thirds will present with one or more associated malformations.

## Associated problems

- Genitourinary.
- Vertebral.
- Alimentary tract.
- Cardiac.
- Neural abnormalities affecting the bladder and bowel.

## Investigations

- Abdominal X-ray—identifies the point at which the bowel ends, determining the extent of the problem.
- X-ray of spine.
- Renal ultrasound.
- ECG.

## Treatment

- Stage 1 (at birth)—a colostomy is formed, in addition to a mucous fistula.
- Stage 2 (at 3–6 months)—a new anus is created. The bowel is pulled down and connected to the anus.
- Stage 3 (at 6–9 months)—closure of the colostomy and mucous fistula.

# Paediatric stoma care

The number of stomas formed in children is much less than in adults. Nevertheless, it is estimated that between 40 and 100 new paediatric stomas will be formed per year and these are almost invariably temporary.

## Paediatric conditions requiring stoma formation

- Anorectal anomalies.
- Hirschsprung's disease.
- Necrotizing enterocolitis.
- Meconium ileus.
- Small bowel transplantation.
- Inflammatory bowel disease (IBD).
- Familial adenomatous polyposis.
- Trauma.

## Considerations during and after surgery

- Informed consent—if under 16 years will need to seek consent for procedure from parents.
- Bowel preparation—varies, generally clear fluids day before surgery, Nil by mouth 4–6 h prior to surgery.
- Stoma siting—child under 7 years generally not sited; parents' consent needs to be sought; principles of procedure same as adult (📖 p. 262).
- Pain control—use of local anaesthetic cream prior to any venepuncture or cannulation, prescribed analgesia, epidurals.
- Stoma management—involve parents wherever possible but encourage independence. Basic care, management, and complications similar to adult. Paediatric appliances available via ostomy companies.
- Schooling and play—important to involve play therapist where possible.
- Body image and self-esteem—support from family and peers.

## Preparation for closure of a stoma

To minimize the risk of perianal skin soreness, the baby's skin can be prepared using the following methods.

- Using olive oil instead of water to clean the nappy area.
- Wipe the nappy area with Comfeel® wipes or Cavilon® (wipes should not be used on sore or broken skin).
- Apply Metanium® ointment as a barrier cream after the above procedures.

## Possible problems following closure of a stoma

- Diarrhoea.
- Perianal skin soreness.
- Stricture.
- Constipation.
- Slow to potty train.
- Problem-solving in paediatric stoma care (📖 p. 654).

## Future considerations

♀ who have undergone corrective surgery to repair an imperforate anus should discuss their past medical history with their doctor before planning to start a family. A Caesarian section at the time of delivery is recommended.

## Bowel management programme

Children with subsequent bowel dysfunction must establish a good regular bowel pattern to avoid faecal impaction or incontinence. The following methods can be used.

- Regular toileting—after meals.
- Toilet training—can begin from ~2 years of age.
- A balanced healthy dietary intake—including fibre.
- Good fluid intake.
- Exercise.
- Self-massage.
- Oral laxatives.
- Rectal aperients, e.g. suppositories or enemas, if necessary.
- Retrograde colonic washouts.
- Pads.
- Psychosocial support for both child and parents/guardians.
- Access to toilet facilities.
- Liaison with the child's school.

# Problem-solving in paediatric stoma care

There are some common problems with children's stomas which vary between age groups. Table 18.1 details some problems and possible solutions.

**Table 18.1** Problem-solving in paediatric stoma care

| Age | Specific need | Stoma management |
|-----|---------------|------------------|
| Infant | Babies' skin tends to be dry | One-piece flexible paediatric, or mini, stoma bags |
| | | Avoid using alcohol-based agents, such as adhesive removers |
| | | Consider adding baby oil to the bath water, ensuring any excess is wiped off the peristomal skin area |
| | Babies grow and develop | Assess regularly as the baby grows and develops, and renew the appliance accordingly |
| | | Inform the parents of potential problems and what to look for |
| | Stomal prolapse (associated with temporary loop stomas) | Manual reduction carried out by a nurse specialist or surgeon |
| 6 months to 2 years | Children at this age prefer familiar faces | Ensure the same family members or staff undertake stoma care |
| | Can become active, beginning to explore and investigate their own bodies | All-in-one jumpsuits or vests ensure the appliance remains covered and intact |
| 2–5 years | Could start to ask questions regarding their bodies and take part in the management of the stoma | Time spent with the child, offering simple explanations, helps their understanding |
| | | A daily routine for stoma management helps parents and children follow a pattern |
| | | Allow the child to be involved in stoma care as they want and are able to |

**Table 18.1** (*Contd.*)

| Age | Specific need | Stoma management |
|---|---|---|
| 6–12 years | Child will start to take on responsibility for stoma management | Assess stoma management needs |
| | | Prompt the child regarding the practical aspects of emptying and changing |
| | | Check the suitability of the appliance |
| | | Advise regarding a stoma appliance that will be sufficiently discreet and robust to maintain security for all school activities, including sports |
| | | Encourage the child to talk about their stoma to family members and friends to gain confidence |
| | | Use websites for additional information for the child and parents |
| Adolescence | Developing a sense of themselves physically, sexually, and emotionally | The focus should be on the adolescent being informed about and skilled in the care of their stoma |
| | Peer pressure | Integrate socially with school friends |
| | | Ensure school activities and socializing with school friends |
| | | Encourage them to talk about how they are feeling |
| | Absence from school owing to ill health and/or surgery | Additional homework might be necessary |
| | | Support from parents and teachers |

# Antegrade continence enema

An antegrade continence enema (ACE) is a possible surgical solution only if all attempts at long-term bowel management have failed. It involves constructing a continent abdominal stoma, often using the appendix. The stoma is then intubated and the bowel washed out with water or saline. If patients are well selected and prepared, up to 80% will report satisfactory outcomes. It is most often used in children with neurological bowel (e.g. spina bifida). For more details on ACE (📖 p. 316).

# Hirschsprung's disease

Hirschsprung's disease is a congenital abnormality of the intrinsic gut nerves (myenteric plexus) which is characterized by the absence of ganglion cells in a segment of the colon, usually the rectosigmoid colon. The affected bowel cannot transmit a peristaltic wave and ∴ meconium accumulates and causes dilatation of the bowel lumen. The ultrasound appearance can be similar to that of anorectal atresia.

Hirschsprung's disease occurs in 1 out of 5000 live births. Most cases will be diagnosed within 1 week of birth, but, less commonly, it might not be diagnosed in childhood. Clinicians should consider a diagnosis of Hirschsprung's disease in adults who present with lifelong constipation.

## Signs and symptoms
- Intestinal obstruction.
- Delay in passing meconium.
- Poor feeder.
- Abdominal distension.
- Vomiting.
- Enterocolitis.
- Risk of perforation/septicaemia.
- Often associated with Down's syndrome.

## Investigation
- Abdominal X-ray.
- Rectal examination.
- Full-thickness rectal biopsy.
- Barium enema.
- Anorectal manometry.

## Treatment
- Rectal washouts.
- Laparoscopic pull-through.
- Removal of the affected segment of the bowel.
- Colostomy.
- In severe cases—total colectomy, with ileorectal anastamosis (which might require a covering or permanent ileostomy).

## Potential long-term problems
- Persistent constipation.
- FI.
- Inflammation.

# Spina bifida

Spina bifida is a congenital abnormality of the neural tube in the nervous system. It occurs in ~1 in 1000 live births in the UK. Before the 1960s, <10% of patients survived infancy, whereas now life expectancy is within normal realms. This means an ↑ number of problems associated with spina bifida are becoming apparent. Most babies with spina bifida have an abnormal nerve supply to their bowel, which alters bowel function.

About a third of children with spina bifida will experience FI. By young adulthood, only 52% of spina bifida patients experience complete continence. Constipation and abdominal pain are also common problems. Up to 85% of young adults require intermittent self-catheterization because of bladder incontinence.

This has clear effects on quality of life and the ability to be independent. In one study, up to 59% of patients who had FI required assistance with toileting.

## Treatment

A good bowel management programme is essential. Constipation should be avoided and management programmes should aim to achieve a regular soft stool. All bowel management will be dictated by the patient's level of independence and mobility. Puberty can bring about changes to bladder and bowel routines.

## Possible management methods

- Regular toileting—after meals.
- Toilet training—can begin from ~2 years of age.
- Ensure the child is supported while sitting on the toilet—which can be challenging if the child has other physical disabilities.
- Balanced healthy dietary intake—including fibre.
- Good fluid intake.
- Oral laxatives.
- Rectal aperient, e.g. suppositories or enemas, if necessary.
- Retrograde colonic washouts.
- Pads.
- Anal plugs.
- Psychosocial support for both child and parents/guardians.
- Access to toilet facilities.
- Liaison with school.
- Antegrade continence enema (Ⅲ p. 656).

## Further reading

Barnes K (2003). *Paediatrics: A Clinical Guide for Nurse Practitioners*. Butterworth Heinemann, Oxford.

Rudolf M and Levene M (2006). *Paediatrics and Child Health* (2nd edn). Blackwell, Oxford.

# Constipation in children: causes

Most constipation in infancy is due to underfeeding or insufficient water intake. Discover what the parent actually means when they complain that their baby is constipated—some parents refer to the hardness of the stool and others refer to its size, but most refer to delay or difficulty in defecation. A breastfed baby might not defecate for >1 week but will then pass a classic mustard-like breastfed stool without any difficulty or distress. If stools are retained in bottle-fed or mixed-fed babies, inevitably the stools will dry up and harden.

## Epidemiology

At some time, ~5% of children have constipation. Constipation affects ♂ more commonly than ♀.

## Normal defecation in infancy

When the rectum fills, it contracts and simultaneously the internal anal sphincter relaxes. This recto-anal reflex is absent in babies with Hirschsprung's disease (a rare cause of constipation). The stool descends and the sensation of the stool in the upper part of the anal canal leads to brief straining of the abdominal muscles, relaxation of the external sphincter, and passage of the stool.

## Causes

Hard stools are difficult to pass along this crooked path and any resulting pain immediately causes a reflex protective tensing of the pelvic floor and external sphincter muscles. This could lead to retention of the stool or painful sticking of the stool halfway out of the anus. It could also lead to tearing of the delicate folds of the anal canal and a fissure that might be persistent because it is reopened by the subsequent hard stool. This vicious circle ↑ while the stool is withheld; stool accumulates, becoming larger and harder to pass.

As the child grows older, reflex tensing of the withholding muscles becomes more voluntary and efficient at delaying defecation. This could be associated with episodes of screaming, hiding, and avoidance of all contact until the offending stool is passed, with even more pain and fear. Parents become ↑ distraught at seeing their child's distress and desperately try all the suggestions given by friends and relatives. Many of these can add to the distress and fear in the child, e.g. holding the child over hot water, pushing in soap 'suppositories', and using real suppositories or enemas provided by health professionals. Parents' anxiety is heightened by fears that the problem is caused by disease of the bowel, especially because many families might have older members who have died from bowel malignancy in which a change in bowel habit was one of the first signs. Other factors may include:

• Congenital anorectal or neurological conditions.
• Developmental problems—learning disability or autism.
• Poor or chaotic diet and inadequate fluid intake.
• Failure to establish a toileting routine during toilet training.
• Social deprivation and maternal depression.

- Behavioural or psychological problems.
- Fear of toilets.
- A cycle of chronic ignoring of sensation, hard stool, and anal pain—
  deferring as long as possible.
- Severe loading—might also result in FI or staining.

## Further reading

Clayden GS and Hollins G (2004). Constipation and faecal incontinence in childhood. In: Norton C and Chelvanayagam S (eds). *Bowel Continence Nursing*. Beaconsfield Publishers, Beaconsfield. Patient information. http://www.digestivedisorders.org.uk (accessed 14.05.07).

# Constipation in children: assessment and management

## History and examination
- Symptoms.
- Onset.
- Pattern.
- Lifestyle.
- Family dynamics.
- Diet—type, amount, and timing.
- Fluids.
- Psychological/behavioural problems.
- Abdominal palpation could indicate faecal loading.
- Avoid rectal/anal examination unless the problem persists because it could alienate the child.

## Investigation
Investigations are not usually indicated unless the child has been constipated since birth (suspect Hirschsprung's disease). An abdominal X-ray should be performed to confirm loading. Occasionally, a history of sexual abuse or neglect is relevant.

## Management
Even with the best advice regarding limiting the amount of cows' milk that toddlers ingest, maximizing fluid and fibre intake, and sympathetic handling of the frightened child, active medical treatment is usually needed. If the stools are hard, softening them with lactulose or docusate might be helpful and, in children >2 years, macrogols can be valuable. Many children rapidly develop their stool-withholding to such a degree that many days could elapse in which nothing is passed. Overcoming this protective response usually requires the use of stimulant laxatives, such as senna, picosulfate, or bisacodyl. The aim is to boost the body's reflex attempts to clear the lower bowel against the child's learned response to tense every muscle in the region at the first sensation of potential stool movement. Because most of these children are between 1 and 3 years of age, it is hopeless to try to reason with them. More success is achieved by softening the residual stool and then creating a softer and more complete daily stool using an evening dose of a stimulant (e.g. senna). Parents are naturally reluctant to start their child on laxatives because they are aware of the myths about causing lazy bowels. However, this can be combated by explaining that a lazy bowel causes diarrhoea, rather than constipation, and the laxative regimen aims to prevent future problems, such as the slow but steady development of the megarectum that can occur with persistent rectal faecal loading.

### Key elements of management
- Explanation—engage the child and parents.
- Ascertain whether the toilet is feared—make the toilet appealing.
- Allow sufficient time and privacy for bowel emptying in the morning.
- Sit comfortably with feet supported—use a footstool if needed.

- Eat breakfast and try toileting 20–30 min later.
- Adequate fibre and fluid intake—not easy with some children.
- Avoid holding breath and straining.
- Push using abdominal muscles and relax anus.
- Consider simple rewards, e.g. a star chart.
- Avoid punishments/reprimands.
- Always respond to 'urge' and do not defer—make an arrangement with the teacher.

## Further reading

Clayden GS and Hollins G (2004). Constipation and faecal incontinence in childhood. In: Norton C and Chelvanayagam S (eds). *Bowel Continence Nursing*. Beaconsfield Publishers, Beaconsfield.
Patient information. http://www.digestivedisorders.org.uk (accessed 14.05.07).

# Constipation in children: other issues

## Severe constipation

In severely constipated children, consider painful anal conditions (e.g. anal fissure). Several months of laxative treatment might be required to force the establishment of a pattern. Senna is most commonly used (for up to 1 year in severe cases).

## Older children

If faecal retention persists, the capacity of the older child's rectum could increase until the residual stool virtually becomes resident, with only overflow faecal leakage preventing intestinal obstruction. However, this leakage causes major psychological and social problems because the child's FI becomes a major embarrassment and life-spoiling feature. If this state develops, it takes many years of laxative treatment, often with in-patient treatment, or surgical disimpaction of stools, intensive medical and nursing follow-up, and intensive psychotherapy for any change to occur and persist.

## Prevention

Apart from trying to prevent the onset of constipation by advocating breastfeeding and plenty of fluid and fibre at weaning, the health professional must take all these worries seriously and share parents' concerns regarding the intensity of suffering that these children endure. Provided micturition is not a problem, most parents can be reassured that the cause of the problem is not likely to be malignancy, which is extremely rare in childhood and usually involves the bladder more commonly than the bowel. Conditions such as congenital anal stenosis, stricture, and Hirschsprung's disease usually present in the first week of life; vomiting with distension and poor weight gain are likely to be major features.

## Further reading

Clayden GS and Hollins G (2004). Constipation and faecal incontinence in childhood. In: Norton C and Chelvanayagam S (eds). *Bowel Continence Nursing*. Beaconsfield Publishers, Beaconsfield. Patient information. http://www.digestivedisorders.org.uk (accessed 14.05.07).

# Toilet training

There are no strict rules for acquiring faecal and urinary continence. Families' expectations are varied, with both extremes of very early or 'wait and see' putting the child at risk of impaired toilet training. Expectations of a child being out of nappies by 2 years of age are bound to lead to disappointment in the majority of parents, with the risk of the use of force or punishment that further delays success. Families that seem to show no interest in helping the child to achieve social continence could be presenting evidence of neglect and are certainly delaying the child's progress in toilet-training education. Society could also handicap the child who normally develops continence late. Because ~10% of 3-year-olds have unreliable continence, the insistence of nurseries and play groups for children to be out of nappies by this age is clearly unreasonable.

Similar to learning other skills, children need the opportunity to learn, rather than strict training. An alert parent will notice the subtle change in activity, contemplative stare or frown, and slight reddening around the eyes that suggests a stool is imminent. If they playfully sit the child on the pot at that stage, a successful stool could reward them. If the child sees the pleasure that this gift generates, a repeat performance is more probable. However, if the stool is greeted with disgust or the placing of the child on the pot is rough or in anger, the learning experience is negated.

There is nothing natural about wearing nappies or having pots and lavatories. It does seem instinctive that children tend to seclude themselves before passing stools. ∴ a degree of privacy in the positioning of the pot is wise, especially if the child has been accustomed to finding a corner or hidden place for defecation when they were in nappies. Making the most of the gastrocolic reflex (the urge to defecate following the ingestion of a meal) ↑ the success rate of a stool ending up in the right place.

The use of structured reward systems, such as instant rewards or stars on charts, is usually unnecessary but could speed the learning process if the child is reluctant to leave other activities to visit the pot or lavatory. Urinary continence is helped by regular visits to the pot/lavatory and catching the child dry, rather than reinforcing the disappointments of being wet. Requests that are too frequent could ↑ resistance in even the most easy-going child.

# Toddler diarrhoea

The most efficient and relaxed pot training can be extremely difficult if the child has frequent, urgent, and loose stools. The term 'toddler diarrhoea' is used for this problem. Many parents might have already consulted health professionals regarding the looseness and frequency of stools in their 12–24-month-old child and should have been reassured if the child's health, weight gain, and relative height are normal.

Simple advice:
- Cut down on the intake of fruit juices.
- Cut down excessive availability of sweet drinks (if the child is using the drinks as recreational sweets).
- Avoid early pot training in these children.
- Provide rapid access to the pot/lavatory to avoid accidents.

Consider:
- Investigate to exclude coeliac disease and cystic fibrosis.
- Investigate cows' milk protein intolerance if misery and respiratory symptoms present.
- Investigate other food intolerance if allergic symptoms of eczema/asthma.
- IBD.
- Older child: frequent loose stool soiling may be retention with 'overflow'.

These toddlers grow well and happily but continue to pass >3 stools/day (the normal defecation frequency range is accepted as being between once every 3 days to three times daily). Pot training challenges the acceptance of this problem as a variation of normal. A child who has several loose stools daily clearly has more opportunity to pass stools on the pot or lavatory, but the urgency rarely gives them a chance to get there in time, even if maximally motivated. Parents are naturally less keen to allow the child to wander around without a nappy if the looseness of the stool poses a risk to clothing and furniture. Fortunately, most children learn to rush to the lavatory in time and most parents learn to avoid giving their child the particular drink or food that further accelerates the stool. Provided there is no evidence of IBD or poor weight gain, a small dose of loperamide might help the child to reach the lavatory in time, especially if otherwise they could miss out on the valuable social experience of a nursery or play group. Parents should be warned to use this only at socially important times, otherwise frequent use could precipitate constipation. In the older child, frequent loose stools in clothing are more likely to be owing to constipation with overflow, especially if there is a past history of dry stools, rather than the classic wet stool of toddler diarrhoea. Bowel-slowing agents, such as loperamide, would make this situation worse, but the history should be the best guide.

# Inflammatory bowel disease in children

## Presentation
The commonest form of IBD in children is ulcerative colitis (UC) or Crohn's disease (CD). The onset could be from the age of 4 years upwards, with an ↑ prevalence with age.

### Ulcerative colitis
The disease presents with diarrhoea, blood and mucus per rectum (PR), urgency, and tenesmus (especially if there is proctitis). It can present with systemic features alone, e.g. weight loss and pallor.

### Crohn's disease
CD might be more insidious and delayed in presentation than UC. Symptoms include abdominal pain, diarrhoea, weight loss, growth impairment, delayed puberty, mouth ulcers, unexplained fevers, perianal disease, and blood and mucus PR. It can present with systemic features alone, especially if the adolescent denies their symptoms, e.g. weight loss, fatigue, and fevers. Look for skin manifestations, e.g. erythema nodosum.

### Other IBDs
Children <4 years of age can also develop IBD, but this is commonly microscopic colitis, indeterminate colitis, or eosinophilic allergic colitis. Symptoms include persistent diarrhoea, rectal bleeding, or failure to thrive, with or without other phenomena relating to food allergies.

## Diagnosis
- Treatment depends on the type of IBD—endoscopic and histological diagnosis is mandatory.
- At diagnosis, most children will have abnormal inflammatory markers:
  - ↑ platelet count, ESR, and/or CRP.
  - ↓ albumin and haemoglobin.
- Supportive radiology includes ultrasound evidence of terminal ileitis for CD and barium follow-through to determine the extent of small bowel involvement.
- All children and adolescents require gastroscopy and colonoscopy, with biopsies, to confirm the type of IBD. Most children <16 years of age will require a general anaesthetic to tolerate endoscopy.
- ↑ use of wireless capsule endoscopy will ↓ the need for repeat X-ray investigations of the small bowel.
- Bone densitometry assesses the impact of disease and treatment on bone mineralization.

## Assessment of growth
- Many children with IBD will have growth impairment if there is a delay in diagnosis or presence of active disease.
- Growth can be assessed by measuring height and weight, plotting these data on paediatric growth charts, and comparing the measurements with the expected centiles.

- Pubertal staging should be assessed to determine whether this is delayed—look at pubic hair, genitalia, and breast development.
- A wrist X-ray will determine the bone age—assessment of pubertal stage.

## Treatment

IBD in children and adolescents often requires intensive treatment regimens. Treatment options differ from adult practice, because there is an emphasis on growth. Multidisciplinary teams, including nurses, doctors, endoscopy staff, child and adolescent mental health services, social workers, teachers, play specialists, stoma nurses, paediatric pharmacists, dietitians, and doctors must work in a coordinated fashion to manage all aspects of the child's care.

## Ulcerative colitis

Special considerations in children:
- Anti-inflammatory products, such as 5-aminosalicylic acid (5-ASA)—requires biochemistry analysis every 3 months.
- Rectal therapies, such as steroids and 5-ASA-based enemas, to ↓ symptoms of proctitis.
- Oral steroids to induce remission, with weaning over 4–8 weeks, depending on the severity of disease.
- Early use of steroid-sparing agents, such as azathioprine, to ↓ risk of steroid toxicity in steroid-dependent children—risk of bone-marrow suppression, needing frequent blood counts.
- Acute severe or fulminant UC requires hospitalization, regular review (with a high risk of colonic perforation), and IV ciclosporin (± IV monoclonal antibody)—there is a >50% risk of colectomy.
- Steroid dependency despite immunosuppression, growth failure, and failure of medical management will necessitate colectomy and formation of an ileostomy. Stoma reversal requires formation of an ileo-anal pouch and carries considerable risk of pouchitis. ∴ stoma closure could be delayed.

## Crohn's disease

Special considerations in children.
- Treatment options depend on the extent and site of disease, degree of malnutrition at diagnosis, pubertal staging, and compliance with therapy.
- Exclusive enteral nutrition for 8 weeks induces remission in small bowel disease and terminal ileitis but requires supervision. This reverses the nutritional and growth sequelae related to CD, but some children find the feed unpalatable. ∴ polymeric feeding is preferred to elemental feeding. Nasogastric tubes or gastrostomy might be required for protracted courses of therapy.
- Steroid therapy induces remission but is avoided in children with poor nutrition and prepubertal children. This should be combined with early introduction of steroid-sparing agents, e.g. azathioprine or 6-mercaptopurine.

- Monoclonal antibody anti-TNF therapy IV every 8 weeks for steroid dependency or failure of steroid therapy. Also indicated in fistulating perianal disease.
- Surgical resection of the affected bowel—most commonly used in patients with terminal ileitis, stricturing disease, failure to respond to medical management, or growth failure.

### Transition to adult practice

The transition from paediatric gastroenterology services (in which the emphasis is on growth, nutrition, steroid-sparing therapies, puberty, and schooling) to busy adult practices needs careful planning and a multidisciplinary transition service to avoid fragmentation of care and continuity as the adolescent moves from home and school.

Some hospitals have set up dedicated IBD clinics for adolescents to manage this transition.

### Further reading

Patient information can be obtained from the National Association of Colitis and Crohn's Disease, which has a group for young people and guidelines on transition clinics.

# Bowel care and vulnerable groups

Bowel care in frail older people  672
Learning disabilities  673
Cultural issues  674
Religious practices and bowel care  676

# Bowel care in frail older people

## Problems

- Constipation (can be 'simple' response to environmental factors, or slow transit, or rectal outlet delay).
- Faecal incontinence (FI)—20–50% of older people in nursing homes.
- Rectal loading (faecal impaction) with 'overflow' soiling in immobile and confused people.
- Bowels are a major concern of many older people—self-report of problems is possibly higher than the actual prevalence.
- Older people who are well are no more likely to be constipated than young adults.
- FI is more common in both sexes with advancing age—can lead to breakdown of community care.
- The majority of residents in care homes have some bowel problems.

Multiple possible underlying problems and potential causes:
- Diet and fluid intake.
- Immobility, loss of independence, and/or inability to toilet independently.
- Polypharmacy.
- Depression, lack of motivation, and intellectual impairment.
- Muscle weakness (anal or abdominal) or diminished sensation (rectal).
- Hormonal (e.g. thyroid problems).
- Multiple comorbidities—neurological, endocrine, or diabetes.
- Loose stools—over-use of laxatives, overactive thyroid, antibiotics, infection, tube feeding, diabetes, or diet.

## Assessment

- History, symptoms, bowel pattern, examination, and rectal examination for faecal loading and anal tone (📖 p. 514).
- Bowel diary.
- Plain abdominal X-ray if colonic loading is in doubt.
- Rectal prolapse possible if there is passive soiling (📖 p. 531).
- If bleeding, weight loss, unexplained change in bowel habit, and anaemia are present, consider investigation for bowel cancer.
- Involve the psychology team if dementia is present.

## Treatment

- Ensure toilet access at suitable time intervals.
- Dementia—patients might need prompting to use toilet.
- Very few intervention studies.
- Constipation—disimpact, if needed; diet, fluids, and change medications, if possible. Suppositories/micro-enemas can be controlled more easily than laxatives.
- FI—disimpact if needed; bowel habit and timing. Loperamide for loose stools (take care not to constipate).

## Further reading

Potter J, Norton C and Cottenden A (2002). *Bowel Care in Older People*. Royal College of Physicians, London.

# Learning disabilities

The patient/client with learning disabilities (LD) can also have any of the other bowel disorders or diseases described in this book. It should never be presumed that symptoms are associated with LD, unless a complete differential diagnosis has been considered.

## Communication

People with LD are known to have poor access to healthcare and many unmet needs. Communication and a mutually understood vocabulary can be difficult or impossible. Social carers might consider it inappropriate to monitor bowel function. It can be difficult to establish the nature of bowel symptoms and presentation can be late.

## Constipation

Might be due to coexisting neurological or behavioural (e.g. ignoring the call to stool) disorders. Could present with vague abdominal discomfort, agitation, behavioural changes (e.g. aggression), or non-specific distress.

## Faecal incontinence

Related to the severity of LD. Affects 3% of mild cases of LD at 7 years of age and 85% of cases of profound LD at 20 years of age: few adults with mild LD have FI; at least 50% prevalence in those with profound LD. FI is usually the result of the following:
• Severe rectal loading and 'overflow' soiling.
• Intellectual impairment or misunderstanding of social rules.
• Failure to systematically toilet train.
• Behavioural disorders.

## Anal digitations

Might be the result of local discomfort (e.g. haemorrhoids or manual removal of faeces); occasionally for pleasurable sensations. Can lead to smearing behaviour, which is difficult for carers to tolerate.

## Toilet training

▶ Start at the usual chronological age. Break down behaviours into manageable steps, and train and reinforce each behaviour individually (e.g. recognition of the need to defecate, getting to the toilet, removal of underwear, sitting, pushing, cleaning, and replacement of clothing). Will often need patience and persistence. Independence might not be possible in cases of severe LD. Various behavioural programmes have been described. The LD team can support.

## Further reading

Smith L and Smith P (2004). Bowel control and intellectual disability. In: Norton C and Chelvanayagam S (eds). *Bowel Continence Nursing*. Beaconsfield Publishers, Beaconsfield.

# Cultural issues

For centuries, people with a variety of histories, cultures, beliefs, and languages have settled in the UK. Although the incidence of disease predisposing to bowel surgery is lower in ethnic communities, there is evidence that the second and third generations demonstrate an ↑ in conditions such as ulcerative colitis, bowel cancer, and familial adenomatous polyposis (Table 19.1).

Cultural background influences a patient's perceptions, behaviour, and concepts of, and attitudes to, disease, illness, and pain. Dietary concerns of those on strict vegetarian diets or fasting as a part of religious practice might lead to difficulties with bowel function or investigation of bowel dysfunction.

Cultural issues must obviously be considered in bowel care, particularly before bowel surgery, in particular when related to stoma formation. Aspects such as clothing, language, and food are all evident, but consideration is also needed with regard to patients' attitudes towards health, illness, and death. Some might have specific beliefs about bodily excretions and consider them as polluting, leading to an unwillingness to care for the stoma. Many patients from ethnic minorities come from extended families where, in some cases, the oldest member of the family is responsible for the decision-making on behalf on the entire family.

Communication can prove difficult because of differences in language. Interpreters are useful, but their use can be difficult during counselling sessions in which a discussion of intimate issues, such as sex and body image, takes place. Arranged marriages remain the tradition in some cultures, and the entire family could be discredited by their community after a bowel surgery that results in stoma formation.

**Table 19.1** Incidence of GI-related diseases around the world[1]

| Disease | High incidence | Low incidence |
| --- | --- | --- |
| Ulcerative colitis | USA (Jews) | Eastern Europe |
| | South Africa (Jews) | Asia |
| | | South America |
| | | Israel (Ashkenazi Jews) |
| Crohn's disease | Europe | India |
| | Scandinavia | Tropical Africa |
| | North America | South America |
| | Australia | |
| Colorectal cancer | Western Europe | Japan |
| | USA | |
| | Australia | |
| Diverticular disease | Western Europe | Africa? |
| | Far Eastern countries and Asia | |

1 Breckman B (2005). *Stoma Care and Rehabilitation* Amsterdam. Elsevier, pp. 261–2.

# Religious practices and bowel care

Some religious groups may have particular issues with bowel care. The most common are listed in Table 19.2.

**Table 19.2** Religious issues in bowel care

| Religion | Religious practice | Considerations |
|---|---|---|
| Hindu | No standard form of worship | |
| | Some fast once a week | Nutritional status |
| | Hindu ♀ are modest and might request ♀ assistance only | Staff skill mix |
| | Some strict Hindu ♂ might not allow any ♂ healthcare professional to assist in wife's care | Staff skill mix |
| | Hindu ♀ should be offered two theatre gowns to ensure they are covered | Dignity/body image |
| | Long hair is important | |
| | Hindus will not eat any food that involves the taking of life | Nutritional status |
| | The cow (beef) is considered a sacred animal; pigs (pork) are considered unclean | Some medications/ creams contain beef or pork extracts |
| | ♀ might need to consult their husbands before signing their consent form | Consent/patient information |
| | Marriages may be arranged | Altered body image/sexual health |
| Sikh | Five religious symbols—uncut hair, comb, steel bangle, dagger, and white shorts | Shaving |
| | Bodily hair should not be removed | |
| | White shorts worn as underwear | |
| | Sikh ♀ often wear a head scarf | |
| | Sikh ♀ prefer to be cared for by ♀ healthcare professionals | Staff skill mix |
| | Could prefer not to eat beef | Some medications/ creams contain beef extracts |
| | Alcohol is forbidden | Some medications contain alcohol |

**Table 19.2** (*Contd.*)

| Religion | Religious practice | Considerations |
|---|---|---|
| Muslim | Set prayers five times/day, including a washing ritual beforehand | |
| | Very particular about cleanliness | Dignity, body image, and spirituality |
| | Faeces are considered unclean | Stoma cleansing/ appliance change |
| | Some prayer takes place lying down on the abdomen | Abdominal wounds/presence of newly formed stoma |
| | The right hand is used for greeting; the left hand is for cleaning | Stoma management |
| | The area above the umbilicus is considered clean and the area below it is considered unclean | Stoma siting |
| | Mostly vegetarian | Nutritional status and bowel function |
| | Halal meat | Bowel function and hydration |
| | Ramadan | |
| | Fatwa ruling | Stoma management |
| Jewish | Sabbath | Stoma management |
| | Mikveh—a ritual bath is taken in relation to the menstrual cycle | Sexuality/body image/relationships |
| | Pork and derivatives are prohibited | Nutritional status |
| | Kosher-prepared foods | Some medications/ creams contain pork extracts |

# Complementary therapies in bowel disorders

Complementary therapies in gastrointestinal
    nursing  680
Irritable bowel syndrome and complementary
    and alternative medicine  682
Colorectal cancer and complementary
    and alternative medicine  684

# Complementary therapies in gastrointestinal nursing

There has been ↑ interest in complementary and alternative medicine (CAM) and there are now an estimated 2 million users of CAM in the UK.

## Definition

Complementary therapies are used in combination with conventional medicine (e.g. massage, aromatherapy, and reflexology). Alternative therapies can be used instead of conventional treatment (e.g. traditional Chinese medicine and homeopathy).

## Common profile of the CAM user

- Educated.
- Higher income.
- Holistic perspective of healthcare.
- ♀.
- Poorer health status.
- Chronic condition.
- Aged 30–49 years.
- Single.
- Urban dweller.

## Commonly used therapies in GI disorders

- Homeopathy.
- Acupuncture.
- Traditional Chinese medicine.
- Herbal medicine.
- Massage/Shiatsu.
- Ayurvedic medicine.
- Reflexology.
- Bach flower remedies.
- Naturopathy.
- Probiotics/acidophilus.
- Hypnotherapy.
- Biofeedback.
- Relaxation/meditation.
- Aromatherapy.

Many patients use more than one therapy, but there is little research evidence to support many therapies.

## Implications for GI nurses

- Must be knowledgeable about CAM.
- Must initiate discussion with patients.
- Must find out which therapies patients are using and advise about the appropriate use of CAM.

## Reasons for using CAM

- CAM complements conventional medicine.
- Safety.
- Serious side effects from conventional medicine.
- Lack of satisfaction with conventional medicine.
- To avoid surgery.
- Lack confidence in conventional medicine.
- Need for greater autonomy/control.
- Desire to feel better.
- Hope for a cure.
- Therapy made more sense.
- Advised by family and friends.
- Recommended by the doctor.
- Read about CAM on the Internet.

## Further reading

Ernst E, Pitler MH, Stevinson C and White A (2001). *The Desktop Guide to Complementary and Alternative Medicine: An Evidence-based Approach* Mosby, Edinburgh.

McGovern K, Lockhart A, Malay P, Palatnik AM, Stiebeling B (2002). *Nurse's Handbook of Alternative and Complementary Therapies* (2nd edn). Lippincott– and Williams & Wilkins, Philadelphia, PA.

Pittler MH, Wider B and Boddy K (2008). *Oxford Handbook of Complementary Medicine*. Oxford University Press.

Rankin-Box D (2001). *The Nurse's Handbook of Complementary Therapies* (2nd edn). Baillière Tindall, Edinburgh.

Woodward S (2005). Complementary therapies in bowel care. *Gastrointestinal Nursing* **3**, 31–4.

# Irritable bowel syndrome and complementary and alternative medicine

In the UK, 16% of IBS patients use CAM. There is evidence to support the following therapies.
- Hypnosis/hypnotherapy.
- Specific food-avoidance diets.
- Probiotics.
- Several herbal medicines.

## Hypnosis/hypnotherapy

There is up to 70% response rate (symptom improvement). Most utilize the suggestion of colonic relaxation. Therapy improves the following:
- Well-being.
- Pain.
- Bloating.
- Bowel habit/gut motility.

The improvement is early and sustained; a Cochrane review is under way.

## Food-avoidance diets

Avoid foods that trigger an individual's symptoms, e.g. milk or wheat. For some individuals, fibre makes symptoms worse, possibly because of abnormal gut fermentation. This has led to the use of probiotics.

## Probiotics

Effects are unique to particular strains; not all probiotics have the same effectiveness. There is recent evidence to support the use of *Bifidobacterium infantis*:
- Stimulates the anti-inflammatory response.
- Inhibits pathogens.
- Prevents bacterial translocation.

However, there is no long-term follow-up evidence.

## Acupuncture

There is some evidence to support the use of acupuncture, but it is mainly descriptive and limited. A Cochrane review is under way.
There is a potential improvement in the following:
- Bloating.
- Well-being.

## Herbal medicine/traditional Chinese herbal medicine

The evidence is conflicting because of the preparations tested. Some good-quality evidence was found in a Cochrane review, but many different herbs were used. Therapy leads to improvement in the following:
- Pain.
- Diarrhoea.
- Constipation.

No adverse events of therapy have been reported.

## Homeopathy
Constitutional and symptomatic remedies have been tried, but there is little evidence of effectiveness except descriptive and anecdotal reports.

## Stress decrease
Attacks might be triggered by stress, so massage-type therapies might help:
- Massage ± aromatherapy.
- Reflexology.

Patients claim therapy helps, but there is little research evidence to support the claim.

## Implications for GI nurses
- Helps patients feel in control.
- Unlikely to cause harm.
- May be expensive as few CAMs available on NHS.
- Current lack of evidence base and ability to select patients likely to benefit.
- Unlikely that any therapy will offer a cure.
- Nurses need to be aware of therapies that have stronger supporting evidence than others.
- Options must be discussed with patients.

# Colorectal cancer and complementary and alternative medicine

Up to 30% of colorectal cancer patients use CAM in the UK. Cancer and palliative care services are at the forefront of integrating CAM services in the UK.

### Predictors of CAM use
- Vegetarian diet.
- Age under 50 years.
- ♀.
- Doctor has recommended its use.
- Changes in bowel habit or fatigue pre-diagnosis.
- Chemotherapy use.

Use of CAM ↑ after the cancer diagnosis.

### Reasons for CAM use
- ↑ hope/hope for cure.
- Belief that CAM is non-toxic.
- Wanting more involvement/control in therapy.
- Improved well-being.

### Commonly used CAM
- Herbal medicine.
- Homeopathy.
- Traditional Chinese medicine (TCM), mainly herbal.
- Vitamins and minerals.
- Alternative diets.
- Aromatherapy/massage.
- Reflexology.
- Acupuncture.

Weak evidence for the effectiveness of TCM from a Cochrane review supports the treatment of chemotherapy side effects with CAM to improve the immune response, i.e. nausea and vomiting, stimulate white blood cell production, and improved appetite. There is no evidence of harm from CAM.

There is limited evidence to support most therapies and the quality of studies is poor, but a lack of evidence does not mean CAM is ineffective.

There is also no evidence that massage, for example, causes metastases.

### Main benefits of CAM
- ↓ anxiety, stress, pain, and fatigue.
- Improved sleep, well-being, and nausea.

### Implications for GI nurses
- CAM is often used without the knowledge of the doctor or nurse.
- Colorectal cancer nurses must provide patients with accurate information about CAM. The aims of therapy are to offer addition support, enhance quality of life, and symptomatic relief. CAM is not curative.

# Further reading

Tavares M (2003). *National Guidelines for Use of Complementary Therapies in Supportive and Palliative Care*. Prince of Wales' Foundation for Integrated Health. http://www.fih.org.uk (accessed 15.05.07).

# Pain management

Introduction *688*
Assessment of acute pain *689*
Drug treatments for pain management *690*
Post-operative pain management *694*
Post-operative nursing care in pain management *696*
Chronic non-malignant pain in gastrointestinal
   disorders *698*

# Introduction

A patient with pain related to a gastrointestinal (GI) disorder is one of the most complicated patients to assess because of the vast number of other complex issues surrounding their care. There could be numerous other factors to consider, such as taking an extensive medical or surgical history, probable long-standing chronic pain, underlying acute pain, short bowel syndrome, or absorption problems. In addition, there could also be other issues to consider, such as the following.

- Previous analgesic history—the patient might not be opioid naive.
- ↑ nausea and vomiting.
- Malnutrition—the patient might be receiving IV nutrition or parenteral feeding.
- Poor IV access.
- A possible history of drug misuse.
- The psychological impact of GI disease, e.g. Crohn's disease or ulcerative colitis.
- The patient might not have a rectal route.

# Assessment of acute pain

There are a number of pain assessment tools designed to identify the type of pain the person is experiencing and to evaluate the analgesic effect of therapy. Pain assessment involves interviewing the patient or relatives and asking questions regarding the patient's pain using the following methods.

• Body charts—to identify the location of pain.
• Scales, e.g. a visual analogue scale (VAS) or categorical scale (e.g. 5-point scale) to assess the degree of pain. A score of 5 is excruciating pain and a score of 0 is no pain.
• Pain diary—to establish the times that pain occurs, duration of pain, whether there is an identifiable trigger before the onset of pain. Used more frequently for patients with chronic pain.
• Pain questionnaires, e.g. McGill Pain Questionnaire.

## Further reading

Melzack R (1975). The McGill Pain Questionnaire: major properties and scoring methods. *Pain* **1**, 277–99.

# Drug treatments for pain management

Analgesia should be given regularly to enable continuous elevation and stability of the blood serum level of the analgesic; on demand medication should be used for breakthrough pain relief.

The oral route of administration should always be considered before using other routes, although IV paracetamol can be administered because of its efficacy in acute pain.

Pain protocols are designed by each hospital trust as a working policy to ensure the safety of both the patient and the staff administering the drug. Refer to your individual hospital policy.

The World Health Organization analgesic ladder[1] should be referred to for guidance in moving the patient from one analgesic stage to another. The analgesic ladder comprises three steps: non-opioid-based drugs, weak opioid drugs, and strong opioid drugs.

The analgesic or pain ladder in Fig. 21.1 is standard for most hospital trusts. However, note that some hospital policies differ slightly in their recommendations for weak and strong opioids (e.g. the use of tramadol in step 2 or 3).

## Step 1: non-opioid drugs

The non-opioid drug used is usually either paracetamol or aspirin. The analgesic effect lasts for ~4 h and ∴ frequent doses are needed to maintain adequate pain relief.

## Step 2: weak opioid drugs

Weak opioids include codeine and dihydrocodeine. These drugs are effective for moderate pain relief and 1–2 tablets every 6 h should provide good pain relief.

## Step 3: strong opioid drugs

These drugs include morphine, diamorphine, fentanyl, pethidine, oxycodone, hydromorphone, and methadone.

1 World Health Organization (2007). *Analgesic Ladder.* http://www.who.int/cancer/palliative/painladder/en/ (accessed 15.05.07).

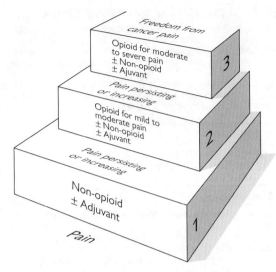

**Fig. 21.1** Analgesic ladder.

**WHO analgesic ladder**

If pain occurs prompt oral administration of drugs should be given, following the guidelines of the analgesic ladder—Step 1: non-opioids, Step 2: weak opioids, and Step 3: strong opioids. To reassure patients and assist in sustaining pain relief, additional drugs (adjuvants) should be used. To maintain pain relief, drugs need to be administered regularly rather than 'on demand'. This is the three-step approach of administering the right drug in the right dose at the right time. NB In acute pain episodes it is important to remember this three-step approach, but also include the right route for efficacy purposes (IV, SC, or IM).

---

**Step 1: mild pain**

Non-opioids (+ additional drugs).
• Simple analgesics: e.g. paracetamol 1 g four times daily.

---

**Step 2: moderate pain**

Weak opioids (+ additional drugs). Weak opioids such as codeine added (not substituted).
• Codeine + paracetamol used separately or as co-codamol (various strengths available).
• Dihydrocodeine + paracetamol used separately or as co-dydramol (various strengths available).

---

**Step 3: severe pain**

Strong opioids with non-opioids (+ additional drugs). Strong opioids— titrate to establish pain control. NB There is no ceiling level for morphine. Refer to pain service for further management.
1. Morphine 5 g–10 mg every 4 h.
   Oxycodone 2.5 g–5 mg every 4 h.
2. Subcutaneous rate infusion (not the same as a palliative care prescription):
   Morphine sulphate 60 mg/19 ml NaCl made up to 19 ml at a rate of 0–6 mm/h.
   Diamorphine 30 mg/19 ml NaCl at a rate of 0–6 mm/h.
   Oxycodone, same regimen as the morphine SC pump.
3. IV morphine PCA 60 mg/30 ml NaCl (2 mg/ml, 1–2 mg boluses and 5 min lock-out).
4. IM (acute pain only for a maximum of 3 days) morphine.
5. Buprenorphine 4 days or 7 days patches in various strengths.
   Fentanyl 3 days patches.
   Durogesic D-trans-fentanyl patch, 12 mcg /h to bridge gaps between fentanyl patches 25 mcg, 50 mcg, 75 mcg, and 100 mcg.

**The following regimens should only be used after discussion with the pain team:**

- Methadone, 5–10 mg every 6–8 h; decrease to once daily for long-term use.
- Hydromorphone 1.3 mg every 4 h increased if necessary.
- Pethidine is not highly recommended because of its side-effect profile. Discuss with the pain team.
- ▶ Avoid prescribing multiple opioids. Use half the dose stated above if the patient is >80 years.

# Post-operative pain managment

There are different options, depending on patient need (Table 21.1).

## Patient-controlled analgesia (PCA)

This enables the patient to self-administer analgesia, usually through an IV route, by pressing a hand-held device. The machine is programmed to provide a predetermined bolus dose when the patient activates the device. A lock-out period provides a safeguard by ensuring the patient can only receive a set amount of analgesia at predetermined intervals.

If the patient has difficulties with absorption, short-term morphine PCA should be considered for acute pain episodes. Oxycodone, fentanyl, or diamorphine can be used instead of morphine. Note that different drug dosages apply for these drugs.

## Subcutaneous injection or continuous subcutaneous pump

SC drugs can be injected but, if required regularly, they can be used through 'Y cannulas', to avoid repeated injections, or SC pumps, to enable continuous infusion.

## Transdermal patches

These patches are applied to the trunk or limbs and are ideal for administering analgesia if the oral route is not always accessible. This route provides minimal fluctuations in the plasma level of the analgesic.

▶ Before commencing administration of a transdermal patch, recognize that the lowest dose of a fentanyl patch (25 mcg/h) is ~135 mg of oral morphine in a 24-h period and the lowest dose of a Transtec buprenorphine patch (35 mcg/h) is ~30–60 mg of oral morphine in a 24-h period.

## Sublingual or buccal route

The sublingual (under the tongue) or buccal (between the upper lip and upper gum) routes can be used. Drugs absorbed through the mouth, rather than swallowed, pass directly into the systemic circulation. This enables drugs to bypass first-pass metabolism (hence eliminating the usual chemical activity that ingested drugs undergo through the gut and liver).

## Lozenges (Fentanyl–Actiq® with oromucosal applicator)

Lozenges can be used for breakthrough pain relief for patients already receiving opioid analgesia. This can be repeated, if necessary, after 15 min, but the patient should not receive >2 doses/pain episode. If there is a need for >2 lozenges, move up to the next dose strength. A maximum of four doses in a 24-h period should be given; however, if the patient requires lozenges >4 times daily, consider ↑ background analgesia.

## Non-steroidal anti-inflammatory drugs (NSAIDs)

NSAIDS must be administered with care. The most common hazard associated with NSAID use is GI intolerance and ulceration. Because NSAID metabolites are eliminated by the kidney, renal toxicity should also be considered. The risk seems to rise with ↑ length of treatment and ↑ doses. Ibuprofen has a low gut toxicity and diclofenac has a medium risk of GI side effects.

### Intravenous paracetamol

Paracetamol is generally noted to be rapidly and completely absorbed from the GIT without any GI side effects but the drug could have effects on renal blood flow under certain circumstances. The drug can be administered IV, orally, or per rectum at a dose of 1 g four times daily.

**Table 21.1** Post-operative pain management

| | |
|---|---|
| **PCA** | Morphine, 60 mg/30 ml NaCl as 1 mg/ 2 mg boluses and 5 min lock-out |
| **SC analgesia pump** | |
| SC morphine | Morphine, 60 mg/19 ml sodium chloride (1 mg/mm) |
| SC diamorphine | Diamorphine, 30 mg/19 ml sodium chloride (0.5 mg/mm) |
| **Transdermal patches** | |
| Fentanyl transdermal patches are available in dose strengths 12 mcg/h to enable dose titration | 25 mcg/h, 50 mcg/h, 75 mcg/h, and 100 mcg/h (there is no upper dose limit) |
| Buprenorphine matrix patches (Transtec®) are available for use after weak opioids in severe chronic pain | 35 mcg/h, 52.5 mcg/h, and 70 mcg/h, which last for 3 days (licensed for 4-day use) |
| Buprenorphine 7 day patches (Bu Trans®) are low-dose opioid patches | 5 mcg/h, 10 mcg/h, and 20 mcg/h, which last for 7 days |
| **Sublingual or buccal route** | |
| Sublingual buprenorphine | 200–400 mcg every 8 h |
| **Lozenges** | |
| Fentanyl lozenges | 200 mcg over a period of 15 min; if no pain relief wait 15 min and repeat dose (some patients might require an initial starting dose of 400 mcg) |
| | Strengths are 200 mcg, 400 mcg, 600 mcg, 800 mcg, 1.2 mg, and 1.6 mg |

# Post-operative nursing care in pain management

In nursing care, anticipating painful procedures following surgical intervention can assist in relieving most episodes of acute pain (e.g. abdominal dressing changes, especially if accompanied by vacuum therapy, transferring the patient from their bed to a chair, stoma bag changes, or physiotherapy input).

Elements of pain management include:
- Explain all procedures to the patient—aim for good pain relief and not the desire of being pain free.
- Ensure the patient's privacy and dignity is maintained at all times.
- Ensure adequate analgesia is prescribed regularly and that on demand medication is administered at least 20–30 min before a procedure.
- Entonox® therapy—inhaled nitrous oxide has an analgesic and amnesic property that is short-acting but not suitable for every patient.
- Use calming words and distraction techniques, if appropriate.
- Light sedation, e.g. diazepam (2 mg three times daily), can be used in the short term for an anxious patient. Administering temazepam (10 mg) or zopiclone (7.5 mg) at night can aid sleeping. Light sedation in addition to analgesia can be beneficial if side effects such as respiratory depression, hypotension, drowsiness, or light-headedness are carefully monitored during treatment. This is especially important if opioids are also prescribed or ↑.

## Other causes of post-operative pain

Acute pain in patients with GI disorders might not always stem from surgical intervention but could be secondary to other symptoms, which can be relieved by different medications or therapies (Table 21.2).

**Table 21.2** Other causes of post-operative pain

| Symptom | Treatment |
| --- | --- |
| Muscle spasm | Hyoscine butylbromide |
| Gut dysmotility | Further medical/surgical investigation |
| Constipation | Laxatives |
| Obstruction (not necessarily owing to ↑ use of opioids) | Further medical/surgical investigation |
| Wind | Peppermint water or antacids |
| Pain related to nausea and vomiting | Anti-emetics |
| Musculosketal pain due to a lack of mobility, disease process, or prolonged illness | Spasms can be relieved by diazepam (5–10 mg/day) and localized pain might benefit from nerve block therapy/TENS |
| Anxiety related to previous unsatisfactory pain experience | Information and support<br>Relaxation therapy, hypnotherapy, or imagery |
| Psychosocial issues | Referral to a psychology department/unit |

# Chronic non-malignant pain in gastrointestinal disorders

Chronic pain (also referred to as 'persistent pain') is defined as pain that has lasted continuously or intermittently for at least 3 months. It usually involves a combination of psychological, physical, and social factors.

The prevalence of chronic pain after laparotomy for both malignant and non-malignant GI conditions 4 years after surgery is 18%.[1] Patients with chronic pain had poorer functioning, poorer quality of life, and more severe symptoms regardless of age, gender, or whether they had cancer. Risk factors for developing chronic pain include ♀ gender, younger age, and surgery for a benign disease.

## Assessment

For all chronic pain disorders, a biopsychosocial approach is required to assess and treat pain. A pain assessment is performed as described earlier (📖 p. 691) but also includes asking about the patient's functioning and psychosocial factors, such as mood and interpersonal relationships.

Acceptance that the patient's pain is real is crucial, but an explanation that the pain has been compounded by psychological and social factors, should also be provided. Pain causes psychological distress because there is a sensory component combined with an emotional element when pain is experienced. As the pain persists, the emotional element becomes stronger. Psychological issues, such as unresolved grief or childhood sexual abuse, can exacerbate the pain by affecting both the patient's ability to cope and their mood. Social issues relate to how the person displays their pain and the effects it has on their interpersonal relationships and employment.

Therefore use of medication as a sole treatment is frequently ineffective and long-term use of opiates can lead to drug dependency and related problems, such as constipation. Use of medication or medical intervention alone can contribute to a patient's belief that their pain is curable (chronic pain is seldom completely resolved). The patient will rely only on this treatment and the prescribing practitioner, rather than developing an awareness of their own role in managing their pain.

## Pain management strategies

The pain assessment is part of the therapeutic process because it helps the patient to understand the precipitating and perpetuating elements of their pain and their role in pain management.

A range of treatments have been used to treat chronic pain, including GI pain:

• Drug treatments—such as simple analgesics (e.g. paracetamol), NSAIDS, tricyclic antidepressants, selective serotonin reuptake inhibitors (SSRIs), and anti-convulsant drugs. Opioids should only be used if other treatments have failed and there is noticeable pain relief from opioids. Regular follow-up should be provided.

---

**1** Bruce J and Krukowski ZH (2006). Quality of life and chronic pain four years after gastrointestinal surgery. *Diseases of the Colon and Rectum* **49**, 1362–70.

- Psychological therapies—such as counselling or group therapy. Cognitive–behavioural therapy is particularly effective for treating chronic pain.
- Massage and manipulation—which might be part of a physiotherapy treatment programme including exercises and hydrotherapy.
- Hypnotherapy—particularly in the treatment of irritable bowel syndrome. Therapy consists of inducing a trance-like state using deep relaxation. Direct suggestion will indicate a ↓ in the patient's pain or explore the cause of the patient's tension.
- Reflexology.
- Transcutaneous electrical nerve stimulation (TENS) machine.
- Acupuncture.
- Relaxation and meditation.
- Imagery.

A comprehensive assessment and the development of a therapeutic relationship are crucial components of pain management strategies because this will ensure that the person who is in pain will receive the most appropriate and effective evidence-based treatments.

# Chapter 22

# Gastrointestinal emergencies

Haematemesis 702
Acute abdominal pain 706
Intestinal obstruction 708
Perforation 710

# Haematemesis

Haematemesis (vomiting blood) can be an emergency, depending on the amount and type of bleeding. Bleeding can be minor or major (which is alarming to the patient), but all forms of bleeding require a full assessment. Emergency resuscitation might be needed. Assess the patient for shock (hypotension, postural hypotension, tachycardia, and collapse). Immediate IV access and blood tests needed. Maintain the airway (suction might be needed). The patient should take nil by mouth until after endoscopy. The nurse must support and reassure the patient and family, who are likely to be very agitated and concerned.

## Mortality

The mortality rate is 10% of admissions overall (the elderly or those with comorbidities are at greater risk). The Rockall score (Tables 22.1 and 22.2) predicts mortality; a low-risk score can fast-track early discharge.

### Fresh blood
Bright red.

### Altered blood (after a few hours in the stomach)
Altered ('coffee ground') appearance. Minor flecks of blood in the vomit might simply be the result of prolonged vomiting.

### Major bleed, shock, or known cirrhosis or alcohol-abusing patient
Immediate IV access and blood cross-matching are sufficient for immediate resuscitation and possible re-bleed. Central venous pressure line and urinary catheter: patients with severe hypotension, older patient, or if this is a re-bleed. The patient might need emergency endoscopy or surgery. Endoscopy should normally be performed in theatre (with support available). It might be possible to inject or ligate a bleeding vessel during endoscopy. However, emergency surgery is necessary if the bleeding cannot be stopped endoscopically.

## Aetiology
- Peptic ulcer—35–50%.
- Oesophageal varices—5–12%, although the mortality rate is >50% if secondary to liver cirrhosis.
- Others—Mallory–Weiss tear, gastric erosion, oesophageal erosion or reflux, gastric cancer, pancreatitis, gallstone perforation of duodenum, swallowing blood (e.g. nosebleeds), swallowed foreign body or poisons, and other rare disorders.
- Children—foreign bodies and the possibility of Munchausen's syndrome by proxy.

## History
- Alcohol abuse.
- Known liver disease.
- Medications—NSAIDs, anticoagulants, or steroids.

## Investigations
### After emergency care
If the source of bleeding is uncertain, perform the following:
- Upper GI endoscopy.
- Liver-function tests.

In 30% of patients, no cause is found.

## Treatment
Depends on cause of bleeding.

### Sclerotherapy or band ligation for varices
Epinephrine, thrombin, fibrin glue, or heat/electrocoagulation, argon plasma coagulation into bleeding ulcer. May need balloon tamponade (▢ p. 192), Sengstaken tube, or use of TIPPS to control bleeding. Surgery is necessary in 20% of patients (the mortality rate is 10%).

### Re-bleeding
30% mortality if re-bleed. IV omeprazole ↓ the risk of re-bleeding in patients with ulcers. If a visible vessel is found in the peptic ulcer at endoscopy, there is a 50% probability of re-bleeding.

### Adherent clot in a peptic ulcer
The probability of re-bleeding is 20%.

### Neither re-bleed nor adherent clot
The probability of re-bleeding is <10%.

## Nursing care
Close monitoring of vital signs. Explanation and appropriate reassurance as patient and family likely to be very anxious.

## Further reading
Palmer K (2004). Management of haematemesis and melaena. *Postgraduate Medical Journal* **80**, 399–404.

**Table 22.1** Rockall score[1] for risk of mortality

| Initial Rockall score | Score |
| --- | --- |
| **Age** | |
| <60 years | 0 |
| 60–79 years | 1 |
| 80+ years | 2 |
| **Shock** | |
| None | 0 |
| Pulse >100 bpm and systolic blood pressure >100 mmHg | 1 |
| Systolic blood pressure <100 mmHg | 2 |
| **Co-morbidity** | |
| None | 0 |
| Cardiac failure or any major co-morbidity | 1 |
| Renal/liver failure or disseminated malignancy | 2 |
| **Initial Rockall score (max. score = 7)** | |
| **Full score after oesophageal gastro-duodenoscopy (OGD)** | |
| **Endoscopic diagnosis** | |
| Mallory–Weiss tear, no lesion seen, and no stigmata of recent haemorrhage | 0 |
| All other diagnoses | 1 |
| Malignancy in upper GI tract | 2 |
| **Major stigmata of recent haemorrhage** | |
| None or dark spots only | 0 |
| Blood in upper GI tract, adherent clot, or visible or spurting vessel | 2 |
| **Final Rockall score (add OGD score to initial score) (max. score = 11)** | |

1 Rockall TA, Logan RF, Devlin HB, and Northfield TC (1996). Risk assessment after acute upper gastrointestinal haemorrhage. *Gut* **38**, 316–21.

**Table 22.2** Relationship between the Rockall score and re-bleeding or mortality[1]

| Rockall score | Re-bleed (%) | Mortality (%) |
| --- | --- | --- |
| 0 | 5 | 0 |
| 1 | 3 | 0 |
| 2 | 5 | 0.2 |
| 3 | 11 | 3 |
| 4 | 14 | 5 |
| 5 | 24 | 11 |
| 6 | 33 | 17 |
| 7 | 44 | 27 |
| 8 or more | 42 | 41 |

1 Rockall TA, Logan RF, Devlin HB, and Northfield TC (1996). Risk assessment after acute upper gastrointestinal haemorrhage. *Gut* **38**, 316–21.

# Acute abdominal pain

Presentation with acute abdominal pain represents the commonest surgical presentation to an Accident and Emergency Department. The potential causes of such an 'acute abdomen' are wide ranging and several factors in the patient history are helpful in identifying the cause. In particular, the site and radiation of pain, aggravating factors, and natural history of pain give pointers to the cause of symptoms. Table 22.3 details the specific patterns of the common causes of acute abdominal pain.

Examination might reveal features of peritoneal irritation, an abdominal mass, the cause of obstruction (especially hernial orifices), and systemic illness. In addition to routine bloods (including amylase), urine microscopy and a pregnancy test (if appropriate) should be performed. If perforation is suspected, an erect chest X-ray will reveal air under the diaphragm.

A supine abdominal X-ray excludes renal stones and bowel obstruction.

Severe pain is uncommon in ulcerative colitis, except in major disease flare-ups. The presence of acute pain in a patient with Crohn's disease requires measurement of CRP and ESR. If these inflammatory markers are elevated, the causes might include an acute inflammatory flare-up, development of an intra-abdominal abscess, or drug-induced pancreatitis. If these markers are not elevated, the possibility of intestinal stricture, adhesional obstruction, peptic ulcer, or renal/biliary colic should be considered.

Management depends on the cause. In general, analgesia should be offered—opiates are often needed for severe pain. If the diagnosis is uncertain, an overnight admission can often clarify the clinical condition.

**Table 22.3** Patterns of the common causes of acute abdominal pain

|  | Site | Radiation | Aggravating factors | Natural history |
|---|---|---|---|---|
| Appendicitis | Central, right iliac fossa | Nil | Movement | Pain shifts from the centre to the right |
| Diverticulitis | Left iliac fossa | Nil | Movement | Older patient, recurrent pain |
| Gut obstruction | Symmetric | Nil | Meals | Severe pain, might start as subacute |
| Gut perforation | Upper | Nil | Movement | Acute history |
| Cholecystitis | Right upper quadrant | Shoulder, back | Inspiration | Recurrent bouts of colic |
| Pancreatitis | Central, upper | Nil | Movement | Severe pain, might be acute-on-chronic |
| Renal colic | Flank | Groin | Nil | Acute severe pain |

# Intestinal obstruction

Intestinal obstruction occurs as a complete or partial blockage of the bowel that results in failure of the intestinal contents to move along the gastrointestinal tract. There are number of causes of bowel obstruction, as outlined below.

## Possible causes

### Crohn's disease

Small-bowel obstruction in Crohn's disease might be due to active inflammation, fibrosis, or stricture formation.

### Ileus

An ileus/paralytic ileus might follow abdominal surgery; the peristaltic action of the bowel, which moves the food or waste along the GIT, stops following handling of the bowel during surgery. The symptoms of an ileus are as follows.
• Abdominal distension.
• Absent bowel sounds.
• Limited abdominal pain.

An ileus can be caused by the following.
• Medication—narcotics.
• Injury to the blood supply.
• Complications of intra-abdominal surgery.
• Intraperitoneal infection.

A paralytic ileus in a newborn might be due to necrotizing enterocolitis and is life threatening.

### Mechanical obstruction

Mechanical obstruction is a physical blockage of the intestine. The causes of mechanical obstruction include the following.
• Hernia.
• Surgical adhesion.
• Impacted faeces.
• Bowel tumours.
• Intussusception—telescoping of the bowel within itself.
• Volvulus—twisted bowel.
• Foreign bodies.

Care must be taken to ensure that the obstruction does not occlude the blood supply and cause tissue death, infection, and gangrene.

## Symptoms
• Abdominal distension.
• Abdominal cramp.
• Abdominal pain.
• Vomiting.
• Constipation or diarrhoea.
• Halitosis.

### Investigation
- Symptom history.
- Medical history.
- Abdominal X-ray.
- Colonoscopy.
- Blood tests for inflammatory markers.

### Treatment
Depends on accurate diagnosis of cause of obstruction (see under each cause listed elsewhere in this volume). A nasogastric tube is inserted and may relieve distension and vomiting if aspirated. Surgery might be required if symptoms do not resolve.

### Bowel cancer
Unfortunately, ~15% of patients who have bowel cancer present with acute obstruction of the colon by the malignancy.[1] There is an added risk that the cancer might perforate, leading to peritonitis and a potentially life-threatening situation.

1 Northover JMA and Kettner JD (1992). *Bowel Cancer: The Facts*. Oxford University Press.

# Perforation

Bowel perforation can occur for a number of reasons. The causes, signs, and symptoms will determine the investigations and treatment required.

## Causes
- Inflammatory bowel disease.
- Diverticular disease.
- Ingested matter, e.g. bones or pins.

## Ulcerative colitis

In ulcerative colitis, perforation can occur as a complication of toxic dilation or delayed surgery or colonoscopy during a severe attack.

The signs of perforation are commonly pain and peritonitis, although these might be masked by steroids. Peritonitis is often characterized by the following:
- Fever.
- Guarding.
- Rebound tenderness.
- Rigidity.
- Absent bowel sounds.

Treatment is with fluid, blood, and electrolyte replacement. When the patient is stable, surgery is indicated—colectomy and ileostomy (usually temporary).

## Crohn's disease

In Crohn's disease, the patient with perforation rarely presents acutely. This is because an abscess cavity often forms and steroids frequently suppress clinical features.

Useful investigations for determining a bowel perforation are plain abdominal and erect chest X-rays. Free gas is shown on the abdominal X-ray. Surgery is indicated if perforation is found on investigation.

## Diverticular disease

There might be signs of peritonitis or a pelvic, paracolic, or subphrenic abscess in patients with a perforated diverticulum. However, in the elderly or debilitated, there might be chronic pyrexia, ill health, and weight loss. Perforation of the diverticulum has a high mortality rate because the signs of peritonitis can be minimal. The risk of perforation, and subsequent mortality, is particularly high in the immunocompromised.[1]

Treatment for a perforated diverticulum might include surgery.

## Foreign objects causing perforation

Signs to observe for ingested foreign objects in children, the mentally disturbed, or elderly are as follows:
- Excessive salivation.
- Regurgitation.

1 Travis SPL, Ahmad T, Collier J, and Steinhart AH (2005). *Pocket Consultant Gastroenterology* (3rd edn). Blackwell, Oxford.

- Choking.
- Distress.

Pain or fever suggests a perforation. Generally, once through the pylorus, the foreign object passes spontaneously. However, ileocaecal perforation can occur.

For ingested objects, the following investigations are suggested:
- Looking in the mouth.
- X-ray.

Chest pain might indicate a perforation, either after endoscopic removal of the foreign object or following ingestion. A small haematemesis might be due to perforation of a major blood vessel. For either symptom, a thoracic surgeon should be urgently sought.

Treatment for ingested foreign objects depends on symptoms and assessment. If the object is impacted in the throat, it can be removed by an ENT surgeon. Endoscopy might be able to retrieve objects that have not yet passed into the duodenum.

# Sources of information and useful addresses

### Barrett's Oesophagus Foundation

University Department of Surgery
Royal Free Campus
Royal Free and University College Medical School
Rowland Hill Street
London NW3 2PF
Tel: 020 7472 6223
Fax: 020 7472 6224
Email: enquiries@barrettsfoundation.org.uk
Web: http://www.barrettsfoundation.org.uk

### Beating Bowel Cancer

39 Crown Road
St Margarets
Twickenham
Middlesex TW1 3EJ
Tel: 020 8892 5256
Fax: 020 8892 1008
Email: info@beatingbowelcancer.org
Web: http://www.beatingbowelcancer.org.uk

### Bowel Cancer UK

7 Rickett Street
London SW6 1RU
Tel: 020 7381 9711
Email: admin@bowelcanceruk.org.uk
Web: http://www.bowelcanceruk.org.uk

### Bristol Cancer Help Centre

Grove House
Cornwallis Grove
Bristol BS8 4PG
Tel: 0117 980 9500
Fax: 0117 923 9184
Email: helpline@bristolcancerhelp.org
Web: http://www.bristolcancerhelp.org

### British Association for Counselling and Psychotherapy

BACP House
15 St John's Business Park
Lutterworth
Leicestershire LE17 4HB
Tel: 0870 443 5252
Email: bacp@bacp.co.uk
Web: http://www.bacp.co.uk

### British Association for the Study of the Liver

http://www.basl.org.uk

## British Liver Trust

2 Southampton Road
Ringwood
Hampshire BH24 1HY
Tel: 0870 770 8028
Fax: 01425 481335
Email: info@britishlivertrust.org.uk
Web: http://www.britishlivertrust.org.uk

## British Association of Parenteral and Enteral Nutrition

Secure Hold Business Centre
Studley Road
Redditch
Worcestershire B98 7LG
Tel: 01527 457850
Fax: 01527 458718
Web: http://www.bapen.org.uk

## British Nutrition Foundation

High Holborn House
Holborn
London WC1V 6RQ
Tel: 020 7404 6504
Fax: 020 7404 6747
Email: postbox@nutrition.org.uk
Web: http://www.nutrition.org.uk

## British Pharmaceutical Nutrition Group

PO Box 5784
Derby DE23 1WU
Tel: 01332 593154
Web: http://www.bpng.co.uk

## British Society of Gastroenterology

3 St Andrews Place
Regent's Park
London NW1 4LB
Tel: 020 7935 3150
Web: http://www.bsg.org.uk

## British Society of Paediatric Gastroenterology, Hepatology and Nutrition

Mrs Carla Lloyd
5 Woodthorpe Drive
Pedmore
Stourbridge
West Midlands DY9 7JX
Tel/Fax: 01384 866446
Email: administrator@bspghan.org.uk
Web: http://www.bspghan.org.uk

## C-Level

268 Bath Street, Glasgow. (Phone 0141 332 2520)
A voluntary organization offering confidential information, advice
and support to those affected by Hepatitis C.
Web: http://www.c-level.org.uk/

## CancerBACUP

3 Bath Place
Rivington St
London EC2A 3JR
Tel: 020 7696 9003
Fax: 020 7696 9002
Web: http://www.cancerbacup.org.uk

## Cancer Counselling Trust

1 Noel Road
London N1 8HQ
Tel: 020 7704 1137
Fax: 020 7704 8620
Email: support@cctrust.org.uk
Web: http://www.cctrust.org.uk

## Carers UK

20–25 Glasshouse Yard
London EC1A 4JT
Tel: 020 7490 8818
Carers' Line: 0808 808 7777
Fax: 020 7490 8824
Email: info@carersuk.org
Web: http://www.carersuk.org

## Children's Liver Disease Foundation

36 Great Charles Street
Birmingham B3 3JY
Tel: 0121 212 3839
Fax: 0121 212 4300
Email: info@childliverdisease.org
Web: http://www.childliverdisease.org

## Coeliac UK

Suites A–D, Octagon Court
High Wycombe
Bucks HP11 2HS
Tel: 01494 437278
Helpline: 0870 444 8804
Fax: 01494 474349
Web: http://www.coeliac.co.uk

**Colostomy Association**

15 Station Road
Reading
Berkshire RG1 1LG
Tel: 0800 587 6744
Web: http://www.colostomyassociation.org.uk

**Continence Foundation**

307 Hatton Square
16 Baldwin Gardens
London EC1N 7RJ
Tel: 020 7404 6875
Helpline: 0845 345 0165
Fax: 020 7404 6876
Email: continence-help@dial.pipex.com
Web: http://www.continence-foundation.org.uk

**CORE**

3 St Andrews Place
London NW1 4LB
Tel: 020 7486 0341
Fax: 020 7224 2012
Email: info@corecharity.org.uk
Web: http://www.digestivedisorders.org.uk

**Digestive Disorders Foundation (see CORE)**
**Education and Resources for Improving**
**Childhood Continence**

34 Old School House
Britannia Road
Kingswood
Bristol BS15 8DB
Tel: 0845 370 8008
Fax: 0117 960 0401
Email: info@eric.org.uk
Web: http://www.enuresis.org.uk

**Face It Hepatitis C awareness campaign**

Hepatitis C information line 0800 451451 textphone 0800 0850859
http://www.hepc.nhs.uk/

**Gastroenterology library**

Web: http://www.library.nhs.uk/gastroliver

**Gastrointestinal Nursing**

MA Healthcare Ltd
St Jude's Church
Dulwich Road
London SE24 OPB
Tel: 020 7738 5454
Web: http://www.gastrointestinalnursing.co.uk

### Gilbert's Syndrome
Action on Gilbert's Syndrome
PO Box 37848
London SE23 2WX
Tel/Fax: 0845 226 2394
Web: http://www.gilbertssyndrome.org.uk

### Haemochromatosis Society
Hollybush House
Hadley Green Road
Barnet
Herts EN5 5PR
Tel/Fax: 020 8449 1363
Email: info@ghsoc.org
Web: http://www.ghsoc.org

### Irritable Bowel Syndrome Network
Unit 5, 53 Mowbray Street
Sheffield S3 8EN
Tel: 0114 272 3253
Email: info@ibsnetwork.org.uk
Web: http://www.ibsnetwork.org.uk

### Ileostomy and Internal Pouch Support Group
Peverill House
1–5 Mill Road
Ballyclare
Co. Antrim BT39 9DR
Tel: 028 9334 4043
Freephone: 0800 0184 724
Fax: 028 9332 4606
Email: info@the-ia.org.uk
Web: http://www.the-ia.org.uk

### Incontact (action on incontinence)
United House
North Road
London N7 9DP
Tel: 0870 770 3246
Fax: 0870 770 3249
Email: info@incontact.org
Web: http://www.incontact.org

### Information on the published Hepatitis C guidelines by SIGN
http://www.hepcscotland.co.uk

### International Foundation for Functional Gastrointestinal Disorders

PO Box 170864
Milwaukee
WI 53217–8076
USA
Tel: +1 414 964 1799
Fax: +1 414 964 7176
Email: iffgd@iffgd.org
Web: http://www.iffg.org

### Joint Advisory Group on Gastrointestinal Endoscopy

c/o JCHMT
5 St Andrew's Place
Regent's Park
London NW1 4LB
Tel: 020 7935 1174, ext. 513
Fax: 020 7486 4160
Email: sarah.carruthers@rcplondon.ac.uk
Web: http://www.thejag.org.uk

### Macmillan CancerLine

Macmillan Cancer Relief
89 Albert Embankment
London SE1 7UQ
Freephone: 0808 808 2020
Email: cancerline@macmillan.org.uk
Web: http://www.macmillan.org.uk

### Mainliners

http://www.mainliners.org.uk

### Marie Curie Cancer Care

89 Albert Embankment
London SE1 7TP
Tel: 020 7599 7777
Web: http://www.mariecurie.org.uk

### National Association for Colitis and Crohn's Disease

4 Beaumont House
Sutton Road
St Albans
Herts AL1 5HH
Tel: 0845 130 2233
Fax: 01727 862550
Web: http://www.nacc.org.uk

### National Nurses Nutrition Group

Lynne Colagiovanni (Chair)
Queen Elizabeth Hospital
University Hospital Birmingham NHS Trust
Birmingham B15 2TH
Tel: 0121 472 1311, ext. 2094
Email: lynne.colagiovanni@uhb.nhs.uk
Web: http://www.bapen.org.uk
National Institute of Clinical Excellence
http://www.nice.org.uk

### Oesophageal Patients' Association

22 Vulcan House
Vulcan Road
Solihull
West Midlands B91 2JY
Tel: 0121 704 9860
Email: opa@ukgateway.net
Web: http://www.opa.org.uk

### Parenteral and Enteral Nutrition Group of the British Dietetic Association

Vera Todorovic
Consultant Dietitian in Clinical Nutrition
Bassetlaw Hospital
Worksop
Nottinghamshire S81 OBD
Tel: 01909 502773
Fax: 01909 502809
Email: vera.todorovic@dbh.nhs.uk
Web: http://www.peng.org.uk

### Patients on Intravenous and Nasogastric Nutrition Therapy (PINNT)

PO Box 3126
Christchurch
Dorset BH23 2XS
Tel: 01202 481625/01933 316399
Email: pint@dial.pipex.com
Web: http://www.pinnt.com

### Primary Biliary Cirrhosis Foundation

54 Queen St
Edinburgh EH2 3NS
Scotland
Tel: 0131 225 8586
Email: info@pbcfoundation.com
Web: http://www.pbcfoundation.org.uk

## Primary Care Society for Gastroenterology
Gable House
40 High Street
Rickmansworth
Herts WD3 1ER
Tel: 01923 712711
Fax: 01923 777275
Email: secretariat@pcsg.org.uk
Web: http://www.pcsg.org.uk

## Scottish National Clinical Guideline
The Scottish Intercollegiate Guidelines Network (SIGN) writes
guidelines which give advice to people who work in the health service
and patients about the best tests and treatments that are available.
http://www.sign.ac.uk

## Society of Gastroenterology Nurses and Associates Inc. (USA)
Web: http://www.sgna.org

## Spinal Injuries Association
SIA House
2 Trueman Place
Oldbrook
Milton Keynes MK6 2HH
Tel: 0845 678 6633
Email: sia@spinal.co.uk
Web: http://www.spinal.co.uk

## St Mark's Hospital and Academic Institute
Watford Road
Harrow
Middlesex HA1 3UJ
Tel: 020 8235 4000
Fax: 020 8869 2936
Web: http://www.stmarkshospital.org.uk

## UK Hepatitis C Resource Centre
http://www.hepccentre.org.uk

## United Ostomy Associations of America
PO Box 66
Fairview
TN 37062–0066
USA
Email: info@uoaa.org
Web: http://www.uoaa.org

**Wilson's Disease Support Group UK**
Mrs Valerie Wheater (information on genealogy)
Email: val@wilsons-disease.org.uk
Ms Linda Hart (contact details for other individuals
with Wilson's disease)
Email: linda@wilsons-disease.org.uk
Web: http://www.wilsons-disease.org.uk

# Index

## A

'544' ILEOSTOMY 264
abdomen, acute 449
abdominal bloating 450
abdominal causes of nausea and vomiting 353
abdominal pain 500–1, 706–7
abdominal rectopexy 531
abdominal ultrasound 47
abdominal X-ray (radiograph) 40, 618
abdominoperineal excision of the rectum (APER) 238, 239
absorption 55, 372
accountability 34–5
achalasia 350–1
acupuncture 682
acute fatty liver of pregnancy (AFLP) 414
adenocarcinoma 384
adhesive removers 272
Aeromonas 463
A-fetoprotein 425
age 704
  advanced and perianal soreness 547
albumin 405, 424
alcohol 67
  abuse 702
alcoholism 60–1
alginate-containing antacids 337
alkaline phosphatase 424
alkaninity and perianal soreness 547
allergies 10, 310–11
alpha-1 antitrypsin 424
alternative therapies 292, 299, 476
  therapies, see also complementary therapies
amino acids 80
aminotransferases 424
amoxicillin 365
anabolism 70
anaesthesia 176–7
anal digitations 673
anal fistula 538–9
analgesic ladder 691
anal sphincter 506, 507, 511, 562

anal stenosis 649
angular stomatitis 16
anorectal agenesis 649
anorectal atresia 649
anorectal conditions and perianal soreness 547
anorectal conditions and pruritus ani 551
anorectum 640
antacids, alginate-containing 337
antegrade continence enema (ACE) 316–17, 588, 656
anterior resection 242, 244, 519
  syndrome 530
anthropometry 143
antibacterials 292
antibiotics 139
anticholinergics 353
anti-emetic drugs and their uses 353
antihistamines 353
anti-inflammatory drugs 615
anti-mitochondrial antibodies (AMA) 424
anti-nuclear antibodies (ANA) 424
antiseptics, topical cleansing 139
anti-smooth muscle antibodies (ASMA) 424
anus see rectum and anus
anxiety and post-operative pain 697
appendectomy 615
appendicitis 449, 707
appendix 449
appliances 270
apthous ulcers 16
artificial anal sphincter (ABS) 572, 573
artificial nutrition support 110, 110–11
ascites 405, 406
aspiration 138, 230–3
Astroviruses 466
auscultation (using stethoscope) 18–19
auto-antibodies 424
autonomic dysreflexia 642–3
autonomic nervous system 39

autonomy 112
azathioprine 634

## B

*Bacillus cereus* 359
bacterial micro-organism 463–5
bacterial overgrowth 376–7
balloon
  dilators 189
  procedure 210
  retained gastrostomy 127
  through the scope (TTS) dilator 190
band ligation 703
barium
  enema 45
  follow-through 44
  swallow/meal 42, 43, 338
Barrett's oesophagus 342–3
basal metabolic rate 70
basket 211
behavioural therapy 64
belts/support garments 273
benficence 113
benzamide, substitute 353
bile 440
biliary duct dilatation 213
biliary stent placement 208–9
biliary system see gall bladder and biliary system
bilirubin 405, 424
biochemical indices 107
biochemical monitoring 143
biodegradable appliances 270
biopsies 230–3
biotin 86
bleeding 12
  ileo-anal pouch 255
  major 702
  rectal 512–13
  stoma care 284–5
  see also re-bleeding
bloating 450
blockages 138
blood
  altered 702
  fresh 702

parameters, abnormal 634
supply to liver 396
tests and liver disease 424–5
body
composition 107
ideal 24–7
image 24, 24–7, 626
mass index 143
presentation 24–7
reality 24–7
bolus obstruction (food/foreign bodies) 344
bowel
cancer 709
care and vulnerable groups 671–8
cultural issues 674–5
frail older people 672
learning disabilities 673
religious practices 676–7
function
colo-anal pouch 246
stoma reversal 259
large 170–2, 553
management programme 653
obstruction, malignant 494–5
retraining 564
see also inflammatory; irritable; neurological; paediatric; small
Bristol stool chart 509
brochoscopy 175
buccal route 694, 695
bulking agents 582
bumps 20
buprenorphine 695
buried bumper 128
butrans 7-day buprenorphine patches 695
butyrophenones, substitute 353

C

calcium 89
Caliciviruses 466
Campylobacter spp. 359, 463
cancer
anal 528–9
bowel 709
cholecystectomy 444
colon, 490–1
colon, follow-up for 526–7
colon, surgical management of 492–3
and constipation 590–1
and diet 66–7

gastric 367
liver, primary 416–17
liver, secondary 418–19
oesophageal 341
rectal 490–1, 516
rectal, follow-up for 526–7
rectal, surgery for 518–19
rectal, tenesmus in 517
see also colorectal cancer
cannabinoid 353
cannula, standard peripheral 152
capsule endoscopy 606
carbohydrates 74–5
carcinoid 384
cardiovascular disease 60–1
catabolism 70
catastrophic abdomen 304–5
catheter
access via central vein 150–1
access via peripheral vein 152–3
care in parenteral nutrition 156–7
damage 157
insertion and parenteral nutrition 154–5
material 112
medina 308–9
midline 152
non-tunnelled 112
occlusion 157
peripherally inserted central venous (PICC) 112
related complications and parenteral nutrition 162–3
tunnelled 112
cauda equina syndrome 641
central vein thrombosis 157
chemotherapy
for cancer of colon and rectum 490–1
and diarrhoea 556
palliative 525
stoma care 320–1
Childs-Pugh score of cirrhosis severity 405
Chinese herbal medicine 682
chlorpromazine 353
cholangiocarcinoma 416–17
cholecystectomy 444–5
cholecystitis 707
cholecystokinin 55

choledocholithiasis 443
cholelithiasis 442–3
cholesterol 73
chromium 93
cirrhosis 702
alcoholic 401
background and causes 401
complications 404–5, 406–7
post-necrotic 401
primary biliary (PBC) 401
symptoms and management 402–3
clarithromycin 365
cleaning and disinfection of endoscopes 224–5, 226–7, 228–9
decontamination 226, 227
disinfection 227
infection transmission 224
ISO symbol for single-use items
management 228
process, management of 228–9
special considerations 229
clinical expert 236–7
clinical governance 36–7
clinical history-taking 10–15
clinical lead 236–7
clinical nutrition 97–172
assessment 106–7
and GI disease 168–72
support 110–11
and the surgical patient 166–7
under-nutrition 102–3
withholding and withdrawing nutrition support 112–13
see also enteral; parenteral
Clostridium botulinum 359
Clostridium difficile 359, 463–4
Clostridium perfringens 359
clot, adherent in peptic ulcer 703
clothing 278
coeliac disease (gluten-sensitive enteropathy) 375
colectomy with ileo-rectal anastomosis 248–9
colectomy, partial and total 496
colitis (radiation enteropathy) 460–1
colo-anal pouch 246–7

colon 6, 447–504
  cancer, follow-up for
    526–7
  cancer, surgical
    management of 492–3
  colonic decompression
    472–3
  dilated 497
  malignant bowel
    obstruction 494–5
  pseudomembranous coli-
    tis (PMC) 458–9
  pseudo-obstruction
    470–1
  structure and function
    448
  see also colorectal cancer;
    infectious colitis;
    intestinal polyposis
    syndromes
colonic disease 610
colonic resection 588
colonic stents 218–19
colonic stimulants 582
colonoscopy 175, 216–17,
  482, 606, 618
colorectal cancer 418, 478,
  478–9, 482
  carcinogenesis 478
  and complementary
    therapies 684–5
  health promotion and
    education 480
  hereditary non-polyposis
    (HNPCC) 488–9
  incidence around the
    world 675
  metastatic 524
  pathophysiology 478
  prevalence 478
  prevention and screening
    480
  risk factors, identification
    of 480
  screening 482
  and ulcerative colitis 616
colostomists 280, 282,
  300–1
colostomy 274, 570
  irrigation 314–15
  percutaneous endoscopic
    318–19
  surgical procedures
    resulting in 238–41
colovesical fistula 541
communication 673
co-morbidity 704
complementary therapies in
  bowel disorders 679–86
computed tomography
  48–9, 50–1, 607
congenital abnormalities
  437, 648–9

conscious sedation 177
consent 34, 180
constipation 14–15, 300–1,
  576–7, 578, 579, 580–1
  biofeedback 586–7
  in cancer 590–1
  in children 660–1, 662–3,
    664
  colostomists 282, 324
  definition 576
  enemas 580
  enteral feeding 140
  examination 578
  and learning difficulties
    673
  management flowchart
    583
  and post-operative pain
    697
  prevalence 576–7
  suppositories 580
  surgery 588–9
  toilet routine, attempt to
    establish 579
consultant 236–7
  clinician 101
continence 12–13
continuous subcutaneous
  pump 694
contraception 254
contrast studies 40
convex appliances 270
copper 92, 425
core-out fistulectomy 538
Creutzfeldt-Jakob disease
  229
Crohn's disease 295
  chronic disease manage-
    ment 626–7, 629
  colonic 600
  environmental factors
    597
  epidemiology 597
  extra-intestinal
    manifestations 604–5
  genetics 598–9
  ileocaecal 610
  incidence 675
  intestinal obstruction 708
  investigation 602–3,
    606–7
  and irritable bowel
    syndrome 668, 669
  medical management
    610–11
  nutritional treatment
    608–9
  oesophageal/gastric/
    duodenal 611
  perforation 710
  perianal 600
  presentation 600–1
  recurrent 251

  short bowel syndrome
    380
  surgical management
    612–13
Cryptosporidium spp. 360,
  467
cuffitis 252
cultural issues 674–5
cyclizine 353
Cyclosporiasis 468
cystic fibrosis 436
cytology 232

# D

defaecation 255, 510–11
Delormes procedure 531
deodorant 273
dermatological causes of
  pruritus ani 551
dermatological conditions
  and perianal soreness
  547
desquamation 321
diabetes mellitus 60–1, 437
diagnostic endoscopic
  retrograde cholangio-
  pancreatography (ERCP)
  206–7
diamorphine 695
diarrhoea 14, 300–1, 552–3,
  554–5, 556–7
  cancer-related:
    management 556–7
  in children 666–7
  definition 552
  dietary causes 553
  differential diagnosis by
    probable site of
    disease 553
  enteral feeding 139,
    140–1
  history and investigation
    554
  management 554
  ostomist 324
  pathophysiology 552
diet 58, 60–1, 64, 564, 627
  see also nutrition
dietary advice for ostomate
  280
dietary assessment 106–7
dietary reference values 57,
  73
dietician 101
digital rectal examination
  (DRE) 20, 514
digital rectal stimulation
  644–6
dilators
  rigid 190
  and stenosis 296–7
  wire-guided 189

Diphyllobothrium latum 381
disaccharides 75
disease recurrence and stoma care 295
dispensing appliance contractor 276
displacement 138
disposal of single-use equipment 232
diverticular disease 172, 476–7, 675, 710
diverticulitis 707
divided colostomy (Devine operation) 238, 240
domperidone 353
double-balloon enteroscopy (DBE) 175
double-lumen feeding tube 121
dressing 156
driving 279
drugs 10, 279
  administration and enteral nutrition 146–7
  and chronic pain 698
  for dyspespsia and gastro-oesophageal reflux disease (GORD) 337
  food interactions 61
  and nausea and vomiting 353
  nutrient interaction 136
  reactions and liver 413
  therapy 64–5, 106
dumping syndrome 169
duodenal ulcers 382
duodenum 372, 373
Dupuytren's contracture 16
durogesic 695
dynamic gracialoplasty (gracilis neosphincter) 572, 573
dyspareunia 26
dyspepsia (indigestion) 332–3, 337
dysphagia (difficulty swallowing) 169, 330–1

E

eclampsia 414
educator 236–7
elderly people 672
electrical stimulation 566
electrolytes 109, 159
  imbalance 16
  mix and intestinal failure 391, 393
embryology 31
emergencies 701–12

abdominal pain, acute 706–7
haematemesis 702–5
intestinal obstruction 708–9
perforation 710–12
employment 279
encephalopathy 405
endocrine causes of nausea and vomiting 353
endocrine cells 9
endocrine function 428
endoscopic retrograde cholangiopancreatography 175
  biliary duct dilatation 213
  sphincterotomy 212
  stone extraction 210–11
  therapeutic 208–9
endoscopy 173–234
  biopsies, aspiration and handling specimens 230, 230–3
  capsule 222–3, 606
  colonic stents 218–19
  colonoscopy 216–17
  foreign-body removal 196–7
  laser therapy 234
  nursing care/procedures 174–5
  oesophageal dilatation 188–9, 190–1
  oesophageal gastro-duodenoscopy 184–5, 186–7
  oesophageal self-expanding metal stent 204–5
  oesophageal varices: banding or injecting 194–5
  photodynamic therapy 234
  polypectomy 220–1
  sedation and anaesthesia 176–7
  sigmoidoscopy, flexible 214,
  ultrasound 234
  variceal balloon tamponade 192–3
  see also cleaning and disinfection of endoscopes; endoscopic retrograde cholangiopancreatography; non-medical endoscopy; percutaneous endoscopic gastrostomy (PEG)

enemas 306, 580
  antegrade continent 316–17, 656
  arachis oil (peanut oil) 580
  barium 45
  microenemas 580
  phosphate 580
  tap water 580
energy 70, 158
  requirements 108
Entamoeba histolytica 360, 468
enteral nutrition 110, 116–17
  at home 144–5
  complications 136–7
  and drug administration 146–7
  GI disturbances 139
  infective complications 139
  mechanical complications 138
  monitoring 142–3
  preparations 134–5
enteric nervous system 3, 4
enterocutaneous fistula 302–3, 613
Enteroviruses 466
environment 16
environmental factors and Crohn's disease 597
environmental pathogenesis of ulcerative colitis 615
enzymes 78
  defects 61
epithelium 9
erythema 321
  nodosum 624
Escherichia coli (type 0157) 359, 464
esomeprazole 365
estimated average requirement (EAR) 57
European Union Directive (2002/46/EC) 68
European Union Directive (2004/27/EC) 69
evacuating proctogram (defaecography; defaecating proctogram) 46
excoriation 310–11
exercise see physical activity
exocrine cells 9
exocrine function 428
external opening 20
extra-intestinal manifestations and ulcerative colitis 616
eyes 16

# F

faecal incontinence 558–9, 560–1
artificial anal sphincter 572, 573
biofeedback 566
bowel retraining 564
colostomy 570
conservative measures 564–5
diet and fluid modification 564
dynamic graciloplasty (gracilis neosphincter) 572, 573
electrical stimulation 566
exercises and biofeedback 566–7
gluteus maximus transposition 572
injectable biomaterials 570
and learning difficulties 673
medication 564
neosphincters 572–3
and obstetric trauma 560–1
patient education 564
post-anal repair 570
products for 565
rectal emptying, effective 564
sacral nerve simulation 524, 571
secca procedure 570
toilet access 564
toilet habit 564
faecal occult blood test (FOBT) 482
faecal soiling 20
faeces
manual removal 644–6
see also stools
familial adenomatous polyposis (FAP) 483, 484
family history 10, 12–13
fasting recommendations 166
fatigue 255
fats 58–9, 67, 72–3
fat-soluble vitamins 83, 87
feeding see clinical nutrition
fentanyl 695
actiq with oromucosal applicator 694
ferritin 425
fertility 626
fibre 76–7
fine-bore feeding tubes 119, 120

fissure, anal 536–7
fistula
anal 538–9
appliances 270
colovesical 541
recto-vaginal 540
fistulating disease 611
fistuloclysis 132
flatus see wind
fluid 109
balance and intestinal failure 391
intake 95
losses 95
modification and faecal incontinence 564
rectal irrigation 584
fluoride 91
flushing 156
folate (folic acid) 86
food allergy 61
food -avoidance diets 682
food contamination 61
food, functional 68
food intolerance 61
food labelling 59
Food Labelling Regulations Act 1996 69
Food Safety Act 1990 69
food supplements 68
foothing 230
foregut 31
foreign-body removal 196–7
foreign objects causing perforation 710–11
fortification 110–11
fruit and vegetables 58–9, 67
functional tests 107

# G

gall bladder and biliary system 18, 439–46
biliary malignancies 446
gall stones: cholecystectomy 444–5
gall stones: cholelithiasis 442–3
primary sclerosing cholangitis 446
structure and function 440
gamma-glutamyltransferase (G-GT) 424
gastric bypass 65
gastric decompression 166
gastric dumping syndrome 368
gastric inhibitory peptide 55
gastric polyps 369

gastric restriction (gastric banding or gastroplasty) 65
gastric ulceration 362–3
gastric varices 346, 404–5
gastritis 361
gastroenteritis 358–60
gastrointestinal smooth muscle 2, 4
gastrointestinal tract 31
gastro-jejunal tubes 120
gastro-oesophageal reflux 169 reflux, disease 334–5, 337
gastroscopy 606
gastrostomy 143
malecot style 127
tubes 120, 126–7, 128–9, 130–1, 131
genetics and Crohn's disease 598–9
*Giardia duodenalis* 378
*Giardia lamblia* 360, 469
giardiasis 378
Gilbert's syndrome 412
Gillick competence 34
glossitis (smooth, shiny tongue) 16
gluconeogenesis 74
glucose 393
gluteus maximus transposition 572
glycogenesis 74
glycogenolysis 74
glycolysis 74
granisetron 353
granuloma 128
gross anatomy 2–3
guarding 18
gut
cross-section 55
dysmotility 697
and its function 1–8
gross anatomy 2–3
gut flora, normal 6–7
structure and function 4–5
obstruction 707
perforation 707

# H

haematemesis 356–7, 702, 702–5
haematological indices 107
haemochromatosis (inherited) 408–9
haemorrhage, recent and major stigmata 704
haemorrhoidectomy 534–5
haemorrhoids 532–3
hand clubbing 16

Hartmann's procedure 238, 239

heavy metals 359

*Helicobacter pylori* 337, 364–5, 382, 383

hepatic encephalopathy 406–7

hepatitis
A 398
alcoholic 400
autoimmune 400
B 398
C 398–9
D 399
E 399
non-viral 400
viral 398–9, 414

hepatobiliary/pancreatic site and diarrhoea 553

hepatocellular carcinoma (hepatoma/HCC) 416, 417

hepato-renal syndrome 407

herbal medicine 682

hereditary non-polyposis colorectal cancer (HNPCC) 488–9

hereditary risk factors and colorectal cancer 480

hernia, parastomal 290–1

hiatus hernia 354–5

hidradenitis suppurativa 549

high-biological-value proteins 79

hindgut 31

Hindus 676

Hirschsprung's disease 657

histamine 337

history of present complaint 10

holidays 627

homeopathy 683

hormones in the gut 55

human lymphocyte antigens (HLA) 614

hydromorphine 693

hydroxy iminodiacetic acid (HIDA)
nuclear scan of biliary system 54

hyoscine hydrobromide 353

hyperglycaemia 136

hypnosis/hypnotherapy 682, 699

**I**

ileorectal anastomosis (IRA) 248–9, 588

ileostomists, hints and tips for 281

ileostomy 242–5, 274

ileum 372, 373

ileus and intestinal obstruction 708

iliac fossa stoma 264, 269

imaging the GI tract 39–54
abdominal ultrasound 47
barium enema 45
barium follow-through 44
barium meal ('upper GI series') 43
barium swallow 42
computed tomography 48–9
evacuating proctogram 46
magnetic resonance imaging (MRI) 52–3
radiological imaging 40–1
scintigraphy (radionuclide imaging or nuclear medicine studies) 54
virtual colonoscopy (VC) or CT colonography 50–1

immunocompromised patients and small bowel infection 378

immunoglobulins 425

immunological pathogenesis of ulcerative colitis 614

immunonutrition 159

immunoproteins 78

immunosuppressants 292
methotrexate 632–3
monitoring 634–5
ulcerative colitis 621

imperforate anus 650–1

impotence 25

incontinence 252
ileo-anal pouch 255
St Mark's incontinence score 13
*see also* faecal incontinence

indigestion 14

indirect calorimetry 108

infection
catheter-related bloodstream 157
ex-site 157
and perianal soreness 547
and pruritus ani 551
skin care 312–13
small bowel 378–9
tunnel 157

infectious colitis 462–9, 463–9
bacterial micro-organism 463–5
viral micro-organism 466–7

infective complications of enteral feeding 137

infertility 26

inflammatory bowel disease 595–638
and appendix 449
in children 668, 668–9
extra-intestinal manifestations 624–5
immunosuppressants: methotrexate 632–3
immunosuppressants: monitoring 634–5
infliximab infusions 630–1
osteoporosis management 636–8
*see also* Crohn's disease; ulcerative colitis

infliximab infusions 630–1

infusion
bags 160
continuous 160
cyclical 160
pump 160

injectable biomaterials 570

inspection 16–17, 20

international normalized ratio 405

intestinal failure
assessment and planning 390–1
definition and classification 387
oral rehydration solution 393
overview 386
pathogenesis 388–9
psychological and social considerations 394
treatment 392

intestinal motility 391

intestinal obstruction 708–9

intestinal polyposis syndromes
familial adenomatous polyposis (FAP) 484
juvenile polyposis (JP) 486
MYH-associated polyposis (MAP) 487
overview 483
Peutz-Jeghers syndrome (PJS) 485

intestine, length of residual 391

intestine as route of enteral nutrition 117

intra-lesional injections 292

iodine 93
based water-soluble and low-osmolar contrast media (LOCM) 40–1

iron 90 saturation 425

irritable bowel syndrome 172, 502–3, 682–3
irritation and nausea and vomiting 353
ischaemic colitis 456–7
Isosporiasis 469

## J

jaundice 422
jaw wiring 65
jejunal extension using percutaneous endoscopic gastrostomy (PEG) 202
jejunostomy 143
jejunum 372, 373
Jews 677
justice 113
juvenile polyposis 483, 486

## K

ketotic breath 16
Kock pouch (continent ileostomy) 250–1
koilonychia (spoon-shaped nails) 16

## L

lactose
  deficiency 376–7
  intolerance 140–1
  tolerance tests 376
lamina propria 9
lansoprazole 365
laparoscopic abdominal surgery 452, 454–5
laparotomy: nursing care 452–3
large bowel 170–2, 553
laser therapy 234
laxatives 582–3
layers 9
learning disabilities 641, 673
left-sided disease 620
leukonychia (white nails) 16
libido, lack of 25, 26
lifestyle issues
  and chronic disease management 626–7
  and colorectal cancer 480
  and ileo-anal pouch 254
  and osteoporosis 637
  and ostomist 278–9
lips 16
*Listeria* spp. 359
liver 18, 169–70, 395–426
  biopsy 422–3
  blood tests 424–5

cancer, primary 416–17
cancer, secondary 418–19
disease 170, 397, 422
disease in pregnancy 414–15
drug reactions 413
flap 16
Gilbert's syndrome 412
haemochromatosis (inherited) 408–9
investigations and findings 422–3
metastases 524
non-alcoholic fatty liver disease (NAFLD) 410
non-alcoholic steatohepatitis (NASH) 410
non-viral hepatitis 400
paracetamol overdose 412
porphyria 413
structure and function 396–7
transplant 420–1
viral hepatitis 398–9
Wilson's disease 412
*see also* cirrhosis
lozenges 694, 695
lumps 14, 20
lymphoma 384

## M

macronutrients 70–1
magnesium 89
magnetic resonance imaging 52–3, 607
malabsorption 170–1, 374
malignancies
  biliary 446
  and bowel obstruction 494–5
  and causes of pruritus ani 551
  and obstruction 324
  pancreas 434–5
Mallory-Weiss tears 349
Malnutrition Universal Screening Tool 104, 105
manganese 92
manipulation 699
massage 699
meat and fish 58–9, 67
mechanical complications of enteral feeding 137
mechanical lithotripter 211
Meckel's diverticulum 383
meconium ileus 648–9
medical history 106
medico-legal issues 34–5
megacolon 497, 498
megarectum 497, 592

mercaptopurine 634
metabolic causes of nausea and vomiting 353
metabolic complications of enteral feeding 136, 137
metabolic complications and parenteral nutrition 162–3
metabolic disorders causing recurrent/chronic pain 501
metabolic syndrome 60–1
metastatic colorectal cancer 524
methadone 693
methotrexate 632–3
metoclopramide 353
metronidazole 365
micronutrients 70–1
midgut 31
milk and dairy products 58–9, 67
minerals 88–93
molybdenum 92
monosaccharides/simple sugars 74, 75
monounsaturated fatty acids 73
morphine 695
mortality 702, 705
motility 372
  stimulants 337
mouth 16, 97
mucocutaneous separation 283
mucosa 9, 448
mucus fistula 256–7
multiple sclerosis 640
muscle spasm 697
muscularis 448
musculoskeletal disorders causing recurrent/chronic pain 501
musculoskeletal manifestations and inflammatory bowel disease 624
musculoskeletal pain 697
mushrooms 359
Muslims 677
myenteric (Auerbach's) plexus 31
MYH-associated polyposis (MAP) 483, 487

## N

nabilone 353
nasogastric feeding route 119
nasogastric tube 122–3, 124–5, 143
naso-intestinal feeding route 118

nasojejunal tube 143
nausea and vomiting 14, 352–3, 697
neck 16
necrosis 286–7
necrotizing enterocolitis 648
needle catheter jejunostomy 120, 132
negligence 34
neosphincters 572–3
neuroendocrine tumours 418
neurological bowel care 639–46
  autonomic dysreflexia 642–3
  digital rectal stimulation and manual removal of faeces 644–6
neurological disorders causing recurrent/chronic pain 501
niacin 82, 85
nipple-valve ischaemia 251
nipple-valve necrosis 251
nitrogen 158
non-alcoholic fatty liver disease (NAFLD) 410
non-alcoholic steatohepatitis (NASH) 410
non-maleficence 113
non-medical endoscopy 178–9, 180–1, 182–3
  consent and sedation 180
  practical and legal risks 231
  practice support 182
  training 182–3
non-opioid drugs 690
non-steroidal anti-inflammatory drugs (NSAIDs) 694–5
nurse prescriber's formulary 37
nurse prescribing 36–7
nurse-prescribing extended formulary 37
nursing care 327–30
  body image and sexuality 24, 24–7
  psychological difficulties 28–9, 30
  stigma and taboos 22–3
  see also clinical history-taking; physical examination
nursing specialties 31–8
  medico-legal issues and accountability 34–5
  nurse prescribing 36–7
  role nurse specialist 32
  training for advanced practice roles 33

nutrients 70–1
nutrition 12–13, 55–96
  cancer and diet 66–7
  carbohydrates 74–5
  diet, influence of on health 60–1
  fats 72–3
  fibre 76–7
  food supplements 68
  functional foods 68
  good health balance 58–9
  minerals 88–93
  nurse specialist 101
  nutrients 70–1
  obesity 62–3, 64–5
  proteins 78–81
  related non-communicable diseases (NCDs) 60–1
  requirements 57
  vitamins 82–7
  water 94–5
  see also clinical nutrition
nutritional complications and parenteral nutrition 162–3
nutritional intake 143
nutritional status and intestinal failure 391
nutritional treatment in Crohn's disease 608–9

## O

obesity 60–1, 62–3, 64–5
obstetric cholestasis 414
obstetric trauma and faecal incontinence 560–1
obstruction 18–19, 251, 697
ocular manifestations and inflammatory bowel disease 625
oesophageal atresia 648
oesophageal dilatation, endoscopic 188–9
oesophageal dilatation, wire guidance for 190–1
oesophageal-gastro-duodenoscopy (OGD) 175
oesophageal manometry 339
oesophageal self-expanding metal stent 204–5
oesophageal varices 194–5, 404–5
oesophagitis 336
oesophagostomy 118
oesophagus and stomach 327–70
  achalasia 350–1
  barium swallow/meal 338

Barrett's oesophagus 342–3
bolus obstruction (food/foreign bodies) 344
dyspepsia (indigestion) 332–3, 337
dysphagia (difficulty swallowing) 330–1
gastric cancer 367
gastric dumping syndrome 368
gastric polyps 369
gastric ulceration 362–3
gastritis 361
gastroenteritis 358–60
gastro-oesophageal reflux disease (GORD) 334–5, 337
haematemesis 356–7
*Helicobacter pylori* 364–5
hiatus hernia 354–5
Mallory-Weiss tears 349
nausea and vomiting 352–3
oesophageal cancer 341
oesophageal diverticula 347
oesophageal and gastric varices 346
oesophageal manometry 339
oesophageal rings and webs 345
oesophageal spasm 348
oesophagitis 336
pH monitoring, twenty four hour ambulatory 340
pyloric stenosis 366
structure 328–9
Ogilvie's syndrome 473
oligosaccharides 74, 75
omeprazole 365
one-to-one nursing 192–3
opioid drugs 690, 690–2
oral intake and intestinal failure 392
oral rehydration solution 393
orogastric feeding route 118
osmotic agents 582
osteoporosis management 636–8
ostomate/ostomist
  dietary advice 280
  discharge planning 275
  pre-operative care 274
  lifestyle issues 278–9
  palliative care 322–3, 324–5
outflow problems 252

# P

paediatric bowel care
647–70
  antegrade continence
    enema 656
  congenital anomalies
    648–9
  constipation 660–1,
    662–3, 664
  Hirschsprung's disease
    657
  imperforate anus 650–1
  inflammatory bowel
    disease (IBD) 668–9,
    669
  spina bifida 658–9
  stoma care 652–3, 654–5
  toddler diarrhoea 666–7
  toilet training 665
pain 12
pain management
  687–700
  acute pain, assessment of
    689
  chronic non-malignant
    pain 698–9
  drug treatment 690–3
  ostomist 322
  post-operative 694–5,
    696–7
  tenesmus 322
palliation of tenesmus
  517
palliative care for ostomist
  322–3, 324–5
palliative chemotherapy and
  radiotherapy 525
pallor 16
palmar erythema 16
palpation 18, 20
pANCA4 614
pancaking 282
pancreas 169–70, 427–38
  congenital abnormalities
    437
  cystic fibrosis 436
  diabetes mellitus 437
  malignancies and tumours
    434–5
  pancreatitis 707
  pancreatitis, acute 169,
    430–1
  pancreatitis, chronic 114,
    432–3
  structure and function
    428
  Whipple's disease 437
pancreatic rupture 433
panproctocolectomy 242,
  245
panthothenic acid 86
pantoprazole 365

paracentesis 406
paracetamol 412, 695
paralytic ileus 451
parasitic micro-organism 547
parastomal hernia 290–1
parasympathetic nervous
  system 39
parenteral nutrition 110,
  148–9
  administration 160–1
  at home 164–5
  catheter access via central
    vein catheters 150–1
  catheter access via
    peripheral vein
    catheters 152–3
  catheter care 156–7
  catheter insertion 154–5
  formulation 158–9
  monitoring 162–3
Parkinson's disease 641
paste 272
past medical history 10
patient-controlled analgesia
  (PCA) 694, 695
patient group directions 37
pelvic abscess 252
pelvic disorders causing
  recurrent/chronic pain
  501
pelvic exenteration, total 523
peptic ulcer 703
peptide hormones 78
percussion 18
percutaneous endoscopic
  colostomy 318–19, 588
percutaneous endoscopic
  gastro- jejunostomy
  132, 133
percutaneous endoscopic
  gastrostomy 126,
  198–9, 200–1, 202, 203
  contra-indications for 199
  indications for 199
  insertion method 200
  jejunal extension using 202
  post-procedure risks 203
  pre-procedure assessment
    198
  pre-procedure clinical
    requirements 200
  procedure 200
  push technique 200–1
percutaneous endoscopic
  jejunostomy 132, 203
percutaneous intestinal
  feeding 132–3
perforation 710–12
perianal disease 611
perianal haematoma 549
perianal skin care 546–7
perianal skin soreness 252,
  255

peristomal granuloma 294
peritonitis 18–19
per rectum (PR)
  examination 20–1
personal history 10
pethidine 693
Peutz-Jegher's syndrome
  384, 485
phantom rectum 299
pharmacist 101, 276
pharmacological reactions
  61
pharyngostomy 118
pharynx 96
phenothiazines 353
pH monitoring, twenty four
  hour ambulatory 340
phosphorus 89
photodynamic therapy 234
physical activity 64, 70, 278
physical examination
  16–17, 18–19, 20–1, 106
  auscultation (using
    stethoscope) 18–19
  environment 16
  inspection 16–17
  palpation 18
  percussion 18
  per rectum (PR)
    examination 20–1
  position 16
physiological stability and
  intestinal failure 392
pigtail gastrostomy tube
  127
pilonidal sinus 544–5
PJS polyposis type 483
polypectomy 220–1, 231
polyps 221, 369
polysaccharides 74, 75
polyunsaturated fatty acids
  72, 73
porphyria 413
portal hypertension 404
position 16, 20
positron emission
  tomography 54
post-cholecystectomy
  syndrome 444, 445
potassium 90
pouch/enterocutaneous
  fistula 251
pouchitis 251, 252
pouch vaginal fistula 252
predictive equations 108
pre-eclampsia 414
pregnancy 254, 279, 414–15
prescribing 36, 158–9,
  276–7
primary sclerosing
  cholangitis 446, 625
probiotics 682
proctectomy 299

proctitis 620
proctoscopy 515
prokinetic agents 582
prolapse 288–9
protective wafers 272
proteins 78–81
  low-biological-value 79
  requirements 108–9
  structural 78
  transport 78
prothrombin time 425
proton-pump inhibitors
  (PPIs) 337
pruritus ani 550–1
pseudomembranous colitis
  (PMC) 458–9
pseudo-obstruction 470–1
psychogenic disorders
  causing recurrent/
  chronic pain 501
psychological care and
  ostomist 324–5
psychological considera-
  tions and intestinal
  failure 391, 394
psychological difficulties
  28–9, 30
psychological therapies and
  chronic pain 699
psychosocial considerations
  and intestinal failure
  391
psychosocial issues and
  post-operative pain 697
pudendal terminal motor
  latency 563
push-dilators 189
push enteroscopy (PE) 175
push technique 200–1
pyloric stenosis 366
pyoderma gangrenosum
  292–3, 624

**R**

rabeprazole 365
radiation enteritis 460–1
radiograph 40
radiological imaging 40–1
radiologically inserted
  gastrostomy (RIG) 126
radiotherapy
  and diarrhoea 556
  palliative 525
  rectum and anus 520
  stoma care 320–1
ranitidine bismuth citrate
  365
re-bleeding 703, 705
rebound tenderness 18
rectal bleeding 512, 512–13
rectal burning/itch 255
rectal prolapse 531

recto-anal inhibitory reflex
  (RAIR) 510, 511, 563
rectocele 574–5
recto-vaginal fistula 540
rectum and anus 505–94
  anal cancer 528–9
  anterior resection
  syndrome 530
  colon and rectal cancer,
  follow-up for 526–7
  defaecation 510–11
  digital rectal examination
  (DRE) 514
  dilated 497
  megarectum 592
  metastatic colorectal
  cancer 524
  palliative chemotherapy
  and radiotherapy 525
  proctoscopy 515
  radiotherapy 520
  rectal bleeding 512–13
  rectal cancer 516,
  518–19
  rectal irrigation 584–5
  rectal prolapse 531
  rectocele 574–5
  recto-vaginal fistula 540
  recurrence, local,
  management of 522
  stools and stool samples
  508–9
  structure and function
  506–7
  tenesmus in rectal cancer
  517
  total mesorectal excision
  (TME) 521
  total pelvic exenteration
  523
  see also constipation;
  diarrhoea; faecal
  incontinence
refeeding problems
  114–15
refeeding syndrome
  114–15, 136
reference nutrient intake
  (RNI) 57
relationships 626
religious practices 676–7
renal colic 707
renal function 48
renal stones 625
renewal rate 9
restorative proctocolectomy
  (ileo-anal pouch) 252–5
retained rectal mucosa 252
retention strips 272
retraction in stoma care
  298
retrograde ejaculation/dry
  orgasm 25

retroperitoneal disorders
  causing recurrent/
  chronic pain 501
Rockall score 702
rod/bridge, management of,
  including removal
  268–9
rotaviruses 360, 467
Ryles tubes 119

**S**

sacral nerve stimulation
  570, 571, 588
safe intake (SI) 57
St Mark's incontinence
  score 13
Salmonella spp. 359, 464
salty foods 67
sarcoma 384
saturated fatty acids 72, 73
scars 20
Schazki ring 345
Schofield equation 108
scintigraphy (radionuclide
  imaging or nuclear
  medicine studies) 54
sclerotherapy 194, 703
scrombotoxin 359
seals/washers 272
secca procedure 570
secretin 55
secretion 55
secretory tumours and
  diarrhoea 556
sedation 176–7, 180, 181
selenium 92
serosa 9, 448
serotonin (5-HT3)
  antagonists 353
seton stitch 538
sex 254, 279
sexuality 24, 24–7, 626
Shigella spp. 360, 465
Shilling test 381
shock 702, 704
short bowel syndrome
  380
sigmoidoscopy 606, 618
  flexible 175, 214, 482
Sikhs 676
silver dressings 139
sinus 20
sip-feeds 110–11
skin 16
  barriers 272
  care 282
  enterocutaneous fistula
  302–3, 303
  excoriation and allergy
  310–11
  perianal 546–7

trauma and infection 312–13
colour 17
damage classification following radiotherapy 321
and inflammatory bowel disease 624
rashes 20
tags 20
small bowel 170–2, 371–94
bacterial overgrowth and lactose deficiency 376–7
coeliac disease (gluten-sensitive enteropathy) 375
and diarrhoea 553
disease 600, 610–11
duodenal ulcers 382
infection 378–9
malabsorption 374
Meckel's diverticulum 383
radiology 606
short bowel syndrome 380
structure and function 372–3
tumours 384–5
vitamin B12 deficiency 381
see also intestinal failure
small intestine 97
small-stomach syndrome 169
smoking 615, 627
'SOAPIER' format 10, 12–13
Soave 238, 243
social history 10
sodium 90
bicarbonate 393
chloride 393
depletion 281
solitary rectal ulcer syndrome (SRUS) 593–4
specimens, handling of 230–3
sphincterotomy 212
spider naevi 16
spina bifida 641, 658–9
spinal cord injury 640
spleen 18
sport 278
Staphylococcus aureus 359
stenosis and dilators 296–7
stents, colonic 218–19
sterility/inability to produce sperm 25

steroids 292
stigma 22–3
stigmata, major of recent haemorrhage 704
stoma
formation 588
site and gastrostomy tube management 128
site, infected 139
see also stoma care
stoma care 235–326
antegrade continent enema (ACE) 316–17
bleeding 284–5
catastrophic abdomen 304–5
chemotherapy and radiotherapy 320–1
colectomy with ileo-rectal anastomosis 248–9
colo-anal pouch 246–7
colostomists 282, 300–1
colostomy 238–41, 314–15
colour 286
disease recurrence 295
end 259
enemas 306
enterocutaneous fistula (ECF) management 302–3
formation of stoma 256–7, 266–7
ileostomists 281
ileostomy 242–5
Kock pouch (continent ileostomy) 250–1
loop 259
medina catheter 308–9
mucocutaneous separation 283
necrosis 286–7
nurse, role of 236–7
ostomate/ostomist 275, 278–9, 280, 322–3, 324–5
paediatric 652–3, 654–5
parastomal hernia 290–1
percutaneous endoscopic colostomy 318–19
peristomal granuloma 294
phantom rectum 299
prescription issues and obtaining supplies 276–7
product choice 270–1, 272
prolapse 288–9

pyoderma gangrenosum 292–3
restorative proctocolectomy (ileo-anal pouch) 252–5
retraction 298
reversal of stoma 258–9
rod/bridge, management of, including removal 268–9
siting of stoma 262–5
skin care 310–11, 312–13
stenosis and dilators 296–7
storage, care and disposal 274
suppositories 306
temperature 286
stomach 97, 117 see also oesophagus and stomach
stone extraction 210–11
stools
characteristics 12–13
cultures 618
softeners 582
and stool samples 508–9
stress 627, 683
striae 16
stroke 641
Strongyloides 469
subcutaneous injection 694
sublingual route 694, 695
submucosa 9, 448
submucosal (Meissner's) plexus 31
subtotal colectomy 242, 247, 588
succession splash 18–19
sugars 58–9
supplementary prescribing 37
support garments and shields 279
suppositories 306, 580
surgical gastrostomy (SG) 126
surgical implant 112
surgical jejunostomy (SJ) 132
swallowing disorder 199
sympathetic nervous system 129

## T

taboos 22–3
tenesmus in rectal cancer 517

therapeutic endoscopic retrograde cholangio-pancreatography: biliary stent placement 208–9
toilet
  access 564
  habit 564
  routine, attempt to establish 579
  training 665, 673
total mesorectal excision (TME) 521
trace elements 92–3, 159
tracheoesophageal fistula 648
Trade Description Act 1968 69
transdermal patches 694, 695
trans-fatty acids 73
transplant, liver 420–1
transtec buprenorphine matrix patches 695
travel 278
trephine procedure 238, 240
Tropheryma whippelii 378
tumours
  colorectal 418
  neuroendocrine 418
  pancreas 434–5
  small bowel 384–5
type 2 histamine (H2) receptor antagonists 337

**U**

ulcerative colitis
  chronic disease management 626–7, 628
  extensive or total 620

incidence around the world 675
investigations 618–19
and irritable bowel syndrome 668
medical management 620–1
pathogenesis 614–15
perforation 710
presentation 616–17
surgical management 622–3
ultrasound 606
  abdominal 47
  endoscopic 234
under-nutrition 102–3
unsaturated fatty acids 72
upper gastrointestinal tract 169

**V**

vaginal dryness 26
variceal balloon tamponade 192–3
varices 346, 703
veins, dilated 16
vestibular causes of nausea and vomiting 353
Vibrio cholerae 359
Vibrio parahaemolyticus 359, 378–9
Vibrio spp. 465
viral micro-organism 466–7
virtual colonoscopy (VC) 50–1
viruses 359
vitamin A 82, 87
vitamin B₁ (thiamine) 84
vitamin B₂ (riboflavin) 84
vitamin B₆ 82, 85

vitamin B₁₂ 85, 381
vitamin C (ascorbic acid) 84
vitamin D 87
vitamin E 82, 87
vitamin K 82, 87
vitamins 82–7, 159, 160
  water-soluble 82, 84–6
vomiting see nausea and vomiting 14
vulnerable groups see bowel care and vulnerable groups

**W**

water 94–5
weight 143
  history 106
Wernicke-Korsakoff syndrome 114
Whipple's disease (intestinal lipodys-trophy) 378–9, 437
Whipple's procedure 434
white cell scan 54, 606
Wilson's disease 412
wind 255, 282, 474–5, 697
wound appliances 270

**X**

X-ray, abdominal 40, 618

**Y**

Yersinia enterocolitica 359
Yersinia spp. 465

**Z**

zinc 91